# PRACTICAL
# ETHICS
*for the*
# SURGEON

# PRACTICAL ETHICS *for the* SURGEON

**Lloyd A. Jacobs, MD**

President Emeritus and Professor
The University of Toledo
Toledo, Ohio

Manuscript Editor
**Patricia A. James, BEd**

The University of Toledo
Toledo, Ohio

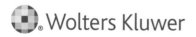

Wolters Kluwer

Philadelphia • Baltimore • New York • London
Buenos Aires • Hong Kong • Sydney • Tokyo

*Acquisitions Editor*: Keith Donnellan
*Editorial Coordinator*: David Murphy
*Editorial Assistant*: Levi Bentley
*Marketing Manager*: Dan Dressler
*Production Project Manager*: Kim Cox
*Design Coordinator*: Elaine Kasmer
*Manufacturing Coordinator*: Beth Welsh
*Prepress Vendor*: TNQ Books and Journals

Printed in China

**Library of Congress Cataloging-in-Publication Data**

Names: Jacobs, Lloyd A., author. | James, Patricia A., editor.
Title: Practical ethics for the surgeon / Lloyd A. Jacobs ; manuscript editor, Patricia A. James.
Description: Philadelphia : Wolters Kluwer, [2019] | Includes bibliographical references.
Identifiers: LCCN 2018002032 | ISBN 9781496388605
Subjects: | MESH: Bioethical Issues | General Surgery–ethics | Surgeons–ethics
Classification: LCC RD27.7 | NLM WO 21 | DDC 174.2/97–dc23 LC record available at
   https://lccn.loc.gov/2018002032

LWW.com

*To the Surgeons of the Departments at*
*The University of Toledo*
*And the*
*University of Michigan*

# ▶ Contributors

**Chandrakanth Are, MD, MBA, FRCS, FACS**
Jerald L & Carolynn J Varner Professor
Surgical Oncology & Global Health
Associate Dean of Graduate Medical
Education (DIO)
Vice Chair of Education, Department of Surgery
University of Nebraska Medical Center
Omaha, Nebraska

**Robert H. Bartlett, MD**
Professor of Surgery, Emeritus
University of Michigan
Ann Arbor, Michigan

**Ramon Berguer, MD, PhD**
Emeritus Professor of Surgery and
Engineering
University of Michigan
Ann Arbor, Michigan

**Shiela Beroukhim, MD**
David Geffen School of Medicine at UCLA
Los Angeles, California

**Steven Bibevski, MD, PhD**
Section of Pediatric and Congenital Cardiac
Surgery
The Heart Institute
Joe DiMaggio Children's Hospital
Hollywood, Florida

**Mark R. Bonnell, MD**
Associate Professor, Division of
Cardiothoracic Surgery, Department of
Surgery
Director, Mechanical Circulatory Support and
ECMO
University of Toledo College of Medicine
Chairman, Life Connection of Ohio Board of
Directors
Toledo, Ohio

**Edward L. Bove, MD**
Helen and Marvin Kirsh Professor
Chair, Department of Cardiac Surgery
University of Michigan Medical School
Ann Arbor, Michigan

**Athanasios Bramos, MD**
Assistant Professor, Department of
Surgery
University of Toledo College of Medicine
Toledo, Ohio

**Francis Charles Brunicardi, MD**
MCO Alumni Endowed Professor and Chair,
Department of Surgery
Cancer Program Director
University of Toledo College of Medicine and
Life Sciences
Academic Chief of Surgery
ProMedica Health System
Toledo, Ohio

**Richard E. Burney, MD**
Professor Emeritus of Surgery
University of Michigan
Ann Arbor, Michigan

**Alexander J. Caniglia, BS**
Medical Student
University of Nebraska College of
Medicine
Omaha, Nebraska

**Annette K. Collier, MD, FACP**
Assistant Professor, Department of Internal
Medicine
University of Toledo College of Medicine
Medical Director
Sincera Palliative Care
Toledo, Ohio

**Anthony J. Comerota, MD**
Adjunct Professor of Surgery
University of Michigan
Ann Arbor, Michigan

**Matthew A. Corriere, MD, MS**
Frankel Professor of Cardiovascular
Surgery
Associate Professor, Department of Surgery
Section of Vascular Surgery
University of Michigan
Ann Arbor, Michigan

**Dee E. Fenner, MD**
Furlong Professor of Women's Health
Departments of Obstetrics and Gynecology
and Urology
University of Michigan
Chief Clinical Officer
University Hospital and Franklin
Cardiovascular Center
Ann Arbor, Michigan

**Amir A. Ghaferi, MD, MS**
Associate Professor of Surgery
University of Michigan School of Medicine
Associate Professor of Business
University of Michigan Stephen M. Ross
School of Business
Director, Michigan Bariatric Surgery
Collaborative
Division Chief, General Surgery, AAVA
Director of Bariatric Surgery, AAVA
Ann Arbor, Michigan

**Jeffrey P. Gold, MD**
Chancellor
University of Nebraska Medical Center
University of Nebraska at Omaha
Omaha, Nebraska

**Benjamin N. Jacobs, PhD, MD**
House Officer VI
Section of General Surgery, Department of
Surgery
University of Michigan
Ann Arbor, Michigan

**Lloyd A. Jacobs, MD**
Professor Emeritus, Department of
Surgery
The University of Michigan
Ann Arbor, Michigan

**Janine E. Janosky, PhD**
Dean, College of Education, Health, and
Human Services
Professor, Department of Health and Human
Services
University of Michigan-Dearborn
Fairlane Center South
Dearborn, Michigan

**Clark T. Johnson, MD, MPH**
Assistant Professor, Department of
Gynecology and Obstetrics
Johns Hopkins School of Medicine
Baltimore, Maryland

**Timothy R.B. Johnson, MD, AM, FACOG**
Arthur F. Thurnau Professor
Bates Professor of the Diseases of Women
and Children
Departments of Obstetrics and Gynecology
and Women's Studies
Center for Human Growth and
Development
Associate, GLOBAL REACH
Center for Bioethics and Social Sciences in
Medicine
Von Voigtlander Women's Hospital
University of Michigan
Ann Arbor, Michigan

**Lisa M. Kodadek, MD**
Chief Resident in General Surgery,
Department of Surgery
Johns Hopkins University School of
Medicine
Baltimore, Maryland

**Joseph J. Lach, MD, FACS**
Assistant Professor, Department of
Surgery
University of Toledo Medical Center
Medical Director
The University of Toledo
Wound and Hyperbaric Center
Toledo, Ohio

**Hollis W. Merrick, III, MD**
Professor Emeritus of Surgery, Department
of Surgery
University of Toledo Medical Center
University of Toledo College of Medicine
Toledo, Ohio

**William S. Messer, Jr, PhD**
Professor
Department of Pharmacology and
Experimental Therapeutics
College of Pharmacy and Pharmaceutical
Sciences
The University of Toledo
Toledo, Ohio

**Christopher S. Chiodo Ortiz, BS**
Bucknell University
Bucknell, Pennsylvania

**Jorge Ortiz, MD**
Associate Professor
Director of Surgical Transplantation
Department of Surgery
University of Toledo Medical Center
Toledo, Ohio

**Jai Prasad, MD**
Advanced GI Minimally Invasive Surgery and
Bariatric Surgery
Fellow, Department of Surgery
Geisinger Medical Center
Danville, Pennsylvania

**Jason L. Schroeder, MD**
Assistant Professor, Department of
Surgery
Chief, Division of Neurosurgery
University of Toledo Medical Center
Toledo, Ohio

**Thomas A. Schwann, MD, MBA**
Professor, Vice-Chair
Department of Surgery
University of Toledo College of Medicine and
Life Sciences
Toledo, Ohio

**Susan M. Shafii, MD**
Assistant Professor of Surgery
Division of Vascular Surgery, Department of
Surgery
University of Minnesota
Minneapolis, Minnesota

**Ashish Sharma, MD**
Associate Professor, Department of
Psychiatry
Director, Consultation-Liaison Division
University of Nebraska Medical Center
Omaha, Nebraska

**Roland T. Skeel, MD**
Professor of Medicine
Chair, Biomedical IRB
University of Toledo College of Medicine and
Life Sciences
Toledo, Ohio

**James C. Stanley, MD**
Professor Emeritus of Surgery
University of Michigan
Ann Arbor, Michigan

**Jonathan R. Thompson, MD**
Vascular Surgery Fellow
Division of Vascular Surgery, Department of
Surgery
University of Michigan
Ann Arbor, Michigan

**James M. Tuschman, JD**
Lecturer in Legal Specialties
School of Social Justice and Director of
Outreach and Community Engagement
College of Health and Human Services
The University of Toledo
Toledo, Ohio

**Rev Andrew T. Wakefield, MMP, JD**
Parochial Vicar
Annunciation Catholic Church
Archdiocese of Washington

**Thomas W. Wakefield, MD**
Stanley Professor, Department of Surgery
Section Head, Vascular Surgery
Director, Samuel and Jean Frankel
Cardiovascular Center
University of Michigan
Ann Arbor, Michigan

**Coleen C. Wening, MBA, JD**
Recent graduate from The University of
Toledo College of Law
Toledo, Ohio

**Kristi S. Williams, MD**
Professor, Department of Psychiatry
The University of Toledo
Toledo, Ohio

**Roman Yusupov, MD**
Clinical Geneticist
Joe DiMaggio Children's Hospital
Hollywood, Florida

**Matthew Ziegler, MD**
Assistant Professor, Department of Surgery
Oakland University
William Beaumont School of Medicine
Royal Oak, Michigan

**Moritz M. Ziegler, MD, MS (Honorary), BS**
Retired
Former: Surgeon-in-Chief & the Ponzio Family
Chair, Children's Hospital Colorado
Professor of Surgery University of Colorado
School of Medicine
Surgeon-in-Chief & Chairman, Department of
Surgery, Children's Hospital Boston
Robert E. Gross Professor of Surgery, Harvard
Medical School
Surgeon-in-Chief & Chairman, Department of
Surgery, Children's Hospital
Cincinnati, Ohio
Professor of Surgery, University of Cincinnati
College of Medicine
Senior Surgeon Children's Hospital of
Philadelphia
Professor of Surgery, University of
Pennsylvania School of Medicine
Philadelphia, Pennsylvania

# ▶Prologue

There are many books on ethics, some by distinguished authors. One may therefore ask: why another? The answer to this rhetorical question is that although there are many books on ethics, there are far fewer devoted to medical ethics and there is a distinct scarcity of books on ethics tailored, or intended to be tailored, specifically for surgeons.

This seems to me to be puzzling, not only because I have the expected surgeon's chauvinism but also because surgeons are, more than members of most professions, makers of decisions about acting in the world. Moreover, the decisions demanded are difficult, the data often inadequate, and the consequences of a wrong decision may be grave. The purpose of this book is to render more accessible to surgeons in training and also experienced practicing surgeons, the paradigms and thought forms of the broad and venerable field of the ethics of decision making, particularly about decisions to action.

It is intended that this book will not only present a surgeon's view of the subject matter but also emphasize the human factors associated with ethical practices. Only a minority of writers on ethics have given emphasis to "psychological ethics"; it is my view that ethics and psychology are inextricable. Moreover, some ethical norms are entirely congruent with current thinking about the structure of the human mind and its functions, whereas other ethical norms are antithetical to the natural tendencies of most human beings. We will emphasize the tension produced by this incongruence and by other forms of incongruence within the field.

Surgeons, uniquely, are called upon to make decisions, the outcomes of which are often immediately obvious and occasionally painful. Their decision-making processes are often unconscious, consisting of a rote following of their mentors, however long past that mentoring may have occurred. In addition, at the risk of getting ahead of ourselves, surgeons who mentor or teach derive great satisfaction and pride from being emulated. I recall distinctly an army major, a surgeon in the medical corps, telling me about an operation to remove the first rib of a young woman patient, a difficult operation in anyone's hands. "I did it exactly as you showed me," he said, "and she did well." I felt a great pleasure at his words.

Although this careful emulation might have been appropriate, particularly in this case, the story does speak to a heavy reliance among surgeons on their training or on a "standard of practice" or on the practice pattern of their peer group. This tendency is not to be derogated; indeed, it is almost always salutatory, but a goal of this book is that alternatives may be more easily thought of and that continuation of past practices be better understood. To have as a goal that every decision, every day, be subjected to such scrutiny is of course unreasonable. We will discuss the making of rules for daily guidance and the departure from those rules, why and how.

It is my hope to write in a language that is accessible to nonspecialists in ethics; I will be forced to use such language because I and the coauthors of this book are nonspecialists in ethics but persons who have in the aggregate practiced surgery for many decades. I will try to illustrate ethical difficulties faced by surgeons by relating actual cases gleaned from 50 years of attendance at mortality and morbidity conferences at a score of institutions. We hope, further, that these discussions will be of some value to those in other disciplines or even to a more general audience, which includes both patients and their surrogates.

Surgeons are, as much as any profession and more perhaps than most, doers. Surgeons act or occasionally decline or fail to act; the very word "surgeon" denotes that fact: "Surgeon" derives from "chirurgeon," a derivative of the word for the human hand. It denotes, therefore, handiwork or the work of the human hand. Surgeons have a unique obligation to pursue and achieve not only practical wisdom (phronesis) but also excellence as a craftsman (techno). In this light, the ethics of action in the world are of first importance. Our actions determine outcomes, an assertion true for every discipline and individual, but of particular force for surgeons. Surgery is about the material world and the difficult medium of bones and flesh and blood.

The discipline of surgery is unique; no other discipline or profession has quite the same requirement for practical wisdom and personal responsibility. No other discipline or profession experiences the emotions provoked by the immediacy of the surgeon's experience. Indeed, the authority of that experience is the foundation for the unique ethical demands on the surgeon. The surgeon's acts are "good" or occasionally "not good" against an intrinsic standard belonging to the centuries-old experience of surgery. As will become clear the authority of the surgeon's experience is the foundation for "deontological" ethics.

The ethics of right action is termed "moral" philosophy; unfortunately, the word "moral" has acquired baggage in modern parlance. Used in this book, "moral" means merely "having to do with actions in the world." Indeed, this topic is of such importance to surgeons that a large part of this book is devoted to the moral philosophy that constitutes the field of a surgeon's ethics. The second half of this book is given to the recounting of actual day-to-day riddles encountered by practicing surgeons.

We mentioned earlier the traditional mortality and morbidity conference. It is our observation that this conference provides the clearest window into the culture of a Department of Surgery and constitutes our discipline's best teaching vehicle, in part because of its immediacy and relevance. In addition, of course, the absence of a mortality and morbidity conference also speaks of a department's culture.

In this context, the culture of an organization comprises the presuppositions and thought paradigms of that organization. It provides the context of everyday acts and utterances, which is often not subject to conscious awareness. Although it may exist largely unconsciously, every department member is affected by it; compliance to it, particularly in departments of surgery, is essential. An organization's culture is notoriously difficult to change, not only among surgeons but also in all societies' structures. Relevant to this discussion, the ethics of an organization, the obligations and values of that organization, are embedded as rules in that culture and provide context to the lives of individual members in that organization.

Finally, there is the issue of belief. What ought one to believe? What is it rational to believe? What beliefs are justified or warranted? To what degree do beliefs determine actions? How do beliefs change? Why do they seem to change so slowly? These and similar questions are relevant to the surgeon, as it is my experience and observation that, to a person, surgeons try to do that which they truly believe to be "right" or "good." But what do these notions mean?

# ▶Preface

As is the case for the world generally, the discipline of surgery has experienced massive and profound changes during the past several decades. These have been salutatory for the most part but have also presented new dilemmas for surgeons and for their patients and families as well as for the Western society broadly. I believe this wholesale change constitutes the strongest rationale for a book such as this one. The practical, day-to-day decisions required of surgeons and the changed emphasis of much of surgical thinking will be aided, we hope, by the pragmatic approach of this book.

A few of the many changes in our discipline include the following:

- A great increase in regulations and compliance requirements, much of which is driven by societal cost.
- The rise of large databases, eg, National Surgical Quality Improvement Program, and their impact on patient autonomy.
- The rapid introduction of new technology has made the surgeons' learning curve a significant issue.
- Surgery is increasingly being split into subdisciplines with special expertise in specific areas.
- There is an increasingly difficult struggle in the Western society between utilitarianism and Samaritanism.
- The training of the next generation of surgeons constitutes our discipline's greatest ethical dilemma.

It would be foolhardy to think that this book, or any book, will or could offer closure on any of these issues. Still, an honest attempt will be made in subsequent pages to find common language for the discussion of issues such as these. Moreover, in this world of rapid change, this book constitutes a search for unchangeable principles for our venerable discipline.

# Acknowledgments

We, the editors, wish first of all to thank the contributors to what we believe will be an important contribution to the discipline of surgery. It seems safe to say that never in the history of our discipline have so many pressing issues been present. We hope this book will meet some of our discipline's needs and initiate meaningful dialogue.

We gratefully acknowledge our readers and are continuously aware of the kindness you give us by your perusal of these essays.

We are grateful to the Departments of Surgery at The University of Toledo and at the University of Michigan. The chairs of these departments have done much to create a milieu in which the surgeon's ethics could flourish. We are grateful to The University of Toledo for the time and resources that have supported this project.

I, Lloyd Jacobs, wish specifically to acknowledge and express my gratitude to one who was perhaps my chief mentor: Dr Alexander J. Walt, President of the American College of Surgeons and Chairman of the Department of Surgery at Wayne State University. I am grateful to my wife, Ola Jacobs, who has inspired me for my lifetime and for this sometimes difficult project.

Patricia James wishes to acknowledge the everlasting support and encouragement of her husband, Brad, and her two sons, Joseph and Stephen, who have taught her the true meaning of joy.

For the Manuscript Editor of this book, Patricia James, it was a labor of love. The months we worked together on this project were among the best times of my life. Thank you Patty.

We are grateful to Wolters Kluwer and its associate TNQ Books and Journals. Specifically, we wish to thank Keith Donnellan and David Murphy. Kim Cox and Kayla Smull have been very helpful. Ramkumar Soundararajan has been both patient and professional.

# ▸Table of Contents

## PART I ▸ THEORY

**xvii**

# PART II ▶ PRACTICE

# PART 1 ▸ THEORY

*Lloyd A. Jacobs, MD*

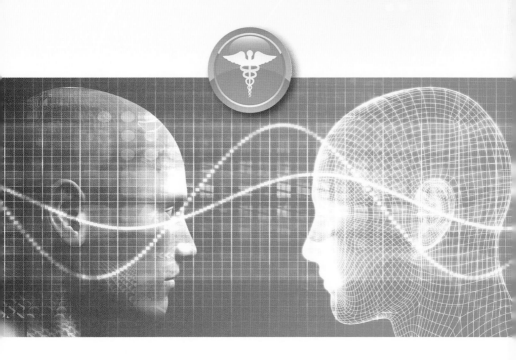

# 1 Introduction

Lloyd A. Jacobs, MD

The field of ethics is about obligations; the obligations of human beings to act in certain ways: to do that which is good, to do that which is right, and to do what one ought to do. Surgeons also, of course, have similar obligations but in a field of narrower scope and greater depth. In choosing a life as a surgeon, one commits to a specific set of ethical norms. And, it is necessary at the outset to note that it is not always easy to know what is the right thing to do or what good will be accomplished by doing what one ought to do. This is particularly true of the acts that surgeons are called upon to do or the decisions they make.

Most of the concepts traditionally used in discussions about ethics are ideals; or at least abstract notions, which do not exist in real life. What surgeons experience is conflict—a tugging in 2 directions. Surgeons struggle consciously or unconsciously with the tension so produced on a daily and continuing basis. We will subsequently discuss the effects of this tension and the lamentable fact that it is often dealt with by avoidance. It may be sufficient to say now that for most surgeons, this tension is not experienced as creative tension; a destructive and enervating effect may also be experienced. There has been much written of late about "burnout" among surgeons and trainees, but only minimal analysis has been proffered concerning the ethical tension that produces anxiety and depression. We will, subsequently, specifically examine burnout as a consequence of ethical tensions.

Most expositions of moral ethics present a taxonomy of ideas or of persons holding certain positions regarding "ethical" actions. In such presentations, notions concerning the morality of human actions are either one thing or another; there is little middle ground. In addition to the presupposition of a dichotomous nature for human actions, being good or not good, at least 2 additional presuppositions should be noted. Of these additional presuppositions the surgeon needs no convincing.

It is assumed that human actions have efficacy, that they are consequential and that they change, however, infinitesimally, the material world. Similarly, the idea of human ethics of action, being important, presupposes freedom of the 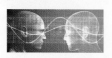 human will; that by taking thought, the acting human being could have caused the material world to be otherwise; that the course of unfolding reality could have been altered in some significant way. Although all the 3 presuppositions have been much discussed by philosophers, they seem obvious to most surgeons who perform or do not perform actions in the world on a daily basis.

On May 12, 2016, a discussion occurred at the Mortality and Morbidity conference of the Department of Surgery at a major academic medical center. Its thrust was as follows. Preparation of the colon for operation on it has often included a "mechanical" preparation and an "antibiotic" preparation. Recent data suggest that there are significant complications of the antibiotic preparation, but fewer such complications with the mechanical preparation. In this discussion a young surgeon was criticized for using neither regimen. She replied, "I believe that one should be 'all in or not at all'." Such categorical thought may be in part the result of the creation of strictly delineated categories in moral ethics and perhaps other areas of life.

All things merge into all; appropriate pride into hubris, prudent frugality into parsimony, and appropriate self-interest into egotism. To array ethical postures as dichotomous has made thoughtful decision-making more difficult for the surgeon, not easier.

It will be necessary to further consider the words "good" and "right" and "ought." An argument is made by some that these concepts are "basic" and need no further foundation beyond intuition. Sidgwick, for example, has written extensively about intuitionism, which implies that these words are indefinable, inscrutable, and their foundations unsayable. We will in this book accept that idea to a significant degree. It seems, however, necessary to expend 1 or 2 paragraphs to go briefly behind the intuition-based notion of "good" and "right" and "ought." Purely biological Darwinism would seem to have little in the way of ethical content. Still there is good evidence of prehistoric women and men displaying altruism in the straightening of fractured limbs, for example. Evolutionary psychologists have postulated an "altruistic" gene and spent several decades seeking evidence of such genetic coding and attempting to rationalize its apparent inconsistency with the hypothesis of natural selection. The great philosopher, Karl Jaspers, pointed out that during the period from about 600 BC to AD 200 humankind experienced a pivot toward social organization and interdependence. Since about that time, nearly every religious tradition and secular philosophy has asserted that "the good life" contains an orientation toward the welfare of others. The Hippocratic physician also possessed this orientation toward altruism, and moderns continue to assume beneficence as a part of our structure of ourselves.

It is important to recognize that questions about "ought" and "good" and "right" have been discussed for centuries and that there is small hope that this book will add anything fundamental in that arena. In what may be only a difference in presentation, we will emphasize that the concepts are leaky and merge into one another and that inclusion of any individual decision within the purview of some category or rule is in itself the act of a fallible being.

A half century of observing surgeons' utterances and acts have convinced me that it is invariably their intent to do that which is "right" or "good." Where surgeons fail to do this is most often due to a failure to see the situation to be addressed as it truly is, which results in the "categorization" errors that occur so frequently in the practice of surgery. It will be necessary, therefore, to think about how the phenomenon of "seeing" is affected by presuppositions and preexisting thought patterns, including those with ethical content. In regard to the work historically undertaken by surgeons, and the societal assignments to them, it may be wise to state here that "health" is for our discipline, a central component of that which is "good" and its pursuit is almost always deemed to be "right."

The notion of "health" is also poorly defined. Narrowly defined, it may be intended to convey soundness of body or to stand opposite illness or trauma. In this context a horse or a guinea pig may be described as being in good health. For purposes of this discussion, I propose to define "Health" much more broadly, to include not only the health that conduces to longevity but also the health of prosperity and pleasure and personal fulfillment. A life deprived of meaning cannot be described as healthy in this context. A homeless person or a refugee is not in good health according to that definition. Shakespeare in *Hamlet* gives this sense to the word when Hamlet admonishes: "Be thou a spirit of health." Similarly, but negatively, *The Book of Common Prayer* uses the word broadly: "…there is no health in us." The surgeon's commitment to a patient's health should be similarly broad and extend far beyond wound healing and resolution of intestinal ileus.

Indeed, perhaps the single, most venerable conflict in ethics is whether the good to be sought is "good for me" or "good for something or someone other than me." It is important to not hastily assign value to either of these conflicting notions.

"Good for others" may include good for patients, their families, or all of the world's sentient beings. And "good for me" may include self-understanding, which promotes my own health or prevents burnout or depression. The surgeon is therefore constantly whipsawed between these conflicting "goods," and statements suggesting a categorical acceptance of only one position drives tension underground to fester subconsciously. In chapter 3, we will label the poles of this dichotomy with names traditionally used in writings on ethics, but first we must consider some of the elements of medical ethics more specifically.

# 2 Foundations

Lloyd A. Jacobs, MD

"Good" and "right" and "ought" are thought by many to be basic notions that do not need additional foundational analysis. We know what they mean, and our everyday use of these words is believed by many to be sufficient to declare their meaning. But even assuming the correctness of that position, what is it that constitutes foundations for obligations to do acts that are right or good?

Ideas about the origin of the obligations that moral philosophy prescribes have at least 2 foundations, 2 back stories. In the aggregate, then what one does with one's life may be analyzed against 3 measures. One widely held foundation for human obligations is that such obligations originate in an external law, a legal statute, or a metaphysical pronouncement. Such ethical declarations of what is good and right and what is evil as well as persons holding that view are termed "deontological." Once enunciated, these ethical norms are believed to be good in themselves and acts conforming to these norms are thought to be intrinsically good. Such actions are thought to be right on their own recognizance. An example might be "one should always tell the truth" or "one should show respect for life." These actions and the rules, which emerge from them, are believed to have intrinsic, deontological value. They are, however, authoritative by virtue of the authority of statute, contractualism, or metaphysical principles.

A separate and distinct criterion for classifying acts as good or evil is from an analysis of their consequences or intended consequences. These ethical norms and those who hold them are called "teleological," a term the surgeon may recall from freshman biology. If the predicted or intended outcome of liver resection is good, then the act is good. Acts are thought not to have intrinsic value but are "known by their fruits." One may speculate whether an act is "good" when its outcome by accident happens to be good. A teleological ethic stresses intention and prediction and seems to me to fail to take into account the indeterminacy that is intercalated between the act and the outcome. There is a space between an act and its consequence into which accident may intrude.

It is important to note that there is a historical progression from a posture, which was entirely deontological to the currently widely held belief that norms should be evaluated teleologically. Earlier norms were based on metaphysics; the *Ten Commandments* are believed by many to have been dictated by God himself. A milestone in the development of an ethical posture more based on experience in the world was the publication of a small book entitled *Utilitarianism* in 1863 by John Stuart Mill. This term is widely used today to designate beneficence measured by the good or evil that occurs as an outcome of a human act. The temporal progression from a deontological base to a teleological base to a humanistic base is as yet incomplete and will be spoken of again in chapter 3.

We are now in a position to expand on what was mentioned in the foreword of this book. The ethics of the surgeon is a deontological ethic, responsible to the authority of the unique experience that surgery provides.

Deontological ethics is based on authority: metaphysical or legal, or intuition based. For the surgeon the authority is the venerable discipline itself. The deontological base of the surgeon's ethic is the spirit of the centuries-long commitment to the unique experience of plunging one's hands into the life of another.

A subset or perhaps a variant of the notion that an act is to be judged by its outcomes deserves a separate analysis. Here the classification of acts or actions is according to a physiologic criterion. If it results in pleasure, it is good; if it results in pain, it is evil. In the abstract, pain or pleasure may be experienced by oneself or by others, but the degree of pleasure or pain is the sole measure of goodness. And for some, pleasure or the absence of pain is the only good; all that is good is so because it produces or is intended 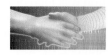 to produce pleasure. This stance is termed hedonism, a term that has entered the language of everyday usage. Since antiquity, hedonism has had worthy proponents, but we have only recently come to understand somewhat better the physiology of pleasure and pain and can immediately think of exceptions to hedonism. Still, the concept has an important place in the discussion of a surgeon's ethics.

This classification or this set of descriptions does not work for the modern surgeon. No life can be guided by a pure ethic from one of these categories, all of modern life is too messy and too complex. That which gives meaning to our lives, namely, the way we attempt to live in the world refuses easy delineations. All merges into all.

The classic example of a deontological ethic: "always tell the truth" must be tempered as every surgeon knows by the impact of that truth on the patient or his family. To always tell the truth, particularly in a single setting, may in fact not be productive of good results. Under a teleological ethic, therefore, always telling the truth may on occasion be evil by virtue of its evil consequences. Once, many decades ago I operated on a 17-year-old girl for presumed appendicitis. At operation, her appendix was normal. Her right fallopian tube was ruptured by an ectopic pregnancy. I bluntly told her and her family of the facts. On her third postoperative day, she jumped from an 11th floor window (this happened before modern window stops) to her death. I have regretted her death now for many years.

As regards a purely teleological stance, in which a good outcome declares an act to be good or right, I remember distinctly being lashed out at by Alexander Walt, subsequently the President of the American College of Surgeons. A young man came to the Emergency Department of the Detroit Receiving Hospital with a stiletto-like knife through his sternum and into his anterior mediastinum. I pulled the knife out; the patient remained absolutely stable and asymptomatic, and after a period of observation was sent home.

Walt spoke angrily to me: "just because you got away with it doesn't make it right." More importantly, I believe, Alex Walt's pejoration surfaces the most important weakness in a utilitarian posture for surgeons. To evaluate every individual act for its contribution to human welfare is not feasible. Rule utilitarianism implies that rules are formulated, which when followed will result in the greatest ratio of good over evil. A rule such as "every injury that penetrates the anterior mediastinum must be explored surgically" is based on that belief. One defines a group of similar situations and enjoins an action, which will result in the greatest human flourishing.

The difficulty, of course, is that nothing is ever the same; similar perhaps, but never the same. The categorization of events and situations becomes the variable. In the case of my stiletto, it mattered not to Alex Walt if the penetration was high or low, into the right side of the sternum or the left; all were to be subjected to surgical exploration. In the aggregate then, absolute adherence to the rule would result, he believed, in the greatest good for the greatest number. He was right, I think.

Surgeons are notorious for giving reasons that their patients, or an individual patient, do not fit the rule's category. "My patient was a young ninety."

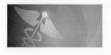 "My patients are uniquely at high risk." The exclusion of an act or situation from a grouping, which is covered by an ethical rule of action, becomes the surgeon's most frequent source of error. It is all too often the result of egoistic or hedonistic thinking.

Opposite this assessment, however, is the recognition that expertise is the very quality that allows one to stretch a category to include events or situations that do not quite fit the rule. The expert decides and performs with seeming ease, seeing the thousands of small steps that constitute an operative procedure in an elastic framework, whereas the beginner displays rigidity. Expertise is the ability to see the appropriateness of inclusion or exclusion into the rules governing moral actions.

Finally, hedonism asserts that pleasure is not only a good, it is the good. This position is unrealistic to those who have studied modern physiology. The difficulty arises, however, with the propensity of some to paint all pleasure as evil and the unnecessary, but incessant self-sacrifice that many surgeons practice risks their own health and their family's happiness. In summary, the historical analysis of moral philosophy as deontological, teleological, and 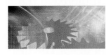 hedonistic offers little day-to-day guidance for the modern surgeon. At the same time, modern surgeons' ethical rules have evolved into a near random list of "do this," "do not do that" which, at first glance, seems unconnected to the historical foundations of moral philosophy. Fortunately, there is a bridge that consists of a compendium of a modern surgeon's moral principles:

1. The surgeon's beneficence is distinctive in its striving for excellence in decisions and skill in craftsmanship.
2. One is to strive to protect and promote the autonomy of patients and other persons who are affected by one's actions.
3. One should strive to distribute the fruits of one's own efforts and the resources of the world in a just fashion.
4. One should strive to avoid conflicts where one's resolution would further one's own interests unduly.

Beneficence, autonomy, distributive justice, and conflict of interest have emerged in the present day as the urgent imperatives for modern health care, and more specifically for the surgeon, practical wisdom and procedural skill have to be pursued.

Let us see if we can enunciate the elements of this bridge to the traditional foundations. Beneficence may be a teleological ethic; it requires acts whose consequences are good in such a way that evil is diminished and good prevails. The sum total of good increases; the sum total of evil diminishes, or at least this ratio moves in the direction of good. This moral philosophy is, however, ancient and is reflected in our own recollected admonition: "first of all, do no harm." A common formulation has it that one should attempt "the greatest good for the greatest number." But many find benevolent acts to be intrinsically good, regardless of their outcome, and the ethics of surgery are fundamentally deontological.

In light of the possible entry of evil into the space between the act and its outcome, some mix of the deontological must be alloyed with this largely teleological stance. That certain acts are obligations intrinsically seems incontrovertible, and the idea of beneficence becomes an amalgam.

Justice seems to be an almost purely deontological ethic. It is mandated as intrinsically valuable by most ethicists, as well as by most religious and secular traditions. Distributive justice seems more complex and seems to have an outcome-based good associated with it. To elevate those who need it most seems on the face of it to intend or predict an increase in the sum total of good in the world.

Autonomy of persons, it may be argued, is a derivative of beneficence. Autonomy is an aspect of human flourishing; its promotion may be predicted to increase the good in the world. However, autonomy can also be seen to have an intrinsic value by placing the human person in a central place, by recognizing that some people assert that humans were created in the image of deity. The distinction is less important than the observation that the autonomy of our patients sits firmly on venerable deontological foundations of our discipline.

The avoidance of conflict of interest can also be seen as derivative. Such conflicts may distribute good in a way contrary to the notion of distributive justice. Moreover, the interests perceived to be in conflict are almost always contrary to the notions of beneficence. The area of conflict of interest is being rapidly expanded, and its concerns are widely debated. The surgeons will have many opportunities to experience such conflict.

The bridge principles of beneficence, conflict, justice, and autonomy are firmly founded. Still there are many riddles here, which we will try to unravel subsequently.

# 3 Deontological Ethics in a Postfoundational World

Lloyd A. Jacobs, MD

The world in which we currently live has been described as "postmodern" or "postfoundational," implying a loss of the certainty and clarity of previous eras. We live, some believe, in a messy world, a world of continuous change and one with no place to plant our ethical feet. The metaphysical base of at least those ethical positions called deontological has been abandoned or marginalized by modern society. This world of constant flux has resulted, in part at least, from the development of a scientific world view. The most widely held ethical stance is utilitarianism. The central assertion of the next several paragraphs is that we are experiencing a return to a deontological base for our ethics. This, however, is a "new deontology" and a "humanistic deontology." This return is of particular interest to the surgeon-ethicist as the central ethic of the surgeon has had a deontological base throughout the centuries.

The rise of modern science has had the ironic effect of simultaneously moving humankind away from a position of centrality and toward such a position of centrality. Humankind is no longer at the center of the physical universe as it once was. The Hubble telescope and the astronomers who analyze the data it produces continue that which was begun by Tycho Brahe and Johannes Kepler and brilliantly synthesized by Galileo, namely, the decentering of our world by the demonstration that our world is a tiny speck of dirt orbiting a very common star.

The revolution precipitated by Charles Darwin when he published *The Origin of Species* in 1859 was vigorously supported by Thomas Huxley in 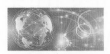 the popular media of that time. The storm of protest with which it was met was not because of its scientific import; similar theories had been extant for years. The revolution had to do with humankind's place in the world and with the importance and sanctity of humankind's unique ways of life. The foundations of those ways of life were shaken.

The rise of science during the last 2 centuries has had spectacular force because of its explanatory power and the way that its technologic spin-offs have improved human life, at least for many segments of the world's population. Science has altered the assumptions concerning what it is to be a human being and, in the eyes of some, has extended itself beyond its legitimate field of endeavor. Currently, scientism is the prevailing world view, and "naturalism," the belief in the ultimate adequacy of scientific theory and practice to all of life's needs, has become the leading world view of contemporary philosophy. What then of moral philosophy?, What of ethics whose deontological bases have been abandoned?, What of surgery's deontological foundations?

Dr John Flynn sat one night in the call room at Riverside Hospital with his personal duffel bag on his knees. He was thinking about suicide and how he would carry out the act and what would be the appropriate time for it. He imagined the upset it would cause to many. After a few minutes contemplating this, he rummaged in his bag for a pint bottle of vodka, thinking all the while of how alcohol possession was a violation of the hospital's rules and how particularly unwise was alcohol consumption while on call for the surgical service. He drank quickly.

Dr Flynn grew up with all of the verities of standard religion and patriotism. He had believed that America was the greatest country ever created; created perhaps by God himself. "God's in His heaven—and all's right with the world!"[1] had been very clear to Dr Flynn. But, at a point that Flynn could hardly pinpoint, he had discovered, as if his beliefs had a mind of their own, that he no longer believed these things. What he had believed was foundational seemed no longer relevant or correct.

John Flynn came to recognize that, somewhere between the beginning of the third year of medical school and the end of the second year of residency, something changes in us. The change occurs subtly, imperceptibly: thought patterns change, jokes change, and relationships with those around us change. We become more Teflon coated. The value of the lives and health of our assigned patients seems lessened by their intransigence, noncompliance, and poor hygiene. Flynn came to hate them. Having recognized this hatred within himself, he went back into his duffel bag for a last sip.

The rise of science has, inadvertently I am convinced, once again moved humankind to the uncomfortable position of ethical centrality; humanism has become the new foundation of moral conduct. But, as Dr Flynn came to know, this ethical posture seems to some to constitute inadequate support for the surgeon. Still, it is necessary for us somehow to find within ourselves an authoritative foundation for the ethics of beneficence, justice, autonomy, and avoidance of conflict. Like it or not, humankind is again at the center, and you are burdened with the freedom to choose your way of life. The ethics of the surgeon provides a resting place. The discipline itself, consisting as it does, of the collected human experience of centuries constitutes our ethical base, a foundation that is largely deontological. This is a humanistic base, with human venturing at its center. This is the way that surgeons "go on"; our commitment is to tread the path that other surgeons have experienced since the dawn of history. Surgeons exemplify a "new deontology" with a humanistic center.

An alternative train of thought may serve to bring us to the same position. An ethical foundation called "contractualism" has been proposed as an alternative form of deontologism. Contractualism is based on a statement of consensus supporting a body of rules, which cannot be refuted or rejected by any reasonable person or persons.[2] Clearly, the ethics and traditions of the discipline of surgery qualify for this foundational support. And, although we will continue to view the surgeon's ethics as deontological and will not speak of contractualism again, contractualism also may provide an adequate base for the surgeon's ethics.

Surgeons, more than any others, are celebrants of humankind's freedom. The practicing surgeon, with his/her own principles of success and failure, cannot see the universe as deterministic. The surgeon, more than others perhaps, possesses a will that is free, free to choose among other things how his/her life's posture will be oriented. Although this freedom is accompanied by its own form of anguish, we have chosen an orientation toward beneficence, justice, and human autonomy.

It matters little to the practical ethics of the surgeon if impulses of beneficence and justice are genetically or societally determined. And, a human-centered ethic need not worry the theist, who generally asserts that man was created in the image of God, or God in the image of man, and may, therefore, be legitimately taken as the central measure of morality. But how do we formulate such a morality, how do we become committed in a postfoundational world?

My first injunction is to try to trust your epistemic apparatus. Trust that what seems right for you to believe and that acts which derive from those beliefs are in fact probably good and right. Try to trust the impulses that seem to be directing you; they are almost certainly valid. This placement of trust may sometimes have a tone of defiance in it. We will do what is good and right even though we have no good reason to do so. One hears this tone of defiance in Dylan Thomas' "Do Not Go Gentle into that Good Night." The 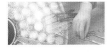 defiance is explicit in the words of de Senancour: "...let us not live in such a way that it [annihilation] would be a just fate." Dr Bernard Rieux is the protagonist of Albert Camus' great existentialist novel *The Plague*. He stays at his duty as he sees it, defying all odds, and with a sort of defiance of the social norms of the plague-ridden city in which he finds himself.

Heretofore, we have described ethical norms as being grounded in an external imperative; such norms are termed deontological. Alternatively, norms have been described as grounded by their consequences in the world; such norms are termed teleological. It is necessary in our postmodern world to assert that ethical norms may rest on a new deontological foundation, namely, their capacity for the creation of meaning in the life of the acting person. Such soul-creating acts will, for the surgeon, invariably include beneficence, justice, and autonomy; they rest now on a new ground, their field of play is the human will and the creation of a life of meaning.

We must therefore recognize a ground for our surgical ethics, which is deontological, derived from the authority of our discipline. This foundation may, in postfoundational parlance perhaps, be described as soul building; ethical action creates the human soul ex nihilo. This third foundational pillar is a deontological pillar far more than a teleological pillar, which would perhaps be weakened by the loose coupling between an action and its consequences.

You may ask, as have many before you, why attempt to act ethically in a world without foundation, a world in which, therefore, "everything is permitted." The answer is clear but not intuitive: one acts ethically for the purpose of creating a meaningful life. Commit yourself to the great ethical traditions of our discipline, and you will become a surgeon who lives and has lived in the light of the discipline's ethical posture.

And, Dr Flynn, there is help available, you need only to ask. Intact reader, perhaps you may become a part of Flynn's support system.

# References

1. Browning R. *Pippa Passes and Shorter Poems*. In: Baker JE, ed. *Odyssey Series in Literature*. New York: The Odyssey Press; 1947.
2. Scanlon TM. Contractualism and utilitarianism. In: Rajchmon J, West C, eds. *Post-analytic Philosophy*. New York: Columbia University Press; 1985.

# 4 Beneficence Versus Egoism

Lloyd A. Jacobs, MD

It is necessary to begin again at the beginning. Surgeons experience ethical issues as tension, as a tug-of-war between competing values and obligations. Surgeons do not experience ethics in relation to normative structural descriptors. Still, because beneficence and its "not quite" opposite egoism, in particular, are widely held to be central concepts in medical ethics, it is necessary to consider from whence they came and whither they might lead us.

We will continue to leave "good" and "right" and "ought" undefined except by intuition and by our common use of the terms. We will decide that, for surgeons at least, self-interest alone as constituting the greatest good has been rejected; egoism as a categorical position is rarely held by surgeons, but egoism as a psychologic force is ubiquitous among surgeons as well as among all human persons.

Our alternative to egoism is beneficence or, if its formulation in modernity is emphasized, it may sometimes be called "utilitarianism." The notion is as follows: We ought to do right and good things for the whole of humankind; indeed in the eyes of some, we ought to do right and good things for all sentient beings or perhaps even all life forms. The idea of utilitarianism is that our acts individually, or the rules of day-to-day conduct, which are formulated, ought to maximize the good produced and/or minimize the evil produced. We ought to, according to this view, by our acts and formulation of rules, pursue by our acts or intentions a maximum ratio of good over evil. In common parlance, our acts or rules ought to produce "the greatest good for the greatest number" of human creatures. This beneficial impact may include oneself, but

**15**

contrary to the posture of egoism, it is not limited to self-interest; its emphasis is, in fact, on "other-ism" or altruism.

It is correct to assert that, currently, the principle of utilitarianism is the prevalent position of many of the world's ethical thinkers. Beneficence is stated to be one of the pillars of medical ethics by most of the texts and other writings in the arena. As may be expected, however, enunciation of this categorical posture leaves the surgeon with many tensions and conflicts on a day-to-day basis.

The two additional principles of a surgeon's ethics are called into our consciousness by a consideration of beneficence. The first of these is "autonomy." To support and celebrate the autonomy of individuals can be seen as a way to maximize the sum total of "good" in the world. It is easier to perceive the impact of the opposite: To practice paternalism or even slavery is to promote that which is not good and clearly does not promote human flourishing. Autonomy, therefore, joins beneficence as a fundamental pillar of a surgeon's ethical stance. Yet another ethical notion constitutes a third pillar of a surgeon's ethical stance, namely, justice. Justice stands nearly opposite beneficence, justice "seasons"[1] beneficence, justice speaks how the fruits of beneficence ought to be distributed. 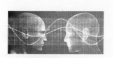 Distributive justice contributes some of the surgeon's most difficult decisions and, therefore, is the source of considerable conflict and tension in the surgeon's inner life. In summary, beneficence, autonomy, and justice constitute the three primary pillars of the ethics of a surgeon. Each will be considered subsequently.

Egoism is a near synonym of self-interest as an ethical posture. Self-interest is a part of living. Although self-interest or egoism is rarely formally subscribed to by surgeons, the notion is best thought of as a powerful and ubiquitous psychologic force. Surgeons in particular must deal with their own self-interests by granting the legitimacy of those interests and by assigning proper weights to them. Consider the situation of Dr Moynihan.

Surgical trainee Moynihan is in his sixth year of residency and has never performed a pancreaticoduodenectomy, a complex and challenging operation. He believes, correctly, that he needs to experience performing this operation.

A patient is admitted to the affiliated Veterans Administration Hospital where Moynihan is rotating with a mass in the duodenum, which biopsy shows to be adenocarcinoma. The kicker, however, is that the patient, 18 months ago, underwent a partial colectomy for a colon cancer at the hepatic flexure. The duodenal mass is, therefore, likely to be a local extension of the colon cancer, now invading the duodenum.

Pancreaticoduodenectomy in this setting is of doubtful efficacy. The patient is 74 years old and frail. On the other hand, he is already experiencing difficulty with gastric emptying.

Moynihan has a difficult decision: to perform a pancreaticoduodenectomy along with resection of adjacent structures found at operation to be involved, or to perform a lesser noncurative operation such as gastrojejunostomy, or perhaps even to only provide palliative care. Moynihan has been assured by his teaching surgeon supervisor that his, Moynihan's, recommendation will be accepted.

Now, Moynihan needs this case; he needs this experience. His stature among his fellow trainees will be enhanced by a successful outcome. His performance at his oral board examination in 2 years may well focus on aspects of cases like this one. Moreover, he loves to operate.

It is easy to state the sterile position, that only the patient's wishes should be honored. It is a little less sterile to state that whatever the surgical literature describes as outcomes for operations, such as the one contemplated, should be determinant, although these elements should be carefully weighed. But it is also important to avoid elements of the situation that do not recognize Moynihan's interests. They are legitimate, and arguments may well be made that this experience will have a salutatory effect on many operations by Moynihan in the future.

In the next several paragraphs, we will consider egoism, the classical label of the "good for me" end of the tug-of-war. Discussions about egoism are found in the writing of Plato. The notion is, therefore, of ancient origin, and, although it is not today the "official" posture of many, it is important to know that egoism is always present in each of us and it weighs on almost every decision we make.

There are at least four claims inherent in the notion of egoism:

*"First, each of us is always and only motivated by our own self-interest. Second, this self-interest may lie in the pride of saving the world, curing cancer or such other seemingly salutatory work. Third, egoism states that one "ought" always to act in one's own self-interest. Fourth, the rational egoist, agreeing with the egocentric contention that all one's interests are interests of the self, argues that minimally it is always wrong to harm oneself."*[2]

I am willing to concede that the polar and categorical brand of egoism described above may be rejected on the outset, on the basis of intuition and the *weltgeist* of today. It is important to note, however, that this ethic of moral action has had and still has a multitude of adherents. Furthermore, egoism is more often manifested by actions in the world than by the profession 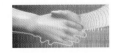 of egoism as one's life position. Many adherents may in action be unconscious of their commitment to egoism, as egoism seems to be the default position for most human beings, the ethical position toward which we all seem to drift.

Surgeons from the earliest recorded history and even before that have rejected egoism as a stated system of obligation and value. Still, surgeons like all human beings drift toward that position if one's commitments are left unattended. It is important for us all not to characterize self-interest as "not good" even though most of us will be unable to embrace the entirety of the 4 components of egoism as enunciated above. To reject self-interest categorically is to reject our humanity and to invite into our lives a rigidity that ultimately destroys.

Although there is a history of medicine before Hippocrates, it is fair to say that the ethics of medicine was established and enunciated by that person or the various writers whose writings constitute the Hippocratic Corpus. Hippocrates is thought to have lived from 460 to 370 BC, and it is he who gave us not only the scientific spirit of medicine but also the ethical ideals of medicine, which still have influence today. And for purposes of this discussion the Hippocratic ethical writings are a clear rejection of egoism.[3] Edelstein points out that in the eyes of the Greeks, "medicine itself imposes certain obligations upon the physician, obligations summed up in the magic phrase 'love of humanity.'" Edelstein points out further that in the writing entitled "On the Physician," it is stated that the physician must be a "lover of man." These statements are interesting not only because they are precisely opposite the notion of egoism but also because they are found in the earliest of the Hippocratic writings and are built on in later writings such as the familiar Hippocratic Oath. That oath clearly commits to "other-ism" and opposes egoism. The obligations spoken of include not only "him who has taught me this art," but go on to castigate behaviors that must, at that historical juncture, have been fairly common elements of self-interest. The oath twice uses the phrase "for the benefit of the sick," a clear repudiation of the categorical egoism described above.

Still, the Hippocratic surgeon must have experienced the inner tension created by strict adherence to principles, which derogate self-interest. The Greek surgeon's motive for developing and practicing his craft was to make a living. Self-satisfaction also must have been a part of the Greek surgeon's psychic life as dressings for the purpose of show are advised against, as are similar evidences of inordinate pride or the advertising of skill. At the same time, although probably at a later date within the Hippocratic period, in the work "In the Surgery," which specifies everything from lighting to the surgeon's posture, the surgeon is told to apply bandages quickly and skillfully "in such a way that it is pleasant to watch."

In summary, the Hippocratic surgeon was admonished to an ideal of altruism, to avoid hubris, and to be generous of his time and skill. However, the Hippocratic surgeon must have experienced ethical tensions similar to the tensions we today experience on a daily basis.

Percival's *Medical Ethics*, published in 1803 by Thomas Percival (1740-

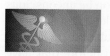

1804), is often dismissed as being composed only of medical etiquette but was published at a critical juncture in the development of modern medicine. It contains several paragraphs, which clearly repudiate egoism as a philosophy that the surgeon may reasonably hold. Among them, one finds:

*"The feelings and emotions of the patients…require…to be attended to, no less than the symptoms of their diseases."*

The comments and descriptions of scores of surgeons, modern and ancient, attest to an altruistic posture. No less an observer of medicine and medical education than Abraham Flexner had much to say about William Stewart Halsted. Flexner was the author of the now famous "Report on Medical Education," published by the Carnegie Foundation in 1910. That work is credited for revolutionizing medical education in the United States. *The Flexner Report* caused the United States to embark on a course, which 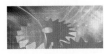 has caused it to be a world leader in medicine. Surgeons, formerly small businessmen, who mentored their understudies for their service or for a fee, became affiliated with institutions as a result of the report. Full-time faculty members largely replaced faculties whose first commitment was often to their lucrative practices.

Although Flexner was not himself a surgeon, nor a physician, his stamp on American Medicine is unparalleled. He was an acute observer, an accurate reporter, and a careful critic. At a point in his life, he became a patient of William S. Halsted, one of the founders of modern surgery.

Halsted majored in athletics at Yale and graduated in 1874. His scholastic success was mediocre. Medical School at the College of Physicians and Surgeons in New York appeared to challenge him more or at least suit him better. He led his class in academic achievement. In 1878, Halsted began 2 years of study in Vienna, but in his second year in Europe he was peripatetic, visiting surgical clinics across Europe. He practiced in New York until he became the professor of surgery at the still developing Johns Hopkins School of Medicine and the Johns Hopkins Hospital.

My purpose in relating this vignette is not only to amuse, but it is meant to illustrate the actions of a surgeon, Halsted, which clearly imply a rejection of egoism. Dr Flexner suffered a slip and fall accident and sustained a Pott's fracture in his left leg. Treatment at a New York hospital only resulted in a recalcitrant wound with exposure of the extensor tendons. It was Mrs Flexner who decided to seek Halsted's care in Baltimore. Moreover, Halsted's actions speak of an ethical dilemma we will consider subsequently, that is, how one may justly distribute time and commitment and material resources. Suffice it to say, Halsted devoted maximal resources to Flexner's wound. Flexner wrote:

> *"Day after day he came in the morning about ten, in the afternoon about four, and frequently at night before bedtime, to dress the wound himself. He said little, but he would sit…After prolonged contemplation…he would ask for this or that. No one else was permitted to touch the foot…"*[4]

These actions seem clearly not to be those of an egoist. But perhaps Halsted's motives are less clear. Pride doubtlessly played a role in his seemingly monomaniac attentiveness. Flexner was a celebrity, perhaps desire for fame was a factor. Ultimately the foot healed with a skin graft, but it was the granulation over the exposed tendons that helped establish Halsted's reputation for greatness. No motives experienced by human surgeons are ever unmixed and include some of the egoism described above.

Egoism in its purest form has become less prevalent as a professed philosophy. It is best thought of now as a psychologic force, a force which is part of us all and part of our humanity. Although the tug-of-war between egoism and altruism plays out in the inner life of us all, it is important not to assume a rigidity of posture in which altruism is good and egoism is bad. Egoism is a part of life, a part of every healthy life. A special variant of egoism has been called hedonism and is the subject of the next chapter.

## References

1. Shakespeare W. *The Merchant of Venice*; vol. IV. New York: George Routledge and Sons; 1885:201.
2. Werhane PH. A normative perspective. In: Peperzak AT, ed. *Ethics as First Philosophy*. London and New York: Routledge; 1995:60.
3. Edelstein L. The Professional Ethics of the Greek Physician. *Bull Hist Med.* 1956;30:391–419. Reprinted in Ancient Medicine. Edited by Owsei, Lillian Temkin C. Baltimore: Johns Hopkins Press; 1967.
4. Crowe SJ. *Halsted of Johns Hopkins: The Man and His Men.* Springfield, IL: Charles C. Thomas; 1957:238.

# 5 Hedonism

Lloyd A. Jacobs, MD

We began thinking about what is "good" and "right" and what one "ought" to do by asserting that these notions were basic, that they had no back story and needed no further explication, and that the everyday usage is sufficient to define them. There is another approach, however, and it is important to discuss and understand what has been subsumed under the rubric of "hedonism."

The fundamental assertion of hedonism is that pleasure is the sole measure of that which is good and that its opposite, pain, stands opposed to the good of pleasure. This very different approach is supported by the observation that hedonism is also teleological, and it depends for its status as "good" on the outcome of the acts described. It is not to be considered a deontological precept because deontological precepts are usually thought of as originating from a statute, commandment, or metaphysical mandate. Pleasure arrives from within us as creatures; hedonism is, therefore, quintessentially humanistic at its core. Hedonism has never, to the best of my knowledge, been the professed position of any surgeon. This is no surprise because the assertion would be nearly tautological. The profession of surgery commits to using one's hands beneficently, not alone for pleasure.

Dr Leonard stepped back from the operating room table and stripped off his gloves. He moved toward the circulating nurse who untied his gown, which he then shrugged off. He stepped back to look over the shoulder of the junior resident who was closing the skin after the multivisceral resection, kidney, liver, small bowel, and colon, for a recurrent but localized colon cancer.

Leonard thought to himself "now that was fun!" He pictured himself at dinner describing the case and the excellent outcome he anticipated. He experienced intense pleasure in his own sense of well-being and the prospect of the future. He experienced and was thankful for pleasure, but he knew very well that pleasure was not the sole good in the life of a surgeon.

Hedonism has a venerable history. A reasonable argument can be made that the pleasure Dr Leonard experienced is good not only for himself but also 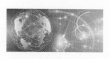 for others. Another supporting argument for hedonism has been that all creatures seem to have intrinsic mechanisms driving them toward pleasure and away from pain. This latter argument can be used to reach other conclusions, however. Surgeons are not hedonists, almost unanimously.

You may ask why then devote a chapter to hedonism? The answer is, I believe, that hedonism connects to multiple other disciplines and thought patterns and that, within us all, at a level, which often remains unconscious, a powerful force for self-preservation exists, along with the pleasure attendant to it. Moreover, because their profession is not a hedonistic one, surgeons have tended to deprecate pleasure and minimize its impact in their lives. The important distinction here is that historical hedonism declares pleasure to be the sole good, while a healthy balanced person perceives pleasure to be one important "good."

There is another face to hedonism, which is known as psychologic hedonism. The notion, which seems to me to be correct, is not that this inner force argues for a general hedonism, but that it has great relevance to what it is to be human. A full understanding of this force, which may be associated with the Freudian id, is necessary to self-knowledge. While the id is that part of the human psyche, which is devoted to pleasure and survival, the concepts of beneficence and justice may more aptly be associated with the ego and superego. Whether this analogy holds or not, psychologic hedonism is a force within us all but does not constitute a logical support for formal hedonism.

A statement of the converse has also been held by some to be true: If it brings pleasure it is good. If it brings pain it is not good. We ought to always act in such a way as to maximize the ratio of pleasure to pain we experience. These statements seem to me to be manifestly untrue. We have learned much about the physiology of pleasure since the notions of hedonism were first enunciated. There are many ways that pleasure-causing endogenous endorphins may be released, including the scourge of opioid drugs. The pain (well controlled) associated with a life-saving operation is at least a concomitant of something good. There is no one-to-one relationship between pleasure and the "good" in the eyes of the modern surgeon.

Some support for the notion of hedonism being an intrinsic force within us all may be derived from Darwin. If, in fact, random mutations are winnowed and culled or encouraged by natural selection, it would be reasonable to argue that there must be pleasure, hedonistic pleasure perhaps, associated with the process. Certainly the procreative portion of the process could be seen in this way. But even if this hypothesis supports the idea that pleasure seeking is an important force within us, the logic that proceeds "therefore, pleasure seeking must be the sole good" seems to me to be weak. Furthermore, evolutionary psychologists have by now spent decades attempting to demonstrate evolution of an "altruistic gene."

Why then have we spent so much time on hedonism, more specifically on psychologic hedonism? Just because of the accuracy of that nomenclature: It provides the link between the field of ethics and the discipline of psychology. The transition from thinking about ethics to thinking about the rate of depression and suicide in physicians and surgeons is to pass across the bridge of hedonism. It is my hypothesis that the absolutism of our profession's commitment to beneficence, justice, and autonomy and our deprecation of healthy nonabsolute hedonism are important causes of the illness of depression and suicide among us.

Thomas Schwenk,[1] in an article that quotes Dyrbye et al, makes the connection between ethics and depression explicit:

> *"...burnout...is associated with higher self-reported rate of cheating on examinations, lying about clinical data, medical errors, and ethical lapses, as well as less altruistic and compassionate care."*[2]

Ethical lapses in this scenario feed back on the resident surgeon to cause greater stress, which in turn exacerbates depression and suicidal ideation. This is a book about ethics, not about the psychology of depression. It is, however, a central hypothesis of this book that categorically idealistic ethical norms are damaging the caregivers' mental health and do the patient little good. A dilute tincture of hedonism may be in order.

## References

1. Schwenk TL. Resident depression – the tip of a graduate medical education iceberg. *JAMA*. 2015;314(22):2357–2358.
2. Dyrbye LN, Massie Jr FS, Eacker A, et al. Relationship between burnout and professional conduct and attitudes among U.S. medical students. *JAMA*. 2010;304(11):1173–1180.

# Autonomy: Concepts

6

Lloyd A. Jacobs, MD

Within the lives of most healthy persons a pattern of individuation may be perceived. Wholly dependent infants become self-confident girls and boys, who become self-sufficient teenagers and ultimately adults who sustain not only themselves but also families and institutions. More importantly, they become, for the most part, psychologically whole, not isolated but whole, with choices and efficacy and freedom of the will. Autonomy emerges as an almost fundamental characteristic, defining what it is to be a whole person. A modicum of self-love and hedonism is a prerequisite for self-sufficiency, which is a necessary quality required for the love of others, and also for the life of a healthy beneficent surgeon.

Illness impairs autonomy. Even minor illness, perhaps a 1-day influenza, occasions solicitude from family members, with tokens of dependency such as traditional foods. Serious illness, and most of all terminal illness, predicts a period of almost total dependency. For many, some of whom may have had a difficult personal journey to autonomy, the fear of this helplessness is more dreadful than death itself. All too often the acts or failures to act by surgeons hasten or worsen the destruction of a patient's autonomy. A brilliant life-saving operation may consign a patient to an institution for life. The referral of a postoperative patient for further care may be seen by the patient as a declaration of hopelessness or abandonment by the surgeon. Symbols such as these may be perceived by a patient as an inadequate trade-off for longevity.

On a day of routine work my friend and colleague Diane, standing in front of my office desk, said casually to me, "I must have a rough edge on a tooth; I find myself lisping." I could barely detect a lisp, but on listening carefully it was distinctly there. Her lisp worsened rapidly. Soon she could not speak or swallow; nor type, nor walk, nor fondle her grandchildren. The diagnosis was amyotrophic lateral sclerosis, and the outlook was for total loss of muscle action, total loss of physical autonomy, and death. What Diane feared most, indeed what prospect she loathed, was the certainty of total dependence. She who had been self-sufficient and the sustainer of her family faced a loss of autonomy.

There are 3 great pillars of the ethical posture of the surgeon: beneficence, justice, and autonomy. Beneficence is practiced every day in our work. Our commitment that every operation or conversation makes the world a better place is beyond doubt. Conversely, we strive to, first of all, do no harm. We pursue the ideal of distributive justice, recognizing the unattainability of that ideal, but using the notion of making our first commitment to our neighbor. But autonomy is different and more complex; autonomy is a chimera that serves an individual's well-being but contains the seeds of that which is harmful. Patients may not want autonomy.

All things merge into all. Autonomy, with its attendant efficacy and freedom, merges in the extreme into alienation, isolation, and loneliness. No patient wants to die alone; human beings need and crave connection with others. Pressing on them too much autonomy may lessen the likelihood of attaining this intimacy. Perhaps seeing these issues as constituting a spectrum with childlike dependence, healthy autonomy and painful alienation as marks along that spectrum will help in the conceptualization of these issues. Moreover, a lessening of autonomy is inevitable under therapeutic circumstances. Autonomy is impossible under general anesthesia!

It is necessary to introduce here the notion of the surgeon as an agent: one who is empowered to act for another. In this role, the surgeon has promised, tacitly or expressly, not to do what is likely to bring about the greatest amount of general good, not to distribute beneficence justly, but to do what the patient wishes or would wish if he/she were competent. Several points are immediately clear: The patient's wishes may be contrary to the dictates of beneficence or justice. The surgeon may, I believe, make certain assumptions regarding what the patient is likely to have wanted but cannot assume that the patient wanted what he/she himself/herself would want. Moreover, the 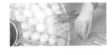 surgeon is saddled with the nearly impossible task of evaluating the surrogacy of others who purport to speak for the patient.

The notion of autonomy is, ultimately, a derivative of beneficence or utilitarianism. The logic is vague, but it is possible to see human autonomy as an aspect of human flourishing, particularly as we watch the child mature to a woman who sustains herself and others. Such human flourishing is "good" for which we "ought" to strive, because we ultimately intend to produce by our actions and utterances the greatest good for the greatest number. But the ideal of autonomy turns on itself when the surgeon is an agent, and what the notion of agency requires may neither maximize the good nor distribute it justly.

This contradictory feedback loop, combined with the impracticality of considering every act individually, demands that we subscribe to the idea of "rule beneficence" when dealing with its derivative "autonomy." There have been, however, few norms developed and fewer rules formulated. Once again, the surgeon may find himself at the locus of tension between conflicting demands.

Sonia Meyerdorf, aged 67 years, drove herself to my office for her initial visit. She had been referred to our vascular surgery practice by her primary care physician who had, upon a routine examination, thought he palpated an abnormally prominent pulse in her abdomen. He appropriately ordered a CT scan, which demonstrated a 5.2-cm abdominal aorta aneurysm that involved both renal arteries. The left renal artery arose from the aneurysm itself and the right renal artery arose from the area of transition of normal appearing aorta to an aneurysmal sac. Her creatinine was 1.7 mg/dL, in spite of her small frame and musculature.

My initial meeting with her showed her to be spritely, active, and acutely aware of her health status. She reported no weight loss, no diminution of muscle strength or walking speed. She believed her energy level to be undiminished. She reported no illness or other deficits, which would contribute to the definition of frailty.[1] Together we decided aneurysmectomy was in order.

The operation went well. The perfusion of the renal arteries was assured. The postoperative course was uneventful. On postoperative day 4, she was transferred to a long-term care institution.

She was brought to her first postoperative visit by an attendant from the long-term care institution, who pushed her wheelchair. She launched into her lament immediately. "When will I drive?" "I want to be back in my own house." "I hate the food; the bathrooms are dirty." And then came her summarizing declaration: "If I had known I'd have to be there, I would never have agreed to the operation. I'd rather have died on my own, at home."

Several observations about autonomy come immediately to mind. There is nothing like a big operation to make a youthful-appearing patient display his 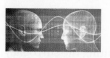 or her chronologic age. Depression is an almost invariable consequence of loss of familiarity, control, and autonomy for the elderly person. Barring very active management of the depression and loneliness, Sonia is very likely to die within the next 12 months. Autonomy is not a luxury; it is not a hedonistic pleasure, it is essential for healthy life.

The concept of the informed consent of a patient to undergo an operation or other intervention is to be distinguished from the formal requirement to obtain the patient's signature on a hospital form. The latter is frequently assigned to a junior member of the trainee team or to a nurse, and great variation has been shown to exist in the process. Far more important is the surgeon's belief that the patient's autonomy has been served with adequate information and voluntary agreement.

James Jones, a cardiovascular surgeon with 4 decades of experience, summarizes the principle of informed consent as well as the extensive literature that exists in this arena.[2] He discusses disclosure of information, complications, and the natural history of the patient's state. He then gives recognition to the variability of understanding a patient may possess. He recognizes that many influences may lessen the voluntary nature of the patient's decision 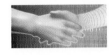 process. Jones recognizes that, like other aspects of ethics discussed in this book, informed consent is an abstract notion, never to be realized in our real world of ill patients.

This unreliability derives from the impossibility of full description of any situation. Operation or procedures can be described or their risk formulated in an infinite number of ways. It is not possible to describe all conceivable courses of action. It is for the ethical surgeon to select those features that are believed to be frequent, to be consequential, and to have an impact on life's quality. It is imperative to recognize that our own biases are impossible to leave behind or even disguise. Surgeons have a bias to action, which may be evident in the framing of a decision. The ethical surgeon will try to ameliorate the effects of an indeterminate reality and his own bias by repeated tellings and by allowing more than one person to inform the patient.

The chief resident was on his way to the operating room at 6:45 AM. He peeled away from rounds, then paused and spoke to Dr Henry Williams, a resident in his first postgraduate year. "Go," he said, "up to five and consent [sic] Mr. Evans for colectomy." Then he was gone.

Williams took the elevator to the fifth floor, found the hospital's consent form in Evan's chart, and went to his room. Williams read from the form: "bleeding, infection, leak occasionally occur." "What portion of the colon will be removed, what extent," Evan's asked. "Will I need a stoma? Will I have diarrhea? What's the frequency of infection?"

Williams assured Evans that he would be right back and went to the operating room, changed, and entered where the chief resident was operating, alone as chance would have it. "The patient wants to know how much colon, what's the chance of infection? I didn't ask him to sign."

The chief resident was distracted, but annoyed. "Damn it, tell him to sign and that I'll talk to him in the pre-operative care area. Don't bother me." Dr Williams followed the chief's orders but was troubled and felt diminished.

It seems a truism that the patient's autonomy is fostered by his possession of information. It matters little from whence the information comes. I remember clearly the first time a patient came for an initial visit to my office with an Internet printout in hand. I confess that I was not only startled but also felt a bit defensive. I, like most surgeons, was accustomed to being seen as the primary source of information, an infallible and complete source even. I have learned subsequently that the Internet gives great preparation for a patient discussion; indeed, more recently I have encouraged patients to seek information and even occasionally supplied them with Internet links.

There was a time when it was thought best or at least convenient to leave the patient ignorant of diagnosis and prognosis and the implication of such knowledge. Oliver Wendell Holmes, for example, wrote condescendingly about keeping patients in the dark. The paternalism, which prompted and fostered such behavior and attitudes, seems now to be directly contrary to the promotion of autonomy.

If one carries this train of thought forward, the idea that ignorance may be in a patient's best interest leads us to the possibility of lying to patients. I assert now, with little fear of contradiction, that there is no more powerful way to undermine a patient's autonomy than to lie to him. Moreover, it taints the caregiver's own welfare at the same time. What then of the comforting lie, the lie the patient may clearly be asking for? As the agent of the patient, are we not bound to give him/her what he/she asks for? This conundrum, like so many when one considers the psychology of human ethics, has no easy answer.

To always tell the truth is the most famous example of a deontological mandate, a maxim often seen as absolute. But, in the minds of some, the telling of the truth always brings rewards, perhaps eternal rewards, to the truth teller but not always to the patient. An outcome-based decision analysis might be more beneficial to the patient. It may be helpful to remind ourselves of the backstory behind the 2 large categories of ethical postures. A deontological backstory postulates the notion that the act, in and of itself, is either good or bad, that one ought to or ought not to act in some particular way because of some intrinsic power of the act itself. A teleological backstory postulates that acts and utterances are to be judged by their outcomes; if the outcome is good, the act was good.

To always tell the truth regardless of the outcome is quintessentially a deontological command. To withhold the truth or to "tell it slant" because of its intended outcome is to assume a teleological posture. A Hippocratic posture, which recommends doing what will benefit the patient, in the judgment of the surgeon, may be the right and good approach. The concept of being an agent for the patient would tend to underscore this outcome-based assessment; the surgeon has covenanted to act in the patient's interest, which, in this situation, may conflict with his own personal interest in being always a person who does not lie.

An examination of Sonia Meyerdorf shows the incision to be clean and dry and healing well. Her legs are well perfused. A call to the laboratory shows her creatinine to be 1.6 mg/dL. There is no "physical" issue. I tell her what I can only hope is true: You will get your strength back quickly; you will be out of there and back home in a very short time. She seemed heartened.

# References

1. Robinson TN, Walston JD, Brummel NE, et al. Frailty for surgery: review of a National Institute on Aging Conference on Frailty for specialists. *J Am Coll Surg.* 2015;221(6):1083–1092.
2. Jones JW, McCullough LB. What is meant by high risk informed consent. *J Vasc Surg.* 2015;62:510–511.

# 7 Distributive Justice: Concepts

Lloyd A. Jacobs, MD

The notion of distributive justice as it relates to the practice of surgery presents great difficulties. Its history is checkered, and the rules of everyday conduct are changing rapidly, and in my opinion, with inadequate thought. Furthermore, the relationship of distributive justice to the other two pillars of surgical ethics is complex. There is no other principle of ethics that will vex the practicing surgeon more than the ideal of distributive justice.

"Distributive justice" is merely an odd locution for the idea of the justice of distribution, the distribution of a surgeon's skill, his/her attention, and the great impact the surgeon may have on the distribution of the goods of a society. The surgeon has had almost sole authority to distribute expensive devices, sutures, heart valves, kidneys, and an array of desirables too long to list. And, although rules for everyday conduct are fairly well formulated, there is still considerable ambiguity in them.

Justice is not a teleological ethic; it is a deontological ethic. By that, it is meant that acts purporting to be just are not judged solely on their outcome or even their intended outcome. Justice is thought to have an intrinsic value; it cannot be derived from the notion of beneficence as can the principle of autonomy be. And, although in more classical writings on ethics, deontological ethics are thought by some to be derived from metaphysics, or perhaps from some statute or command, most ethicists agree that its current basis is intuitional: "that it just seems right."[1] The notion of distributive justice stands away from beneficence, and it places boundaries on one's ability to practice beneficence. Justice limits beneficence. And although beneficence and autonomy are teleological ethics, in that they may be evaluated by their outcomes, deontological nature of justice demonstrates that a mixture of ethical infrastructures is unavoidable. And justice militates against egoism and hedonism, which, as we have seen, are also teleological, in that they are evaluated by their outcomes. It is not surprising, therefore, that an inevitable tension exists between justice and beneficence and even between the dictates of justice and autonomy.

The basic notion of the justice of distribution is that stuff of value ought to be distributed according to some model, which is perceived by one's intuition as equal and therefore just. This formulation contains much ambiguity. Is to each according to his need an acceptable model of justice? Is to each according to his merit or societal contribution an acceptable model of justice? Or is to each according to his race or accidental place of birth an acceptable model of justice? Clearly, our notion of an acceptable model of justice rests on both political and metaphysical foundations. Some of the ambiguity in the notion has been ameliorated by a slightly more specific formulation: "Treat equal (or similar or like) cases alike." This formulation moves the ambiguity to the concepts of "equal" or "similar" or "like." A more recent contribution to the discourse on justice includes the formulation: "Treat unequal cases unalike."[2] This addition adds considerably to the flexibility of the imperative. However, what is "like" or "unlike" in any given situation?

To consider the distributive justice implications of every individual act of a surgeon would be impractical, indeed impossible, although there are those who are proponents of "act" ethics. "Rule" ethics involve the formulation of everyday rules of thumb for guidance. Even with this softening approach, the mandates of distributive justice are unattainable; the surgeon is after all subject to "being one traveler." Ultimately, even though true distributive justice is an unattainable ideal, its psychologic impact is significant on the practicing surgeon, and its principles "ought" to guide the surgeon's everyday behaviors. Not all the stuff to be distributed justly is material. One's presence is also of value, and its distribution is subject to ethical considerations.

Robert Marsh is a resident in his sixth postdoctoral year of surgical training. He has been planning a trauma fellowship beginning in a few months, a prospect he is excited about. Tonight, however, he is looking with anticipation toward something else—a long-planned dinner out with his wife with whom he is all too conscious of having spent inade- 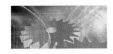 quate time in recent months. And spending time with her was not a duty for Marsh, but a pleasure that sustained him. He was to leave the hospital in 1 hour.

Marsh seeks out the resident to whom he is to sign out and sits down with him. He runs through a list of routine patients and learns that the staff surgeon on call that night will be Dr Thomas and that a level I trauma patient is en route from a hospital nearly 50 miles away. The patient is a 43-year-old man who fell 6 stories from an industrial scaffold.

Now, Dr Thomas is notorious among the residents for leaving them alone for long periods during operations at night and the resident to whom he has just signed out, a third year on one of his first nights on call, is not interested in trauma and has had only one rotation in the trauma service.

Where does Marsh's duty lie? He could call his wife and cancel; she would understand; God knows he has had to do that many times before, or he could try to put the unknown, unnamed trauma patient out of his mind and enjoy the evening. Moreover, the recently enacted limitations on resident work hours require he leave the hospital.

The official institutional stance is that Dr Thomas and the third year are "credentialed" for this type of case. They may in fact be annoyed if Marsh intrudes. Marsh knows, however, that the patient's chances would be greatly increased if a person with more trauma experience participated.

There is no answer to this dilemma. Marsh will be wrong whatever choice he makes. There are no rules, at least not applicable rules, as the limited work hour rules have only recently been promulgated.

It may not be immediately obvious that the case of the falling worker is an example of distributive justice. It is important to note that what Marsh has to distribute is not only his skill and his experience but also his very presence and his contribution to the stability and well-being of his marriage.

Marsh's own well-being and pleasure are not to be seen as mere egoism or hedonism. He has a duty, he knows, to care for himself and for others. He chooses to sign out and go home, but he is preoccupied throughout dinner and felt unmoved by his wife's amorous advances later that night.

The principle of distributive justice has many faces. So many, in fact, that it seems difficult to see them all at once. One obvious issue receiving much attention currently is health care disparities.

Health care disparities are widespread in this country and even more marked around the world. Infant birth weights vary widely from zip code to zip code in many American cities. Rural and urban health statistics favor the urban population outcome. Thirty-seven percent of African American women have hypertension. Sixteen percent of Native American women have been diagnosed with diabetes. Such disparities may be related to race, ethnicity, disability, or sexual orientation. It is easy to think that this is a problem only for third world countries, but, in fact, it is widespread in the United States. Many of these issues are due to biologic or social and environmental factors, but some fraction of them is related to the availability of surgical care. What ethical posture does the profession of surgery take toward these pressing issues? Some surgeons respond as individuals and seem oblivious to global disparities, whereas others are obsessed and distracted by them.

## References

1.  Phrase by Alvin Plantinga, an American analytic philosopher.
2.  Hart HLA. *The Concept of Law*. Oxford: Oxford University Press; 1965: 155.

# 8 Distributive Justice: Proximity

Lloyd A. Jacobs, MD

At the end of the last chapter we left Dr Marsh heading home for a dinner and evening with his wife. A number of forces may have influenced his decision: he had at this time no formal duty to the injured man, he was properly hesitant to encroach into the sphere of the covering resident and the attending surgeon, and, I believe, he considered that he had no relationship to the injured worker. He had, of course, a relationship to him as a fellow human being but had no special relationship, no relationship of intimacy, or even closeness in what we have come to call "the doctor-patient" relationship. He did not feel that he had the special duty, owed by virtue of proximity; the injured man was not his "neighbor."

The requirements of distributive justice have posed special difficulties for the surgeon, in part because of the intense need for focus when performing a procedure. Every surgeon has experienced the tension that occurs when, in the midst of a complex procedure, colectomy perhaps, or aneurysmectomy, a junior resident or nurse transmits a message from the intensive care unit (ICU): "Your patient Mister Jones has severe hypotension, anuria, and inadequate oxygenation." My own experience is one of significant distress in this circumstance. If we grant that the principles of distributive justice are adequately enunciated by the precepts "Treat equal cases alike" and "Treat unequal cases unlike," we see that the ICU and the operative cases are not similar or "like" one another. However, both patients are "yours." Arguably, the ICU patient has the more urgent need. Neither case can be described as

**33**

"futile," at least on the information in your possession. The parameter that best declares that they are "unequal" is proximity. You send an intern to attend the ICU patient.

The duty of proximity is not a duty asked only of the surgeon but is perceived to be a duty of all persons attempting to live an ethical life. It must be seen as a rule of thumb for the guidance of decisions on a day-to-day basis, and, therefore, an implementation strategy for the more abstract, deontological notion of distributive justice. Like every rule of thumb, it has pitfalls, however.

Dr Marsh, who left the hospital while a trauma victim was en route, recognized a special form of duty that derived from yet another rule: "One should keep one's promises or covenants." And, as Marsh doubtlessly considered, certain covenants create proximity. In the case of marriage, the proximity created is of a physical kind; other covenants create proximity of a nonmaterial nature but are as binding nevertheless.

The covenant most relevant to our current train of thought is the time-honored physician-patient relationship. And although the duty to proximity is best seen as an implementation strategy for the deontological principle of justice, the sanctity of the surgeon-patient relationship rises nearly to the level of a principle in its own right.

When health care disparities are considered in the context of the modern forces of globalization, the problem is literally staggering. Good health, and surgery as a means of its attainment, no longer has either knowledge or technology as its limiting steps. When seen from a global perspective, logistics and resources emerge as the limiting factors. It seems likely that even current therapies in daily use in the United States and other advanced countries will never be fully implemented in sub-Saharan Africa or other indigent areas of the world due to resource constraints. How then may one operate in an air-conditioned suite, with laminar air flow and excellent lighting, with modern technologies including robots and ceiling-mounted X-ray machines? The all too easy answer is in the duty to proximity. The patients receiving this kind of care are literally in proximity and possess, furthermore, the created proximity of the doctor-patient relationship. The surgeon's need to earn a living and experience a successful career are usually classified under the headings of egoism or even hedonism and, therefore, often deemed to be of lesser weight or even reprehensible.

The duty of proximity has historically been discussed as the duty to one's neighbor. This rendition of the duty of proximity has biblical overtones related 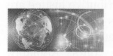 to the story of a Samaritan giving aid to an injured traveler. The confrontation of the Samaritan with the injured man seems, however, to have been a purely random occurrence. There is no indication that the Samaritan knew that an injured man lay ahead, at best he might have known that injuries by robbers were frequent in this stretch of road. The scenario he encountered could not have been anticipated, and the general thrust of the story seems to emphasize the chance nature of the encounter. However, the surgeon is in a consciously created relationship with his patient; for his part the surgeon has voluntarily created the proximity: first, by binding himself to the profession and its ethics and second by covenanting with the patient to accede to the duties of a special relationship. The surgeon's contracted beneficiary should prevail.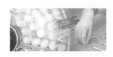

Equality of distribution implies a random distribution. All of a class are showered with the surgeon's beneficence randomly and, therefore, equally. However, the surgeon-patient relationship modifies the fundamental randomness of distribution of the fruits of the surgeon's beneficence and stands nearly opposite the duties of an ideal distributive justice. The physician-patient relationship is a covenanted, special relationship in which value is exchanged in a way that is contrary to a random and, therefore, equal distribution.

The ideal of perfect distributive justice is impossible to attain. A rule for day-to-day living declares the duty one has to persons in proximity and which takes into account the special covenantal proximity created by the surgeon-patient relationship. A surgeon must focus on the task at hand.

Although the concept of a duty to proximity, which limits the application of an ideal of distributive justice, is essential to the surgeon, it is fraught with potential for misuse. In this context, it is important to remember that we ourselves arrange much of what seems to be happening to us. It is, therefore, all too easy to allow a legitimate desire to live comfortably with one's family, which becomes an obsessive pursuit of wealth. We ourselves may, at times, court distraction by covenanting with too many patients, or creating unrealistic expectations in their family surrogates, or, like Dr Marsh, at least considering an intrusion into a situation for which he had no obligation.

Many surgeons and other physicians have spoken eloquently, extolling the physician-patient relationship as giving meaning to one's life. That highly valued relationship does not occur in isolation, however. It has a social context, with presuppositions, preexisting thought forms, and competing aspects of life. It comes to exist with ethical tensions as an inherent part of the relationship itself. Consider the situation of Dr Sanders.

Dr Sanders has only recently been appointed a member of the Medical Devices Evaluation Committee of St. Raphael's Hospital in the Midwestern town where he practices. He is pleased with the appointment, as he enjoys committee work and the camaraderie that often develops by regular participation. In addition, it is his hope to become involved in hospital administrative work and intends someday to obtain an MBA degree and focus his career in that direction.

Although he performs the occasional operation elsewhere, Dr Sanders does more than 90% of his work at St. Raphael's Hospital. The operating room personnel know and respect him and often give him preference for early operating slots. Moreover, he rents a suite in the St. Raphael's office building at very competitive rates. In short, he is a St. Raphael's surgeon.

The charge to the Medical Devices Evaluation Committee is to assess the value of implantables and to guide the administration in the choice of purchases of these very expensive items. Hips, knees, pacemakers, and vascular prostheses are among these items, but the list of implantables for purchase or potential purchase is very long. Although the designation "evaluation" suggests an assessment of quality, it becomes obvious to Sanders even in the first meeting he attends that cost is also a very important part of the assessment expected from the group.

Dr Sanders is a busy vascular surgeon, operating nearly daily. His most 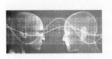 frequent procedure is open carotid endarterectomy; his colleagues are convinced that this operation is superior to catheter-based stenting. Dr Sanders is skilled at the operation and has an excellent record of good outcomes. He shunts every case and closes every arteriotomy with a patch.

At Sanders' third meeting at the committee, a visit was received from a hospital legation led by St. Raphael's Chief Operating Officer (COO) and that included the chief medical officers (CMOs) of the hospital.

The COO began by thanking the committee for their commitment to the institution's welfare. He then turned the conversation over to the CMO who outlined a proposed new program for cost savings. He asked the committee to evaluate every class of implantables and to choose 1 hip prosthesis, 1 knee prosthesis, and 1 implantable in every category. The COO chimed in that this program was projected to save St. Raphael's several million dollars annually.

As the discussion proceeded, Dr Sanders became suddenly aware that one of the implantables to be considered was the gusset material that he routinely used to patch the carotid artery. Sanders' routine choice of material was the most expensive among those available and seemed the likeliest candidate for elimination.

Sanders reflected on this cost-saving proposal almost obsessively for weeks. He came to dread the next monthly meeting of the committee. Not only was he familiar with the feel and characteristics of the gusset material he used, but also he was convinced that the material contributed to his manifestly excellent results. Sanders' reflections included, sometimes at 2 AM, the recollection of St. Raphael's COO saying how important the projected cost savings was to the institution and its ability to budget significant amounts each year to charity care. Soon the issue would come to the need for a firm recommendation from the committee.

Dr Sanders recognized that he was spending more time reflecting on this situation than it perhaps deserved, but he could not get it out of his mind. He noted, of course, that there existed no surgeon-patient relationship in an immediate sense and no potential neighbor recipient of whatever beneficence his good actions might produce. There existed, to be sure, vague references to "other patients" to be served by the hospital's fiscal welfare. Sanders was aware that the arteriotomy patch he preferred had not been demonstrated to be superior; it was most agreed, in "equipoise" with other less expensive materials. Sanders himself was convinced, however, that it was superior, but he was also sufficiently self-aware to know that his believing it was so did not make it so. In the end, Sanders abstained from this discussion and finally abstained from a vote, which did in fact support the recommendation that the hospital stop purchasing "his" gusset material. Sanders did not, however, feel satisfied, nor did he believe he had behaved well in the face of an ethical dilemma. He recognized that his feelings were almost all self-centered and that his position was one of egoism or perhaps even hedonism and felt that there was something reprehensible about the way he had dealt with the committee's work.

The neighbor theme has frequently been central to various statements pertaining to the achievement of a meaningful life. We have discussed the neighbor theme in the context of a duty to physical proximity and the idea that the surgeon-patient relationship is an example of the creation of proximity or the status of neighbor by covenant. It remains to speak of an even more difficult notion: the solemn confrontation of a woman or man with another creature that represents a symbol of the rest of the universe. Mankind's encounter with the "wholly other" has a certain force that creates and binds one creature to another. A consequence of that bonding is to create a neighbor relationship. In doing so, the bonding process also creates a special difficulty for the application of a distributive justice obligation.

Such encounters should not be seen as random events. We all have experienced random passings in the night in which no eye contact is made nor is there the moment in which one apprehends the existence of another mind. There is no entry into a creative reciprocity. However, the Samaritan and the injured traveler "saw" one another. They participated in that solemn event that binds creatures in their humanity to a singleness where before there had been a separateness. The surgeon-patient relationship at its best is of this nature. The surgeon and the patient "see" one another, and their lives and fates are inextricably bound together. Such is the nature of this nearly mystical relationship between surgeon and patient.

Historically, surgeons have written little about this relationship, and although I know it to exist frequently, most surgical writings describe a one-way relationship. Three quarters of the paragraphs in one translation of the Hippocratic Oath have "I" as their central subject. The patient is referred to with the general "the sick." Perusal of the writings of surgeons during the intervening centuries reveals almost uniformly a similar emphasis. Surgeons have not often grappled with the notion of one's neighbor as a way of rationalizing the impossible to achieve the ideal of distributive justice, nor have they often spoken of the creative reciprocity of their relationship to patients.

# 9 Autonomy: The Good Death

Lloyd A. Jacobs, MD

We have significant choice about many aspects of our lives and, once having chosen, we live happily or unhappily with the consequences. The concept of death is almost opposite to this; our choices are severely limited. Everybody dies. The notion of a good death is very much contrary to the current norms of thought in the discipline of surgery. The ubiquitous morbidity and mortality (M&M) conference that constitutes the best window into the culture of a Department of Surgery serves to establish nearly subconscious paradigms and presuppositions in its participants. Even at its origin, the M&M conference contextualized death as evil. Allen O. Whipple, an originator of the conferences, grouped death with a list of other unhappy occurrences:

> "...regular surgical conferences once a week to discuss the errors in diagnosis, the mistakes in technique, and infections of clean wounds and deaths..."

This negative framing has been continued in the recent classification of complications by Clavien and Dindo: Death defines Grade V, after other complications requiring intervention. The perception of death as an integral part of the gift of life can hardly emerge in the milieu. To see the good death as something to be achieved moves from the notion of death as something to be avoided.

We may be able to exercise some autonomy regarding the time and place where we die, but in truth, except for martyrs, we have little to choose. The idea that for most choices we live with the consequences is clear; regarding death we know not of the consequences, nor do we have any understanding of how subsequent events or perhaps nothingness will be experienced. It is important, therefore, to separate the dread of death as an unknown from the legitimate fear of the experience of dying. The most salient feature of that experience is for many a loss of personal autonomy.

Sherwin B. Nuland, who called himself "Shep," was a well-trained surgeon. Shep was also an essayist who wrote dozens of essays for a column in *The American Scholar* under the heading: "The Uncertain Art." Shep's greatest impact, however, may result from his book entitled *How We Die: Reflections on Life's Final Chapter.*[1] The thrust of the book might be summarized: We die in loneliness, with pain and dyspnea and dread, in a noisy place, surrounded by unfamiliar machines and people, long after any pleasure or value can be experienced from continued life. There may be some hyperbole here; however, a new syndrome has emerged called withering syndrome. It is frequently seen in the postoperative period and is often related to wanting "everything" done. It consists of the following:

- Prolonged intubation and ICU stay
- Tube feedings or parental nutrition and muscle atrophy
- Depression and lethargy
- May involve hemodialysis
- The patient is discharged to a nursing home or other institution

The 1-year mortality of this syndrome is high, and the quality of life is low. For a nonagenarian to die well is not tragic, but for a nonagenarian to develop the withering syndrome is tragic.

In the interval, since Shep's book, there has been considerable new thinking about death, and the hospice movement and palliative care units have made Shep's description a bit less accurate. Still it is all too commonly entirely accurate, and, I deeply regret to state that surgeons have not been leaders in this movement. Fortunately, the American College of Surgeons along with other professional groups has undertaken to support the movement toward a less burdensome death in the fullness of time.

A central theme of Shep's book is that there exists an art of dying, an *ars moriendi*, which, like every art, is subject to times and places, fads and fashions, and perhaps most of all, is subject to what it is we believe about the nature of the human condition. Currently, Shep implies that quantity has become nearly the sole measure of life's value; every minute no matter 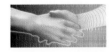 how miserable, in which the function of a few cardiac cells and a few neurons is detectable, is considered to be of value. There is a movement, as we stated, which contravenes this view.

The way we die is determined largely by the culture of the times. Drew Gilpin Faust, now president of Harvard University, recently authored a book entitled *This Republic of Suffering: Death and the American Civil War.*[2] She uses the phrase "the good death." The phrase has been used by authors before and after Faust; she, however, forcefully makes the point that the perception of death and its confrontation is socially determined.

Most of us will recall that the American Civil War was ghastly in that more than a half million young men died. What is less well known and what Faust argues convincingly is that the Civil War altered how death was perceived both in prospect and retrospect. Faust's description of "the good death" relies heavily on the correspondence of soldiers with their families in which the soldier pledges faith and fearlessness and declares his unceasing love for his parents and siblings. The good death included the courage derived from having made peace with God and a sort of noble resignation. There are echoes here of the connection to others, which moderates autonomy. The human need for succor must not be derogated or ignored in a very strenuous commitment to autonomy, the end result of which may be alienation. What is important to our train of thought here is that a good death may be conceived of and strived for. Nuland and others, including Dan Hinshaw[3] who is also an accomplished surgeon, make clear that it is part of the surgeon's commitment to beneficence and autonomy to help the patient experience a good death.

Faust's work also makes clear that for the Civil War soldiers, the good death had at least 2 salient features that correspond precisely to Nuland's ideas about the good death. The soldier was unafraid and, therefore, died with dignity. The soldier loved his parents and loved his duty to his country and possessed a sense of his life having had meaning. Nuland and others go on to assert, correctly I believe, that our patients want the same: death with dignity and the certainty of having had a meaningful life.

The American College of Surgeons and the Cunniff-Dixon Foundation has published an excellent handbook for residents dealing with end-of-life issues entitled *Surgical Palliative Care: A Resident's Guide.* In it is discussed practical advice for pain control and changing the goals of the care provided for the patient and his family to comfort as opposed to longevity. Many others have similarly provided both philosophical and practical guidance for caring for patients in this phase of life. *Skeel's Handbook of Cancer Therapy* briefly summarizes the position of the oncologist on the therapeutics of this focus of care. Chapters 15 and 22 will expand on these themes.

It is not my intent to repeat the excellent regimens or advice of these 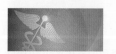 authors nor even to offer a synopsis of their work. Instead, it is my hope to argue that a surgeon's ethical posture requires of his/her attention to those aspects of care, which increase the likelihood of a good death for his/her patients. The logic is straightforward: Beneficence is intuitively of value and is the centuries-old commitment of the discipline of surgery. Autonomy for individual patients is a logical derivative of beneficence. The good death is heavily dependent on serving the personal autonomy of your patient.

Surprising is the historical lack of commentary by or about surgeons and their care for patients at the end of life. Modern surgeons too have largely abdicated responsibility for moral acts in this arena. It would be unfair to lay responsibility for this abdication solely at the doorstep of the physician and surgeon. The deep and widespread ethos of value in the Western world currently has replaced the good death with the postponed death. Our attitude is, "Yes, everyone must die, but not today, not me today!" Our phraseology under- 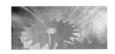 scores this: The postponed death is spoken of as "a life saved." One might reasonably ask, "Saved for what?" The appropriate answer many believe is, "saved for exercise of autonomy, saved for the beneficence of which our discipline is constituted. Saved for dignity and meaning, or at least the striving toward these. Saved for a good death, an important ingredient of which is a sentient peace."

Nuland goes on to say, as does Drew Gilpin Faust, that the good death has increasingly become a "myth." Both imply that it may always have been a myth and that pain and dyspnea are inevitable. However, the modern surgeon, oriented as he/she is toward efficacious action, can be as active in this arena as in the areas more often historically assigned to the surgeon. Surgeons are themselves, more than almost any other group, autonomous; they should strive to extend that gift whenever possible.

Autonomy is a milestone in the lifelong process of individuation and the pursuit of meaning. To die with dignity is to ratify the meaning of one's life and to continue to sustain loved ones and the world. To give inadequate attention to this goal, even though it be ultimately unobtainable, is to fail in our responsibilities to beneficence and its derivative autonomy.

The dying person must make his/her own decisions or have complete faith in the commitment of agency binding a surrogate. But the clear logic rarely applies and the practical day-to-day events regarding surrogacy are nearly always imperfect.

At the institutional Ethics Committee of the University of Toledo Medical Center, the case of a 56-year-old man was discussed on June 16, 2016. The unfortunate man had suffered a major stroke and was described as "unresponsive" and "in a vegetative state." At the time of the Ethics Committee discussion the patient had been in the hospital for more than 3 months. An impasse had been reached in the communication with the patient's family: They resisted plans for extended care transfer and continued to believe that more could and should be done for their loved one. The presentation stated, "Family not participating in pt [sic] care conferences," and later, "We are unable to reach family and the family has repeatedly not attended family meetings that have been scheduled…"

As was believed even in retrospect to be entirely appropriate, the institution approached the Lucas County Common Pleas Court for the appointment of a guardian, where appointment was made promptly. However, no relief was gained: The guardian was unavailable, did not visit the patient, and did not even return phone calls. At the time of the discussion, the staff was considering a return to the judge who appointed the guardian.

The discussion that ensued emphasized a number of points we have already made. The practice of ethics is a pursuit of an abstraction; it is never 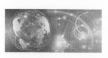 an endpoint to be achieved. Our patient, lingering as he was in a vegetative state is not, of course, likely to experience a "good death," nor is his family. The surgeon is always positioned between the patient's wishes and the institution's mandates, between the principles of autonomy and those of distributive justice.

In the case described previously, the dilemma arose in large part because linguistic ambiguity created unrealistic expectations. Before the family had disappeared they had stated: "We want everything done." The caregivers, in trying to perform their roles as agents, as advocates, believed this statement bound them to unreasonable goals.

Whenever phraseology like "everything" is used the surgeon should always follow up by saying, "what do you mean by everything?" We will certainly do everything reasonable, everything a prudent surgeon would do in similar circumstances. But "everything" is unbounded; we must discuss the boundaries you envision. This response, of course, takes time the surgeon may not have, but it will save time in the long run. At a minimum, the surgeon should always clarify, "of course we will do everything, everything reasonable for your loved one."

In the late 2014, Brittany Maynard was diagnosed with a terminal resectable glioblastoma. She was 29 years old. At that time the state of California had not yet passed legislation that would allow physicians to assist patients in suicide. Brittany Maynard moved to Oregon to avail herself of the "Death with Dignity" law of that state.

I have described this case to several dozen medical school applicants, asking their opinion as to how her California physician should advise her regarding this action. The degree of uniformity in their answers was truly remarkable. Everyone began by discussing alternatives and counseling about the availability of such alternatives. Everyone of the applicants transitioned to a discussion of patient autonomy and ultimately came to state that in the end it was up to the patient; he/she would be encouraged to freely choose. Not a single applicant cited a metaphysical principle as overarching; all stressed Brittany's autonomy.

In volume 415 (8944) of *The Economist*, the worldwide trend to legalize physician-assisted suicide is discussed. At the time of that writing, 16 countries had specific laws allowing support for assisted dying. As mentioned above, California has recently passed legislation in this arena. It is likely that this trend will continue to grow.

A comprehensive review of the issues related to physician-assisted suicide was recently published in the *JAMA*.[4] The report focused specifically on attitudes and practices and may be summarized as follows: The number of states or countries where physician-assisted suicide is legally condoned is growing slowly, reflecting a likelihood that the "market" for this service has already been saturated. A very small number of physicians have been asked for or have practiced physician-assisted suicides. There is virtually no evidence of abuse of this service; most patients are appropriately selected patients with terminal cancer.

Once again the surgeon is faced with a choice for which there is no correct answer: to approve and perhaps participate in this activity or to categorically condemn it. The tension between respect for life and the respect for human autonomy pulls one in 2 directions. Worse, there is no easy resting place between them. Consistent, however, with my repeated admonition, surgeons should, in my opinion, avoid taking categorical stances, particularly when those postures consist of impossible to reconcile ideals. The absence of resting places between the poles of a dichotomy often causes the surgeon to experience a sense of being locked into a course of action.

## References

1. Nuland SB. *How We Die: Reflections on Life's Final Chapter*. New York: Knopf; 1994.
2. Faust DG. *This Republic of Suffering, Death and the American Civil War*. First Vintage Civil War Library Edition; January 2009.
3. Hinshaw DB. *Suffering and the Nature of Healing*. Yonkers: St. Vladimir's Seminary Press; 2013.
4. Emanuel EJ, Onwuteaka-Philipsen BD, Urwin JW, et al. Attitudes and practices of euthanasia and physician-assisted suicide in the United States, Canada, and Europe. *JAMA*. 2016;316(1):79–90.

# 10 Distributive Justice: Changed Expectations

Lloyd A. Jacobs, MD

Both the principles of proximity and the notion of agency often cause the surgeon to believe that the fruits of his/her beneficence are owed first or even exclusively to the patient with whom he/she currently has a surgeon-patient relationship. There is, of course, much to recommend this: the notion is considered by many to be one of the very few unambiguous rules in our ethics. Second, the surgeon must have the ability to focus, concentrate on the duty at hand, and not be distracted by the multitude of human needs the world contains. Thomas Percival (1740-1804) underscores an extreme of a position of agency when he writes:

> "...surgeons should not suffer themselves to be restrained, by parsimonious consideration, from prescribing wine, and drugs even of high price..."

Try telling that to a hospital administrator! In another place Percival takes a more balanced view:

> "Medical Ethics should be concerned with the ultimate consequences of the conduct of physicians toward their individual patients and toward society as a whole,..."

Percival casually sets up yet another tension: the individual patient verses society as a whole. The balance between the claims of these 2 potential

**44**

recipients of the surgeon's beneficence is changing rapidly in the Western world. This changing pattern has been strongly promoted by governments becoming invested in the health care industry. It is fair to generalize that the view a government may take of distributive justice is significantly different from the view of a small businessman, which is what surgeons have been. Good and poor arguments can be made regarding this movement.

A majority of surgeons are now employed by institutions, which, traditionally at least, have taken a broader view than the individual patient advocacy model. What seems incontrovertible to many is that modern health care is too complex, expensive, and needful of safety provisions to be left to the small business model. The pure advocacy model is already nearly obsolete; the era in which the surgeon saw his/her duty only to his/her patient and peers is disappearing. The list of clambering voices is long. Medical staff organizations promulgate rules concerning antibiotic stewardship, clearly a beneficent behavior toward the public at large as well as for future generations.[1] Credentialing committees and quality review committees concern themselves with safety and excellence not only for individuals but also for the institution at large.

However, an even more fundamental change is underway. The idea of shared risk and shared expense and the evaluation of outcomes for populations have all but abolished the notion of advocacy for the individual patient. The utilitarian formula of "the greatest good for the greatest number" has already prevailed in most of the Western world's medical and surgical circles, without regard for the mitigating force of a duty to proximity, without the concept that beneficence is owed first to one's neighbor, and without honoring a "neighbor" relationship called the surgeon-patient relationship. Population health is in ascendancy.[2]

What should be the attitude of the ethical surgeon toward this trend? It would be naive to think that one voice, your voice, could stem this tide. However, we have repeatedly noted that the value of an ethical ideal is in the striving, even when the attainment is unrealistic. Your voice is important in the debate concerning the balances within your hospital and within your government, between the claims on the surgeon's beneficence by his/her individual patient and the society at large. The future will continue to cause this tension to become more prominently felt and more productive of stress.

## References

1. Spellberg B, Srinivasan A, Chambers HF. New societal approaches to empowering antibiotic stewardship. *JAMA*. 2016;315(12):1229–1230.
2. Washington AE. Academic health systems' third curve: population health improvement. *JAMA*. 2016;315(5):459–460.

# 11 Epistemology

Lloyd A. Jacobs, MD

Epistemology is the branch of philosophy that concerns itself with questions of what is permissible for one to believe. How are beliefs justified; how do we know anything; how do we know what beliefs are justified or warranted? There is an aspect of ethics involved in one's epistemology. A surgeon, or any person for that matter, may not believe any irrational thing but must subscribe to some structure and rationality of belief. Our profession also has its own ethics of belief.

In an earlier chapter, I related the vignette of a young surgeon presenting a case at that institution's mortality and morbidity conference. The presentation caused debate about the value of antibiotic bowel preparation for colon surgery. The case was discussed in an earlier chapter as an example of dichotomous thinking. However, later in the discussion the emphasis shifted when the young surgeon stated that she had received knowledge of antibiotic use in her training from a trusted mentor. It was, at that juncture, that the chairman first entered the discussion. He was pejorative. A higher complication rate following antibiotic colon preparation was supported by data, he said. He strongly implied the epistemological superiority of "data" over what was "taught in her training." Surgeons, he implied, have a duty to what they believe and an obligation to an epistemology of surgery. There are ethical rules of belief in the discipline of surgery. These rules are, one hopes, tactics of application for utilitarianism: Follow the rules to achieve the greatest good for the greatest number.

There are at least 2 corollary points to be made immediately. They are both statements of belief themselves but are accepted as rational beliefs by most surgeons and many other thoughtful people. The first is that beliefs guide and, in an ideal world, determine actions. What a surgeon believes about cholelithiasis in large part determines what will be his/her actions toward a patient with cholecystitis and influences the conduct of the operation, if one is performed.

The second corollary is that there exists a hierarchy of beliefs; some beliefs are more justified and more rational than others. Here surgeons differ significantly, most significantly concerning the place of reproducible data in that hierarchy. Finally, it should be noticed that the body of beliefs that constitute surgical knowledge is not optional for acceptance; there is a powerful societal force supporting acceptance of beliefs about surgical issues.

The entire body of knowledge contained in standard textbooks, such as Greenfield or Schwartz, constitutes only a portion of what a surgeon is required to believe. In addition, there is a large body of unwritten behavioral knowledge for the conduct of an operation, for the management of patients, and important for our current train of thought, the ethics and their derivative rules of everyday conduct. Young surgeons as well as older surgeons are right to be skeptical of some of these required beliefs: many will be modified in our own lifetimes. Moreover, in the last several paragraphs, we have been relying on the authority of mentors, chairpersons, and others to give warrant to surgical beliefs. It is important to note that one should examine the criteria for the granting of such warrant and to continuously hold one's surgical beliefs up against criteria such as reproducibility, intersubjectivity, or the likelihood of achieving a meaningful life.

Recent decades have seen an increase within the discipline of surgery concerning a certain tension or polarity regarding what one may reasonably believe. The story of the young surgeon and her chairman's admonition about antibiotic data illustrates the tension that derives from belief in evidentialism as preferable to, say, belief in the authority of the mentorship experienced. Respect for and acquiescence to the authority of one's mentor have a long tradition in surgery. The Hippocratic Oath contains a statement of respect for and fealty to one's teacher, and the impulse remains strong within our discipline: "I was taught by Alfred Blalock; I was taught by Frederick Coller," and so on. I spoke to a young surgeon only yesterday who asserted that, at a training program in Florida, things are done "the Michigan way."

Prudent women and men will, from time to time, reexamine even their most firmly held beliefs. This is particularly important for surgeons, as experience unfolds and data become available that may cast doubt on the transmitted beliefs of the most warranted nature. The place in one's hierarchy of justifiable beliefs for recent experiences is more complicated. "Experience" 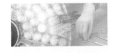 is an exceedingly broad concept: at one end of a spectrum may be the experience of reproducible numerical readings on a spectrophotometer, whereas at the other end may be the inexplicable, unreproducible, fleeting glimpse of something undefined. A surgeon must find a place on this spectrum, on this hierarchy for each of his/her clinical experiences.

Experience is never purely objective; all experience is interpreted experience. Much of our inner life centers on mental models of reality; all experience is force-fitted into those models until a kaleidoscopic shift discards the old model and, hopefully, substitutes a new one. Experience, therefore, always contains the projected presuppositions of the person who experiences and is always subjected to the processes of human memory. Still, the surgeon must accumulate experience, and the patient must be benefited from it.

Reproducibility is the most important safeguard against the malleability of memory. Beliefs held in memory that are not reproducible by others must be seen as relatively low on an epistemic hierarchy. A reinforcement as casual as "Yes, I've seen that too" from a colleague elevates the warrant of a surgeon's belief that, for example, "the aorta is friable near the origins of the visceral vessels." The surgical case conference is invaluable for the development of that intersubjectivity, which creates epistemic justifiability.

Intersubjectivity falls short, however, in at least 2 circumstances. The first is when there is widespread consensus about something untrue, and although philosophers have argued for centuries about the epistemic status of such beliefs, surgeons want to eliminate them. The notion that duodenal ulcer disease could be cured or mitigated by an acid-reducing operation was a widely held belief in our discipline for decades and invited hundreds of surgeons to experiences that corroborated that belief. Ultimately, there is a strong predisposition to experience what we think we will experience.

Another instance in which the test of intersubjectivity may fall short is the truly important paradigm shattering but difficult to reproduce experience, perhaps, such events as the CERN collider may provide. Here most of us are constrained to rely on testimony, which, of course, introduces a whole new world of epistemic uncertainties. Moreover, some of life's most important realities, essential for the well-lived life and for prophylaxis against burnout, depression, and substance abuse, are in this category of events that are not always immediately reproducible. In the end, each of us must develop an epistemology of our own regarding some of these issues. It has seemed to me, however, that there must ultimately be some seamlessness, some congruence to one's structure of beliefs. It has seemed to me to produce stress and tension to hold simultaneously 2 incompatible beliefs.

Surgeons owe their fundamental epistemic method to Francis Bacon (1561-1626). He had a noble predecessor in Vesalius (1514-1564) and able 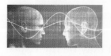 successor in René Descartes (1596-1650) who was to achieve more lasting fame than Bacon himself. Francis Bacon repudiated the deductive reasoning, which had enjoyed precedence since Aristotle, and promulgated an inductive method: reasoning from accumulated facts to generalizations. This is precisely the method mentioned earlier in speaking of the accumulation of a surgeon's experience. Reasoning, Bacon asserted, was to be from the specific to the general by accumulations of concrete facts. There has been much refinement of this method during the years intervening since Bacon's enunciation. Statistical analysis, estimates of power, and blinded trials all are refinements of Bacon's original thought.

Andreas Vesalius must be seen as a stage setter for Bacon, although it is not known if Bacon was familiar with Vesalius' great work: *On the Fabric of the Human Body.* This earth-shaking work contained, for the first time, accurate drawings from actual dissected material and details of anatomy that were unprecedented. 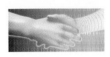 Relevant here is that the depictions were of actual experiences in the world, unlike the products of contemplation that were common at that time.

Rene Descartes acknowledged his debt to Bacon for his emphasis on inductive thought. Descartes followed with incisive thinking about verifiability. He was a doubter and wrote of stringent requirements for acceptance of conclusions of inductive thinking.

Bacon, Vesalius, and Descartes created a new epistemology now frequently referred to as evidentialism. Evidentialism is the prevailing epistemic method for all of modern science, including surgery, and is thought by many to be the only method to warrant any given belief. Others insist that large segments of the human experience are ignored by this epistemic exclusivity, pointing specifically to relationships, acts of mercy, and other experiences that seem difficult to subject to the criterion of evidentialism for verification.

The current ethic for belief by surgeons is evidentialism. Implementation strategies for evidentialism were given by the great bacteriologist Robert Koch in 1890 when he published criteria that, in his mind, clearly linked a bacterium with a disease. To prove that linkage, Koch required the following:

1. The constant presence of the organism in every case of the disease.
2. The preparation of a pure culture, which must be maintained for repeated generations.
3. The reproduction of the disease in animals by means of a pure culture removed by several generations from the organism first isolated.

Koch's postulates are of historical interest only to modern-day bacteriologists, but they demonstrate the degree of rigor that came to be applied to Francis Bacon's inductive methodology. Koch's postulates should be seen as establishing warrant for knowledge about disease-causing bacteria, knowledge obtained by Bacon's inductive method. Modern-day surgeons have an obligation to epistemology; they cannot believe just anything and must consider the ethical norms for beliefs held by the discipline to which they have committed themselves.

An excellent example of careful epistemic methods is to be found in Supplement S of Volume 61 (March 2015) of the *Journal of Vascular Surgery,* which presents the "Society for Vascular Surgery practice guidelines for atherosclerotic occlusive disease of the lower extremities: Management of asymptomatic disease and claudication." Great care was taken to observe a pristine epistemic methodology with emphasis on intersubjectivity as these 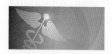 guidelines were developed. This excellence of method is to be distinguished from the equal excellence of the guidelines produced. A duty of the modern surgeon is to strive for some level of discernment regarding the integrity of epistemic methodology. And the guidelines, although carefully stated as recommendations, represent a compendium of warranted beliefs for the vascular surgeon. The surgeon has a duty to consider the ethical norms for belief of our discipline.

There persist, until the present day, doubts and alarms about methods for establishing warrant for surgical knowledge. Wenner et al[1] have acknowledged the many weaknesses in the "prospective randomized trials," which currently constitute the gold standard epistemic norm. Observer bias, inadequate skill, and conflict of interest are all still epistemic weaknesses in our standard methods.

In spite of these weaknesses, the double-blinded randomized controlled study has become the modern grail for the acknowledgment of surgical truth. It is fundamental to note that reality tends to display itself in ways that are highly dependent on the model and method of its interrogation. Only a very narrow slice of the massive spectrum of reality reveals itself in studies of this kind. Surgeons have long recognized other aspects of warrant for belief, particularly for practical wisdom, and cannot exercise their discipline and cannot make fully ethical choices with only this narrow slice of reality at their disposal.

There are fiscal incentives for granting warrant only to the narrow slice of reality whose evidence can be rated to be in Category I of evidence-based practice. The Centers for Medicare and Medicaid Services regularly convene "Medicare Evidence Development and Coverage Advisory Committees" to advise the agency on coverage for specific health care services. These committees are strongly committed to and orientated toward evidentialism.

In addition, because of the narrow scope of studies of this kind and the need to extrapolate their finds to other groups or situations, the surgeon's judgment requirements are merely shifted. The surgeon now makes a judgment concerning whether a specific patient fits, or nearly fits, a study category. This tends to blur the decision point unnecessarily.

In recent years, there has been increased usage of meta-analyses of data already in the surgical literature. This approach to establishing warrant for a principle of surgery has its own special pitfalls, often related to grouping together disparate data sets. A summary of the issues related to this method is printed in Volume 308 of the *JAMA.*[2]

Surgeons generally display a healthy skepticism about new experiences, whether their own or those of others reported in the surgical literature. However, 2 points need to be made. First, surgeons appear to be eager to use new technologies including laparoscopes and robots while incorporating new knowledge more slowly. Second, resistance to new knowledge has historically constituted some of the darkest history of our discipline. Bloodletting as therapy persisted well beyond the time when solid knowledge existed to render the belief anachronistic. The history of the resistance to belief in antiseptic or aseptic surgery is too notorious to be recounted here. In summary, adoption of the new and abandonment of the old are generally based on beliefs about the modality involved, and beliefs are never purely abstract but are always produced by a mix of presuppositions and experience. An awareness of these issues, in the context of frequent self-examination, is a part of the ethical commitment of our discipline as surgeons.

# References

1. Wenner DM, Brody BA, Jarman AF, et al. Do surgical trials meet the scientific standards for clinical trials? *J Am Coll Surg*. 2012;215:722–730.
2. Mills EJ, Ioannidis JPA, Thorlund K, et al. How to use an article reporting a multiple treatment comparison meta-analysis. *JAMA*. 2012;308(12):1246–1253.

# 12 The Surgeon-Patient Covenant

Lloyd A. Jacobs, MD

The central obligation of a surgeon, or other physicians for that matter, is implicit in the relationship of the surgeon with the individual patient. This relationship has evolved and is evolving. The relationship has roots that are distinct from the moral philosophy of ethics and arises ultimately from a contract, not from a deontological or teleological base. The relationship has evolved, however, partly in response to those ethical forces and, to a degree, has come to be defined by them. Certainly, the nature of the surgeon-patient relationship is influenced by the ethical norms that surround it. The surgeon's central obligation, therefore, reflects the broader ethical norms of society but is not derived from them. The "surgeon's ethic" is the establishment and maintenance of a relationship of nearly sacred trust with the patient as an individual person.

It is interesting to consider the primitive origins of the covenant; however, there exists no clear record of the first such covenant between a surgeon and an ill person. Perhaps, the oldest evidence of the commercial nature of the covenant is found in the "Code of Hammurabi," which included a fee schedule for surgical procedures and a list of draconian penalties for failed interventions. For example, "If a man has destroyed the eye of a patrician, his own eye shall be destroyed." Retaliation was the appropriate remedy for contractual breeches. The following paragraphs closely follow Sigerest.[1]

Surgical fees depended on successful operations and on the social status of the patient. For the successful surgical treatment of a broken bone, the fee was 5 shekels if the patient was a patrician. If the operation ended fatally, the surgeon's hands were cut off! Moreover, the procedures and methods were treated as trade secrets, owned by the surgeon. It is easy to see that the fees, penalties, and ownership of procedural information defined a relationship best described as a commercial contract.

The evolution of this commercial relationship toward a sacred trust truly deserves the appellation: The "surgeon's ethic" began with the writings of the Hippocratic Corpus and the practice of the ancient Greek physicians.[2] The early Hippocratic writings show little evidence; however, the surgeons of that era were moved by "the love of humanity." The surgeon was advised on how to make a living and how to avoid blame or other unwelcome consequences. It was later in the Hippocratic era that the first movement occurred in which the commercial contract began its evolution toward a sacred trust. That evolution begins to be reflected in the oath that was composed in about the fourth century BC. The evolution continues through the period of Aristotelian and Platonic writings and is clearly influenced by them and may also have been influenced by early Christian metaphysics.

The evolution of the surgeon's central obligation was well under way by the time the work of Galen (AD 131-201) marked the end of the classic era. Galen spoke then of the "love of mankind" as the motivation of the Hippocratic surgeons, an assertion that Edelstein disagrees. The use of the phrase does, however, signal a milestone in the evolution we have posited. The influence of the Hippocratic writings continued for nearly a thousand years, through the vicissitudes of translation to Arabic and back, as well as the transport first to the east and then back to the west in what came to be known as the 12th-century Renaissance.

During its thousand-year sojourn to the East, our ethic absorbed influences from eclectic sources, including medieval Christianity and the birth and spread of Islam. During the early portion of its sojourn, the ethic was under the protection of Christians of the Nestorian heresy whose expulsion from Edessa in AD 489 precipitated a diaspora, which sent Nestorians to as far as China and India. That diaspora caused the ethic to absorb aspects of the Eastern doctrine of ahimsa, which forbids harm to any living being; there is a clear echo of our Hippocratic aphorism here. The history of the migration was chronicled by none other than Allen O. Whipple of pancreaticoduodenectomy fame.[3] There is, subsequently, evidence that a certain Leonard 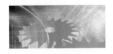 of Bertipaglia of the 15th century was influenced by his reading of Galen's "Commentaries on the Aphorisms of Hippocrates," now again in Western Europe, having been translated back from Arabic.

The next great milestone in the evolution of the surgeon's ethic came with Sir William Osler (1849-1919), whose sojourn at the Johns Hopkins medical institutions, and his textbook, and his later career at Edinburgh had great impact on us all. Although Osler was not a surgeon, his biography was written by one of the world's greatest surgeons and humanists: Harvey Cushing. Osler is credited by some for the founding of scientific medicine. Relevant to our train of thought are his respect for his patients and his recognition that the surgeon's ethic is a trust, not a contract.

> *"...we... [are] the immediate agents of the Trust, [and] have but one enduring corrective—the practice toward patients of the Golden Rule of Humanity..."*

And finally this brief sketch of the evolution of the surgeon's ethic was celebrated by Alexander J. Walt, later President of the American College of Surgeons, when he said:

> *"Today the word 'contract' has too many commercial connotations for comfort, so I prefer to use the word 'covenant' which has inescapable moral implications."*

Clearly, Walt acknowledged the evolution of our ethic and its culmination in a moral "trust."

The surgeon's central ethic is then the product of evolution from what originated as a commercial contract. This ethic finds itself distinct from several prevailing ethical norms of modern society and even occasionally in conflict with the stated norms of the modern renditions of more general medical ethics: beneficence, justice, and autonomy.

In this setting the surgeon's conceptual norms are not, however, so specific as to be without their own ambiguity, and a lifetime of a surgeon's acts and utterances are rarely without regret. Ethical ambiguity is believed to increase the likelihood of regret, and regret is a precursor to surgeon's dysphoria. The frequency of symptoms of burnout among surgeons is truly astonishing, even if we grant that the estimating methodology is imperfect. A study by Elmore et al estimated that symptoms of burnout are present in 68% of general surgery residents.[4] Similar but somewhat lower estimates have been published for practicing surgeons. As is well known, depression, substance abuse, and even suicide 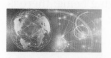 are hazards for surgeons. Writers analyzing burnout and its sequelae point to inadequate work-life balance as causal and to improved work-life balance as preventative and corrective. A central hypothesis of this paper, however, is that ethical ambiguity and the regret caused by it are important stressors for surgeons and are frequent causes of burnout and depression.

I want not to be naïve here: there are many contributors to surgeon dysphoria, to point to only one would be naïve. At the same time, I assert that too much emphasis on life's balance ignores the ethical dilemmas inherent in the modern surgeon's life.

There appears to be an almost irresistible urge to categorize ethical principles and to state which ethical norms are primary, which are derivative, and from whence they emanate. These attempts have almost uniformly failed and have been of minimal help to surgeons. Still a very brief nosology may be helpful. Historically, in the Western world at least, most ethical norms rested on a metaphysical foundation. In the spirit of the 18th and 19th centuries, parallel with a less metaphysical and more objective view of reality, Jeremy Bentham (1748-1832) and John Stuart Mill (1806-1873) created or 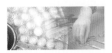 at least promulgated a more worldly foundation for ethics ultimately called "Utilitarianism." The aim of an ethical act, they said, was its utility, and successors such as Herbert Spencer and Henry Sidgwick further developed the principle that the description of an act as good or not good depended not on some intrinsic value of the act itself but on its intended, predicted, or actual consequences in the real world.

In a somewhat parallel time frame, the foundation previously described as metaphysical came to be known as "deontological," a concept originally belonging to the Stoics. Finally in the current day, called by many a postmodern period, the foundation of ethics is reflexive: an act is good or evil, as its creative impact on the actor is good or evil.

So we have 2 broad categories: deontological ethical norms arise from the intrinsic value of the act and teleological ethical norms whose value is determined by their consequences. It is correct to say that the most widely held ethical foundation today is utilitarianism: the act is good if it produces the greatest good for the greatest number of humankind.

The problem for the surgeon is that most of our day-to-day moral choices do not fit neatly in this categorization. The most central ethic of the surgeon (and the medical profession generally) has arisen outside this nosology, derived as we have said from contract law and evolved to be a distinct ethic governing or at least influencing most of what a surgeon does daily.

The forced choice between 2 conflicting ethical alternatives makes regret virtually inevitable. In many circumstances faced by surgeons, no matter what you do, you will experience regret. I would like to discuss briefly 3 surgical scenarios in which the "surgeon's ethic" conflicts with or is at least distinct from the prevailing ethical norms of the present day.

1. Standard decision analysis derived from utilitarianism and from the principle of autonomy is an inadequate model for surgeon's and patient's decision making.
2. A decision to withhold all or part of the "truth" is consistent with the surgeon's ethic but conflicts with current day orthodoxy.
3. Our society currently undermines the surgeon's agency, which has a major impact on the well-being of the surgeon.

Standard decision theory is a formalized derivative of the "utilitarianism" of John Stuart Mill, which he championed in a little book of that name published in 1863. Utilitarianism states that the outcome of an act or utterance is what determines whether the act or utterance is good or not good.

The act or utterance has no intrinsic goodness or evil; if its consequences are good, intended to be good, or predicted to be good, then the act is good. Classic decision analysis derived from this idea readily accommodates the choice between a certainty of winning $50 and a 45% chance of winning $100. Such analysis fails, however, to be of value when a surgeon is discussing an operation or end-of-life or other significant issues with a patient. A classic 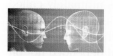 requirement of decision analysis is to be purely objective, and the ethic of promoting patient autonomy says to let the patient decide. Neither is feasible. First, the choices are almost always incommensurate; no rational comparison can be made between the likely outcomes. Jean-Paul Sartre spoke of the choice between joining a just war and staying home to care for aging and ill parents. No reasonable comparison can be made. Similarly, life with bilateral above-knee amputations versus the certainty of death presents incommensurable outcomes. Pascal's famous wager can be criticized on the same ground of incommensurability.

It is impossible to describe all the possible outcomes of an operation. This "inexhaustibility of description" drives us to discuss outcomes with which we are most familiar, outcomes for which we have language, and outcomes of prior experience that have caused us the most regret. Classic decision theory, in the face of this multiplicity, fails to anticipate which outcome will constitute "the greatest good."

Standard decision theory requires that decisions should be made without contamination by emotion. This criterion is impossible to achieve for human creatures, including either the surgeon or the patient. We are creatures of emotion as much as, or perhaps more than, creatures of reason. Emotion does not follow the rules of utilitarianism; it does not follow the rules of classic decision theory. A patient may wish to live or die as her mother lived or died; certainly the patient's belief about the meaning of life and the patient's own sense of meaning or lack thereof is involved in every decision.

The ancient and venerable surgeon's ethic requires active guidance at least, and the ideal to be pursued is, I believe, that the surgeon join with the patient in true reciprocity and in full appreciation of a life's context. Somehow the separate inner lives of the patient and the surgeon become one; forces are joined for the decision. One cannot discharge one's obligation by a sterile recital of facts, leaving the patient to decide. The notion of compassion speaks of *suffering with.*

It is fair to say that utilitarianism and its derivative decision theory is the prevailing ethical posture in the Western world today. It will work, however, neither for the surgeon nor for the patient.

The notion of advocacy presents an ethical norm that conflicts with utilitarianism. Under this norm we are bound to participate in or at least accept not what we ourselves want or would want but what the patient wants or would want, even when that desire does not conform to the utilitarianism of the classic decision theory. The ethic of advocacy conflicts with the ethic of utilitarianism.

A second scenario that occurs to the surgeon nearly daily has to do with truth telling. You recall, of course, the Hippocratic aphorism "first of all do no harm." However, the current orthodox ethical stance is professed to be "tell the truth, the whole truth." Can truth telling cause harm? Can one predict that it will or may cause harm?

The absolutism, which requires that we tell the truth always and completely, derives from Immanuel Kant's "On a Supposed Right to Lie Because of Philanthropic Concerns." He wrote the following:

> *"To be truthful in all declarations is, therefore, a sacred and* unconditionally commanding law *of reason that admits of* no expediency *whatsoever." (Italics added.)*

Among surgeons, all are aware that the truth can harm; it can cause dejection, despair, and defeat. A Kantian ethic obliges one to a complete telling of the truth; the Hippocratic ethic and the surgeon's ethic, which evolved from it, demand that we do no harm. Clearly a conflict may on occasion exist between the Hippocratic ethic and the Kantian ethic. I have observed surgeons in the family waiting area outside the operating room, in the clinic, or at the bedside for well over 50 years. All, in navigating between this Scylla and Charybdis, choose a description from the inexhaustible possibilities, which is optimistic and on occasion is near to nondisclosure. All, in the words of Emily Dickinson, "tell the truth but tell it slant."

Dietrich Bonhoeffer was a spy involved in a plot to kill Hitler who was himself later killed by the Nazis. He was also a highly principled person who anguished over the deceit required by his role in the German resistance. He justified his deception by pointing to a deeper truth when he wrote the following:

> *"He dons the halo of the fanatical devotee of truth who can make no allowance for human weaknesses; but, in fact, is destroying the living truth between men."*

Bonhoeffer was aware also of the dangerous slippery slope on which these thoughts placed him. The consequences of a misstep on this slippery slope are described in a recent essay that appeared in "The Economist," titled "The Art of the Lie."[5]

A short but poignant essay entitled "Nondisclosure"[6] appeared recently in the *JAMA*. In this, Abby Rosenberg tells her own struggle with this ethical conflict while caring for a 13-year-old boy with incurable terminal cancer. Ultimately, Rosenberg came to believe that "nondisclosure" was the right thing, 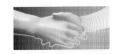 the good thing, and the thing that, in that specific circumstance at least, one "ought" to do.

Here an interesting aside may be apropos. Telling the "whole truth" unburdens the teller, at some risk of harm to the patient. Nondisclosure, if the circumstances demand it, places a greater continuing burden on the surgeon in service to the Hippocratic ethic to cause no harm.

Historically, one of the few unambiguous rules in our ethics compendium has been the surgeon's ethic that beneficence is owed first and perhaps solely to the patient. We are currently immersed in another field of tension: the individual patient versus society as a whole. The balance between these positions is changing rapidly in our society. Thomas Percival (1740-1804) enunciated one extreme:

> *"...surgeons should not suffer themselves to be restrained, by parsimonious consideration, from prescribing wine, and drugs even of high price..."*

You will immediately recognize this posture as running afoul the "antibiotic stewardship committee" and the "implantable device selection committee," as well as the institution's chief fiscal officer. The idea of agency dictates that the surgeon has a singleness of view, a singleness of concern: the patient and the patient only. Of course this ethic of agency was, appropriately, applied less in wartime, plague years, or other emergency situations. Still most surgeons choose to use biological mesh for hernia repair when they deem it appropriate. My own pacemaker is not the one that the hospital's implantables committee has standardized. It is the most expensive on the market.

The surgeon's ethic of agency requires that the surgeon do what is best for the patient here, even at the expense of the rest of society. But the hospital, it is said, will be able to allot more funds to charity care if you will use 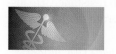 the standardized, lowest priced implantables. The ethic of utilitarianism demands acts and utterances that produce "the greatest good for the greatest number"; our ethic of agency requires that our beneficence should be directed to the patient now in front of us. The surgeon is left with ambiguity and probably with regret.

The allocation of funds is often an accurate surrogate for the justice or injustice of distribution of benefit. I have attended surgical case conferences for well over 50 years. Until a decade ago, I cannot recall ever hearing "cost" mentioned. In recent years, I had been counting the mentions of "cost" in surgical conferences at 2 academic medical centers, but I have long since lost count of the mentions. A recent publication concerning intraoperative costs was discussed in a letter to the editor of the *Journal of the American College of Surgeons*.[7] The letter writer called the surgeon's knowledge of costs a "deficit" to be remedied by "education"; the clear inference was that surgeons were somehow ethically deficient in this regard. The surgeon's ethic of advocacy is being diminished in strength, and the surgeon is being buffeted by the change.

Please allow me to quote again from Alexander Walt who was a mentor and friend.

*"The long tradition that care of the sick is not primarily a business has been unsentimentally demolished...as the hard-eyed men of finance decree that survival depends on rapid conversion..."*

However, even more fundamental change is under way. The idea of shared risk and shared expense and the evaluation of outcomes for populations have all but abolished the surgeon's ethic of advocacy for the individual patient. The utilitarian formula of "the greatest good for the greatest number" has already prevailed in most health-care settings. Population health is in ascendancy.

The well-being of surgeons is very much promoted when ethical obligations are clear and unambiguous. However, currently, surgeons are racked by at least 3 ethical dilemmas in which the ancient and venerable surgeon's ethic conflicts with prevailing ethical norms. They are the failure of classic decision models in the face of the ethics of utilitarianism and autonomy, and also the conflict between the Hippocratic and the Kantian ethics regarding truth telling, and finally, the rapid erosion of the ethic of advocacy by a form of utilitarianism.

You may ask, as have many before you, why attempt to act ethically at all, particularly in this modern world in which, it seems, "everything is permitted." The answer is clear but not intuitive: our acts and utterances create the meaning of our lives; indeed, they create us as human beings. If we commit ourselves to the great ethical traditions of our discipline, we become surgeons who have lived in the light of the discipline's ethical posture.

# References

1. Sigerest HE. *Primitive and Archaic Medicine*. New York: Oxford University Press; 1967.
2. The William Osler Lecture in the History of Medicine. December 9, 1955. Reprinted in Edelstein L. *Ancient Medicine*. Baltimore: Johns Hopkins Press; 1967.
3. Whipple AO. *The Role of the Nestorians and Muslims in the History of Medicine*. Princeton: Princeton University Press; 1967.
4. Elmore LC. National survey of burnout among U.S. general surgery residents. *J Am Coll Surg*. 2016;223(3):440–451.
5. The Economist. Leaders—post-truth politics. *Art of the Lie*. September 10–16, 2016;420(9006):9.
6. Rosenberg AR. Nondisclosure. *JAMA*. 2016;316(8):821.
7. Dempsey DT, Furukawa A, Salasky V, et al. Correcting surgeons' knowledge deficit. *J Am Coll Surg*. February 2016;222(2):213.

# PART 2 ▶ PRACTICE

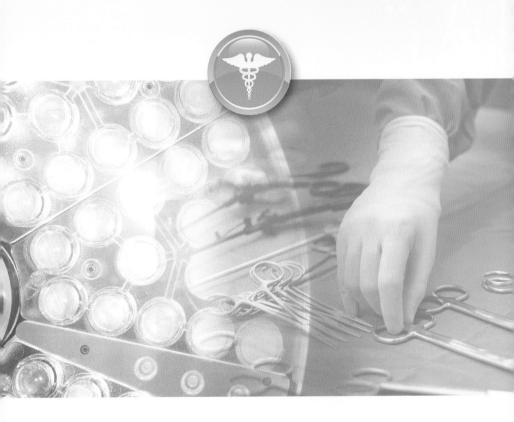

# 13 Ethical Decision Making in Neurologic Surgery

Jason L. Schroeder, MD

PROLOGUE ▶ Neurosurgery constitutes a field that is at once ancient and modern. Prehistoric skulls show evidence of a crude operation, trephination, in which an opening is created in the skull for purposes we do not fully understand. Modern neurosurgery, however, dates from the late 19th and early 20th centuries.

Harvey Cushing was born in Cleveland, Ohio, in 1869. He may perhaps single-handedly be credited for the development of the field of neurosurgery, including innovative techniques for the excision of brain neoplasms. Interesting for our current train of thought are the evidences of a true humanism in Dr Cushing. He wrote the voluminous official biography of Dr William Osler, who is often credited for uniquely mixing the sciences of medicine with a deep humanism. Cushing also expressed his own ethical posture in his "Consecratio Medici," a series of essays enunciating his ethical views.

Dr Jason L. Schroeder is an assistant professor of surgery and the division chief of neurosurgery at the University of Toledo College of Medicine. He has experienced both the world of private practice and the academic practice of neurosurgery. He has had special training in bioethics, having received a Master of Arts degree from Case Western Reserve University. He chairs the Institutional Ethics Committee at the University of Toledo Medical Center.

**63**

## What Is Neurosurgery?

Neurologic surgery is a specialized field of surgery involved with treating diseases that affect the central, peripheral, and autonomic nervous systems. In practicality, this means that neurosurgeons are responsible for treating a wide variety of ailments, potentially in patients of all ages, which range from congenital anomalies of the brain and spinal cord to traumatic and degenerative diseases that primarily or secondarily impact the functioning of the nervous system. The amount of requisite knowledge that is encompassed in the field of neurosurgery is growing exponentially—in a way similar to that which is seen in essentially all fields of modern medicine. Generally, neurosurgeons are called on to be technically capable in the diagnosis and medical and surgical care of these disease processes, including the preoperative, intraoperative, and postoperative care required by their patients. Sadly, the human side of neurosurgery has often been lost or ignored as the technical portion of the field has continued to develop. As a result, many practitioners feel inadequately prepared to deal with the nonmedical, or at least less medical, parts of caring for their patients.

Neurosurgery is a diverse field, and in the age of subspecialization within neurosurgery, this may be truer than at any time in the past. There are neurosurgeons who treat only children, who treat only tumors, who only operate on the spine (or even a subsection of the spine), and even who do not perform any procedures that would classically be considered surgery (ie, radiosurgeons). Interestingly, despite the many potential differences between neurosurgeons and individual neurosurgical practices, there remain significant similarities that should not be dismissed. Some of these similarities include (1) the notion that patients are typically not well informed about their disease process—including the diagnosis, potential treatment options, and prognosis; (2) that patients tend to come to the doctor/surgeon when they feel ill and hope to be made to feel well through the physician-patient interaction; and (3) the fact that in virtually all medical situations, there exists a deficit from complete knowledge and a resulting ambiguity about what treatment can or should be done. Each of the 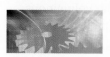 just listed examples of similarities exposes a potential area in the doctor-patient relationship where technical mastery of diagnosis and surgery alone will be inadequate to reach the best outcome possible for the patient. These examples help to illustrate the need for humanism in medicine—the need to understand neurosurgical problems within the context of a patient's life—to deliver the best possible care to the patient.

## How Is Neurosurgery Potentially Different From Other Surgical Subspecialties?

Perhaps neurosurgery is different from other surgical subspecialties for a couple of reasons. First, despite a recent decrement from the traditional high standing afforded to medicine in general, neurosurgery remains a field of medicine where much is unknown or at least unclear to the general public. The potentially "mystical" aura surrounding brain surgery, the frequent uncertainty of outcome in cranial trauma, and even the generally unclear reputation of spinal surgery over time leave much within the realm of neurosurgery as foreign to most medical and nonmedical people alike. Beyond this general lack of familiarity with most of the elements of clinical neurosurgery, there is also the reality that the locus of the 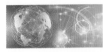 "true essence of self" or one's "personhood" is for many people felt to reside in the brain. Neurosurgery may seem to be more fraught with ethical dilemmas because "[n]eurosurgeons alone have the training and education to operate on the organ that constitutes the locus of humankind's consciousness, emotion, and intelligence."[1] For some, there remains a strong pull to consider the "wants of the heart" versus the "thoughts of the mind"—but as cultural, psychologic, and medical knowledge have grown through time, there is a fairly strong consensus that no matter how it actually works, the brain is the organ within individual humans that gives them the ability to think and thus provides substantial determination as to who a person is from a thought and personality standpoint. Seen from the patient's vantage point, consideration of surgery on the brain thus carries with it not only risks that are similar to other types of surgery—loss of specific functions (with brain surgery, functions such as sight, hearing, and speech)—but also potentially more existential concerns such as "will I be able to think, will my memory be changed, will my personality be different, and will I even be myself."

## Neurosurgical Codes of Ethics

Multiple neurosurgical societies have enumerated codes of medical ethics for their constituents. The American Board of Neurological Surgery (ABNS) has its Code of Ethics, as does the American Association of Neurological Surgeons (AANS), whereas the World Federation of Neurological Societies (WFNS) has produced a longer Statement of Ethics in Neurosurgery. In reviewing each of these documents, there are multiple similarities that help to point to some of the most important concepts related to ethics and neurosurgery.

The overriding principle that guides each of these documents is that the patient's interests and well-being are paramount. This is stated in the ABNS document: "The issue of ethics in neurosurgery is resolved by a determination that the best interests of the patient are served."[2] Similarly, the AANS document calls on its members to "be dedicated to the principle, first and foremost, of providing the best patient care that available resources and circumstances can provide and shall treat the patient's best interests as paramount."[3] Finally the WFNS Statement of Ethics in Neurosurgery describes the relationship between neurosurgeons and their patients as being based on "ethical principles developed primarily for the well-being of patients."[4]

Beyond this call to keep patients' well-being and interests at the center of the surgeon-patient relationship, these documents all call for neurosurgeons to commit to continuing education and to "practice only within the scope of … personal education, training and/or experience."[3] Neurosurgeons are called on to communicate openly and honestly with their patients (regarding risks, benefits, and alternatives to treatment) 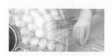 and the public (regarding advertisement of services, professional competence, and public education regarding neurologic disease). Each surgeon is required to respect patient privacy and to safeguard patient confidence—understanding that at times information may need to be disclosed for the safety of the patient or the community. Informed consent must be obtained before nonemergent operations, and neurosurgeons "must take time to get to know our patients as individuals, and share with them information and perspectives suited to their personal needs, enabling them to understand their own medical situation, and to knowledgeably participate in decisions about their own care."[4] Surgical intervention "shall be recommended only after careful consideration of the patient's physical, social, emotional, and occupational needs … [p]erformance of unnecessary surgery is an extremely serious ethical violation."[2] Neurosurgeons "must not exploit patients [financially]" and "should provide those aspects of postoperative patient care within the unique competence of a neurosurgeon."[2] Neurosurgeons should also "work collaboratively with colleagues and other health care providers to reduce medical errors, increase patient safety, and optimize the outcomes of patient care."[3] Members of the neurosurgical community collectively have "a social obligation to be involved in community and world activities"[3] and "to support international efforts to raise the standard of care in all areas of the world."[4]

It truly "is the duty of all neurological surgeons to place the patient's welfare and rights above all other considerations."[2] However, these ideals are lofty and important, but by themselves they do not provide clear guidance for the day-to-day challenges that individual surgeons and patients face. For example, what exactly constitutes the best interests of a patient in deep coma on hospital day 7 after a severe traumatic brain injury (TBI)? Or, for those who find too much difficulty in thinking about questions of continued life versus death, what constitutes the best interests of a patient with neurodegenerative problems (degenerative spine problems or neurodegenerative problems of the brain [such as Alzheimer disease, Parkinson disease, and so forth]) who has expectations that are bordering on being unreasonable for neurologic function either with or without surgical treatment? As the field of neurosurgery has become more sophisticated, so too have neurosurgical patients raised their expectations for outcomes after neurosurgical procedures. Where once patients may have been happy to arrest deterioration of function after surgery, now many patients are hoping for restoration or possibly even enhancement of function as an expected surgical outcome.[5-7]

## What Types of Ethical Issues May Reasonably Be Expected to Arise in Neurosurgical Practice?

As outlined earlier, neurologic surgery is a varied field—covering many different parts of the human body and potentially encompassing care episodes from the earliest times in life until the end of life. As such the ethical challenges that may arise in the course of practicing neurosurgery are also significantly varied. Some types of ethical dilemmas that might reasonably be expected to present themselves within the practice of neurologic surgery include ethical challenges related to end-of-life decision making; ethical issues at the beginning of life; ethical issues regarding reproduction; questions about the efficacy versus futility of treatment; ethical issues related to pain and the potential role that pain plays as a motivator for medical/surgical intervention; ethical issues that may be made more challenging because of the impact of neurologic (cognitive) deterioration; ethical issues that stem from problems with systems of care and resource usage; and ethical issues that stem from working with patients who may be considered a part of a vulnerable population (Table 13.1).

Clearly some of these types of ethical dilemmas are likely to be more common than others—for instance, at first glance it may be difficult to know why neurosurgeons could have interactions with patients affected by ethical issues surrounding reproduction, but in fact a variety of potentially neurosurgical disorders can impact patient's thoughts about the appropriateness or desirability for childbearing. This is probably most obviously illustrated by patients afflicted with tumor syndromes that affect the nervous system (consider neurofibromatosis types 1 and 2 [NF1 and NF2] and von Hippel-Lindau [VHL] syndrome as examples). Additionally, some may argue that ethical dilemmas arising out of questions regarding systems of care or resource usage are not dilemmas that only neurosurgeons must face. Although that is true, it is also important for neurosurgeons to realize that our individual contributions to problems within the general systems of care and our 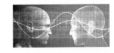 own gluttony or restraint with regard to resource usage do contribute to the overall impact of these factors on medicine and society in general. As such, neurosurgeons must do their part to help systems/practices improve and to be more resource conscious.

## What Are the Ethical Obligations of Neurosurgeons to Their Patients?

It seems that each neurologic surgeon has at least the following ethical obligations to his/her patients. First, the neurosurgeon is called to be truthful, honest, and as unbiased as possible. As a corollary to this first point, neurosurgeons

**TABLE 13.1 ▶ SOME EXAMPLES OF DIFFERENT TYPES OF ETHICAL ISSUES IN NEUROSURGERY**

| | |
|---|---|
| End of life | Withdrawal of care, decision for trach/PEG in severely neurologically injured patients |
| Beginning of life | Intrauterine treatment of myelomeningocele, congenital hydrocephalus |
| Reproduction | Inheritable tumor syndromes (NF 1 and 2, von Hippel-Lindau), surgical complications that may lead to impotence |
| Futility | Difficulty of prognosis early in severe traumatic brain injury, quality-of-life considerations in malignant middle cerebral artery stroke syndromes particularly on the dominant side |
| Pain | Chronic poststroke pain, medication management and pain contracts, use of illicit substances |
| Systems of care/ resource usage | Use of evolving technologies in the operating room and imaging suites |
| Vulnerable populations | Patients with neurocognitive disorders and their ability to comprehend diagnosis and/or proposed treatment, research subjects |

are obligated to educate their patients and their patients' families in an effort to help them understand the diagnosis and the potential positive and negative implications of individual treatment options—whether the options are primarily medical or surgical, palliative, or intended to be curative. Additionally, the surgeon is bound to work as an advocate for the patient—this is even more true when the patient has impaired decisional capacity or when the patient is not capable to act as his/her own best advocate (the family also has a significant burden in this regard). Fourth, a good and competent neurosurgeon owes technical prowess and is engaged in continuing education and technical skill development to his/her patients—in an effort to maximize positive outcomes and to limit suboptimal outcomes. Again as a corollary, beyond showing technical mastery at diagnosis and medical and surgical management of neurosurgical problems, neurosurgeons need to recognize their own limitations. "A neurosurgeon must maintain qualification by continued study, performing only those procedures in which he or she is competent by virtue of specific training or experience... [t]his competence must be supplemented with the opinions and talents of other professionals and with consultations when indicated."[2] Finally, neurosurgeons have an ethical obligation to admit when situations are not clear and to help themselves and their patients (and patients' families) understand that ambiguity is a part of clinical medicine—that not knowing everything is a reality, which must be faced, likely with significant frequency.

## Principles of Medical Ethics in Neurosurgery

Do the commonly quoted principles of medical ethics—nonmaleficence, beneficence, autonomy, justice[3]—apply well to neurosurgery as a discipline? Are there other principles of medical ethics that should also be considered—"totality," the principle of double effect, distributive justice, a preferential option for the poor and vulnerable, and so forth? Although none of the 4 classic principles of medical ethics are specifically mentioned in the documents regarding medical ethics and neurosurgery reviewed earlier, each of the 4 principles was called on in the drafting of these treatises. The principle of beneficence forms the basis for always seeking to provide for the betterment of the patient—"providing the best patient care that available resources and circumstances can provide"[3] and holding the patient's best interests as paramount. The principle of nonmaleficence underlies the prohibition that "[p]erfomance of unnecessary surgery is an extremely serious ethical violation" as explicitly delineated in the ABNS Code of Ethics. Nonmaleficence also underlies the positive duty of respecting patient confidentiality and patient privacy. Autonomy is strongly alluded to in the individual charges to get to know patients as individuals and to obtain "a fully informed consent prior to any operation."[4] Additionally, the World Federation of Neurosurgical Societies statement specifically points out that "[w]e must remember that the patient has the right to choose between treatments, or to refuse treatment altogether. We must respect this right." The principle of justice is the foundation of the neurosurgeon's duty to work collaboratively, to work to improve patient safety within the realms of medical and surgical care in general, and to elevate the standard of care in our local, national, and global communities. Often multiple principles work collectively to support ethical duties—for example, nonmaleficence, beneficence, and justice all underlie the prohibition against financial exploitation of patients.

Following are 2 case examples that have been adapted from recent real-life experiences. Each case is meant to provoke thinking about how medical ethics, principles, or duties as outlined earlier help to shape thinking in real-world situations. Often there are multiple potential ethical dilemmas that could arise in any given case, and as a result, there are also multiple potential ways to work through the challenges that may present themselves.

## Case Examples

**Case 1**—An octogenarian presents to the emergency department (ED) as a new trauma patient after falling at home with medical history significant for coronary artery disease (s/p coronary artery bypass for revascularization and treatment with dual antiplatelet agents), prior ruptured abdominal aortic aneurysm (s/p open repair), and multiple falls with overall deterioration in function over the prior year. Initially after the fall, the patient was awake 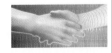 and conversant but complained of hip pain. The patient could not move the painful leg well because of the severity of the pain and could not get up off the floor. Within 30 minutes, the patient began to display a decreased level of consciousness and 911 was activated by the family. The admission radiologic workup included a head computed tomography (CT) scan that revealed a 2.5-cm subdural hematoma with a midline shift of 2 cm as well as additional imaging that showed a hip fracture. His admission neurologic evaluation revealed midsized, minimally reactive pupils, with positive cough and corneal reflexes and bilateral decerebrate posturing.

From this case, a variety of important questions begin to emerge.[1] What is the neurosurgeon's role in helping to evaluate an elderly patient with multiple comorbidities and multiple acute traumatic injuries, which will definitely be life altering and may become life limiting?[2] How should the neurosurgeon on call respond when asked to "come and evaluate" a patient whose statistical chance for meaningful recovery is in serious doubt? Here, as in most cases in medicine, the best choice is to go to the patient's bedside and evaluate the patient via history (whatever can or cannot be obtained) and physical examination. There is no substitute for examining the patient. Radiology, electrophysiology, laboratories, and the like are all useful adjuncts in the overall patient workup. However, the axiom that radiographic evaluation and additional ancillary tests are meant to be supplemental to the direct examination of the patient is astute in its simplicity.

Patients (and the families of patients) presenting with significant acute neurologic deficit(s) deserve the opportunity to have competent evaluation by providers specializing in neurologic or neurosurgical disorders. Practically speaking, even at 3 o'clock in the morning, it is the neurosurgeon's duty to assist with and/or to guide the evaluation of patients who present to their attention and to investigate the potential for improvement from timely neurosurgical intervention. In this regard, evaluating the patient means to obtain reliable data related to the patient's current medical problem and past medical and surgical problems and reliable data regarding the patient's current physical condition (ie, perform a history and physical examination). In an appropriate clinical setting, evaluating the patient may mean to review the findings of and to help direct a history and examination completed by a competent proxy. Furthermore, the patient's evaluation includes reviewing ancillary testing results that have already been completed and if necessary, helping to direct further workup of the patient. Importantly, this duty to evaluate patients appropriately does not mean and should not imply that every patient is entitled to an operation nor does it mean or imply that other persons (other physicians or staff or the patient/family) are entitled to mandate the scope of

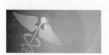 the evaluation or to decide what tests will be considered. Decisions regarding the scope and type of evaluation and those regarding the treatment options that are appropriate are made on a case-by-case basis with contributions from the neurosurgeon, the patient or surrogate decision makers, and consultants (on an as-needed basis) so that a comprehensive understanding of the problem at hand as well as the impact of other comorbidities and/or other simultaneous new conditions (if present) is obtained.

Generally speaking, people (lay persons, other physicians from nonrelated fields, patients, and the like) have relatively little understanding of

how and why decisions are made by neurosurgeons. This does not necessarily arise from neurosurgery being too difficult or too obtuse a subject. Rather, it is simply a reflection of the reality that decision making in neurosurgery (as in much of medicine) requires competence in the appropriate subject matter combined with an individual practitioner's personal expe-rience and the specific facts of the case at hand (medical history/comorbidities, patient's stated goals for treat-ment, resources available to provide specific types of care 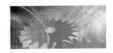 in the local setting, and so forth) to distill an appropriate treatment plan for the given situation. This portion of the decision making is completed primar-ily by the neurosurgeon attending to the case. This individual plan or group of options is then presented to the patients or their decision maker(s) to see how it does or does not support the patients' wishes and goals. The patients deserve and must get appropriate information to be able to make an informed decision about whether to go forward with or to reject the proposed plan. The process of delivering this information to the patients consists of educating the patients about their condition, helping them to understand the potential risks and benefits of the proposed treatment as well as the alternatives to that treatment, and explaining the potential outcomes associated with the indi-vidual treatment options. Explanation and discussion continue until the pro-vider and patients can agree on an acceptable treatment paradigm—it is very possible that the final treatment algorithm does not resemble that which was proposed or expected at the outset.

For the specific example listed earlier, there appear to be many of the duties that the attending neurosurgeon owes to this acutely injured patient. First, it is important to come to the bedside and to evaluate the patient. If the patient cannot provide information, then alternative sources of infor-mation are sought—ED nurses, life squad personnel, family members, and records. In addition, a review of the ancillary testing that has been completed (trauma CT scans as well as laboratory data and previously completed docu-mentation from the trauma team and ED physicians/nurses) helps to give a broader understanding of the patient's overall health condition. Then taking into consideration the patient's comorbidities (premorbid coronary artery disease, active platelet inhibition by dual antiplatelet treatment, report of progressively declining health over the past year, and new diagnosis of hip fracture) the neurosurgeon uses the collected information from history, physical examination, and ancillary testing to formulate a potential treat-ment plan as well as alternatives to that treatment plan. The duties listed earlier could collectively be considered the primarily *technical* portion of the evaluation. These data must then be presented to the patient or his/her surrogate to provide education regarding the patient's diagnosis as well as the prognosis and the options for treatment and the likely outcomes for the treatment options (likely presented as the preferred treatment option ver-sus other options—and if so, why one option is preferred over others from the neurosurgeon's perspective). As this discussion unfolds, new information may become available, and through continuing education, the patient/surrogate may come to better understand the potential severity of the health care 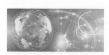 situation—in this example the situation is dire (octogenarian with hip fracture—potential high morbidity and mortality—as well as with acute TBI with expanding intracranial mass lesion in the presence of coagulopathy and significantly impaired neurologic status—again with significantly high potential morbidity and mortality).

Personal experience reveals that during these discussions, the patient or family sometimes desire one treatment paradigm but may also simultaneously want to avoid certain parts of that treatment course that may be inevitable. As an example, consider the family member who expresses a desire for craniotomy to relieve mass effect and to hopefully preserve "life" but who simultaneously states that mechanical ventilation is not acceptable for any period of time. Alternatively, in the same situation the family may not only want treatment but also state that the patient could not live with any new impairment or would never accept consideration of trach/PEG/rehab or nursing home placement. In this type of situation a disconnection exists between what seems to be desired and the reality of what is likely to be needed to attempt to attain the stated goal. This disconnection between desire and reality would then lead to a need for further education, discussion, and reflection between the neurosurgeon and the decision maker to try to arrive at a treatment plan that is fully acceptable and also has reasonable potential to come to fruition.

**Case 2**—Another case to consider involves a previously healthy woman in her mid-20s. She was involved in a significant trauma and suffered brain damage but does not have a mass lesion as the cause of her new incapacity. She does not have other significant, life-threatening injuries. Her family consists of a husband of less than a year, no children, 2 surviving parents, and a sibling. Clinically she is nonresponsive with Glasgow Coma Scale score of 3 and is intubated and requiring full ventilator support in the intensive care unit.

In some ways, this seems to be a nonchallenging clinical scenario. The patient has severe neurologic impairment, does not have other confounding injuries to consider, and has multiple relatives who can be asked to help make decisions on her behalf. Unfortunately, however, she does not have any documented advance directives, and as a younger patient, she is not likely to have discussed end-of-life wishes with her family. Legally her spouse is her decision maker; however, they have only been married a relatively short period of time. Additionally, given her relatively young age, her parents still feel a strong feeling of responsibility for her overall well-being.

In this specific example case, there is no chance for the patient to improve; however, in many real-life cases, it may be difficult to tell how a patient's condition will evolve over time. Prognosticating outcome, survival versus nonsurvival, or potential future quality of life—especially early after TBI—can be very difficult; and as a result, this particular challenge often presents itself as another layer of difficulty when counseling patients' families. The level of certainty about the patient's current condition and the level of confidence regarding the patient's ultimate prognosis often increase over time. As a result, the timing of family conferences and the level of detail and information discussed should be tailored to the individual circumstances of the given case. Families typically need time to process what has happened to the patient and to begin to prepare for decisions they will need to make moving forward. This reality is true for scenarios in which the patient is likely to die but is also true in cases where the patient will hopefully survive but full neurologic recovery is not expected. Understanding the adaptations that are likely to be needed if the patient survives is important for families to begin making preparations for post–acute care needs. Some examples include a wheelchair ramp if the patient is not likely to regain ambulation; assistance with patient monitoring/care if the patient will be dependent for activities of daily living or unsafe to leave without supervision; and provision for care in an extended care facility if the patient will not be capable of returning home.

As in all acute clinical scenarios, one of the most important assessments to make for patients who present with severe injury is whether or not the patient remains legally alive. Sometimes this determination is easy—a patient found with no pulse and no respiratory effort and who is already cool to the touch with rigor mortis meets the criteria for death.[9] However, even in nonneurologic injuries, there can be difficulty in determining the patient's vitality. For example, patients who have been exposed to extreme cold can present with no clear heartbeat and no obvious respiration, but they still require rewarming before pronunciation of death. Alternatively, patients with a left ventricular assist device will continue to have a "heartbeat" even if respiration ceases, which could be confusing for family members or practitioners not familiar with this technology. Regardless, in the case presented earlier, the potential confusion for many physicians, nurses, and other medical personnel typically stems from a lack of familiarity regarding the evaluation and management of patients in extreme neurologic distress—more specifically, lack of familiarity with the appropriate components of a neurologic examination and lack of facility with the criteria for brain death testing. For neurosurgeons and neurologists, difficulty with neurologic examination should not be a problem—training programs for both provide opportunities for the evaluation of neurologically devastated patients, some of whom would meet the criteria to be declared brain dead and others would not, so that expertise can be developed in determining how to differentiate these two groups of patients. Unfortunately, clinical expertise in 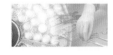 the determination of brain death does not guarantee significant familiarity with how to clearly document its occurrence nor does it guarantee facility with how to best convey the diagnosis to the patient's family.

The origin of modern brain death criteria began to be developed in the 1960s by the Harvard Commission.[10] The elements of a brain death examination include (1) certifying that no other potentially reversible cause of impairment is present (examples include cold temperature, presence of neurologically depressing drugs/substances, significant electrolyte abnormalities, and so forth), (2) documentation of the lack of brain stem function as evidenced by lack of brain stem reflexes (lack of pupillary reaction to light, corneal reflexes, occulocephalic reflexes, and the cough and gag reflexes), (3) documentation of a lack of motor reaction to deep central pain, and (4) documentation of a lack of respiratory drive through completion of an apnea test. Patients may require a variety of treatments before brain death testing— to correct electrolyte disturbances, to bring core body temperature into a normal range, and to ensure adequate oxygenation and ventilation through adjustment of respiratory parameters on the ventilator. The time it takes to make these changes in the patient's overall condition also provides time to meet with the patient's family and to begin to discuss the perceived severity of the brain injury and to explain the purpose of proposed treatments and assessments. During this time, it is especially important to be empathetic and compassionate because particularly in acute traumatic injuries, there was no time for the family/friends to prepare for this difficult new reality—where someone they care for deeply is in mortal danger and the prognosis is not yet certain for survival or death.

Even this early phase of caring for the patient and for the patient's family can give rise to a variety of difficult ethical dilemmas. These may include uncovering a previously developed lack of trust in the medical enterprise, lack of previously documented advance directives, or potentially a complete lack of prior discussion regarding the patient's wishes with regard to this type of situation, difficult family dynamics that may inhibit a consensus understanding of the diagnosis and prognosis, competing demands for hospital/societal resources, and questions about how quality of life is to be determined and/or balanced against potential future quantity of life. These dilemmas can affect all parties involved with the patient's care—physicians, nurses, mid-level providers, ancillary staff (social workers, nurse aides, radiology personnel) as well as the patient and the patient's family and friends. As such it is important to understand that misunderstandings or even truly irreconcilable differences may emerge and may significantly hamper successful provision of care to the patient. As previously outlined in this book, there are guiding principles that can be considered in trying to rectify these ethical dilemmas (nonmaleficence, beneficence, autonomy, and justice), and when such dilemmas arise, a real and honest effort should always be made to work through the issues. Importantly, it should be noted that the health care team does not always intrinsically represent the appropriate solution to the problem—more succinctly "the doctors and nurses do not always have the right answer."

Consider just one of the ethical dilemmas mentioned earlier—that of competing demands for hospital and/or societal resources. It is not difficult to see that there are many ways in which this ethical problem could relate to the care of an acutely brain-injured patient as outlined in case 2. Patients with severe neurologic injuries require resource and labor intensive care. Furthermore, depending on the evolution of the patient's condition, this demand on resources

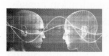

can be long lasting. The hospital resources dedicated to caring for such a patient include bed space in an intensive care unit; nursing care often on a 1:1 ratio (1 nurse to 1 patient); respiratory care including use of mechanical ventilation; radiologic resources including serial neuroradiologic examinations (time on the CT and magnetic resonance imaging scanners as well as time for the radiologist to interpret the completed studies); pharmacy services for everything from electrolyte replacement to preparation of medication drips (cardioactive drugs, pain and sedative medications); and physician resources for serial neurologic evaluations, critical care management, and time for family meetings. Other hospital resources include social worker coverage, potential use of interpreters, waiting room space, and a host of other resources, which are too numerous to list. Resources that are used from the family's side include time away from competing interests (employment, paying bills, other missed family obligations such as schoolwork, children's activities, and so forth), a significant detriment to quality and quantity of sleep, use of monetary resources (for travel to and from the hospital, accommodation, nutrition), and probably most importantly, use of emotional resources as the family attempts to grapple with the now suddenly changed reality of their individual and collective lives in relation to the status of the injured patient. Hospital resources are finite, and as such the resources expended to care for any one critically injured patient are equally important for the care of any other critically injured patient. As one patient approaches the point at which no further care will be able to maintain or improve life, there is a moral obligation to limit the care delivered, especially when system resources are taxed to the point of lacking the ability to care for other patients when these other patients have a better chance of survival or are more likely to have improvement in quality of life. Similarly, within the sphere of the family and friends who are affected by the patient's critical illness, there are finite resources available for all aspects of daily living, and those resources directed toward care for the patient come at the cost of opportunity to direct them (time, thought, energy, finances) toward the remainder of life's obligations. As the patient's care team and family progress through the process of potential brain death determination, it is important to remain objective in the midst of trying to show compassion and empathy toward the patient, the family, and the situation.

## The Difficulty of Death

Because of new challenges in determining the potential vitality of patients, multiple groups have worked to codify criteria for the declaration of death. As alluded to earlier in this chapter, in the past the determination of death was based solely on the irreversible cessation of cardiac and respiratory functions. In contrast, for contemporary medicine new innovations have blurred 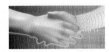 the line between life and death to at least some degree. This decrement in clarity between life and death has occasionally spurred not only controversy but also sarcastic humor. "The methods for diagnosis and treatment have today reached a degree of refinement and efficacy which tends to make them too powerful tools in our hands, when dealing with critically ill patients. In top-equipped hospitals, it is not quite uncommon to witness processes of dying more extended than what should be natural in a biological, psychological as well as ethical perspective. To use our formidable diagnostic and therapeutic capacity in a reasonable fashion is indeed a challenge, not least to the less experienced doctor or nurse. With a scent of black humour, someone in my country recently made this very pertinent remark: 'The progress in medical research has increased the average age of man, by lengthening the process of his dying.'"[11]

Despite potential misgivings by some regarding the manner in which patients can now be declared dead, the reality of modern medical practice and life in general still require a principled approach to determining when death has occurred. Socially, death remains important to justly terminate contracts, debts, and individual rights. Medically the determination of death remains equally important to release the medical team from further fiduciary responsibilities to the patient and to allow the medical system to reorient its resources toward the care of other patients. To help establish clarity that brain death and cardiopulmonary death are equivalent, the concept of a uniform determination of death came out of the President's Commission on Ethical Problems in Medicine (1981)[12] and recommended the following language become statutory in all states.

## Uniform Determination of Death Act

*"An individual who has sustained either (1) irreversible cessation of circulatory and respiratory functions, or (2) irreversible cessation of all functions of the entire brain, including the brain stem, is dead. A determination of death must be made in accordance with accepted medical standards."*

The impetus for consideration of this new standard for the determination of death arose from what the commission called a "new category" of "artificially maintained bodies"—those patients where "because of new advances in medical technique.... [physicians can] generate breathing and 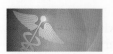 heartbeat when the capacity to breathe spontaneously has been irretrievably lost .... [and] certain organic processes in these bodies can be maintained through artificial means, although they will never recover the capacity for spontaneous breathing or sustained integration of bodily functions, for consciousness, or for other human experiences."[12] To put this more succinctly, criteria for brain death were needed because some patients with no opportunity to regain the capacity for life—the integration of bodily functions (including sustained, spontaneous cardiac and pulmonary functions) and consciousness—might otherwise have been maintained in a state between life and death relatively indefinitely. Furthermore, one of the central conclusions from the President's Commission was "that death is a unitary phenomenon which can be accurately demonstrated either on the traditional grounds of irreversible cessation of heart and lung functions or on the basis of irreversible loss of all functions of the entire brain."[12] Though 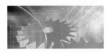 it seems that the modern determination of death may be fraught with more difficulty than in the past, this concept of a uniform determination of death is meant to bridge the gaps between past, present, and future and to provide for common language across jurisdictions at the end of life.

*"Dying has, during the history of man, fundamentally and always been a common event, a completely natural part of human life. This is clearly a positive and very important factor. It is crucial that any one person is competent to judge whether a fellow-man is alive or not. When situations of dying and death have to be met, there is a definite human value in communicating what is happening in simple and adequate layman's terminology. The ability to understand and recognize that a person has 'lost his life' should not be an issue for experts. But this does not mean that the state of death should not be* confirmed *by an expert. Under all circumstances, one must by all means avoid turning the state of 'being dead' into a* diagnosis, *which can only be recognized by qualified experts, after examination. The death of a human being is, and must remain, an event familiar to the common people."[13]*

## Conclusion

As outlined in the introduction, neurosurgery is a subspecialty that focuses primarily on the surgical treatment of diseases affecting the nervous system. This encompasses a large diversity of disease process and covers doctor-patient encounters that can commence before birth and last until the end of life. That wide spectrum of care can lead to difficulty in trying to determine exactly what ethical dilemmas are specific to or most frequently encountered in neurosurgery. It should, however, be clear from the preceding text that neurosurgeons may be called on to help resolve ethical dilemmas relating to end-of-life decision making and questions surrounding the concept of brain death, incapacitated patients who cannot act as their own decision maker (and thus dilemmas associated with surrogate decision makers), and challenges that come from injuries that may not be fatal but will nevertheless result in significant neurologic morbidity (and thus questions about quality of life and even questions regarding whether or not a patient will still "be himself or herself" after the acute disease process has run its course).

Unfortunately, most neurosurgical training programs lack any direct, specific instruction related to these topics. Often neurosurgeons in training and those in practice are left without many personal or institutional resources to help resolve these ethical dilemmas. As a result, many of these surgeons feel uncomfortable with working through these types of challenges. Formal neurosurgical education, as well as surgical and medical education in general, needs to renew its dedication to the development of curricular activities that will help to fill this void in training. The formal declarations of ethics compiled by the ABNS, the AANS, and the WFNS are all useful documents, and they help to codify many of the broad principles of the profession of neurosurgery and the ethical obligations of the members of each of these societies. They do not, however, provide clear practical advice about how to resolve individual ethical dilemmas that may arise during the practice of neurosurgery. In the end, neurosurgeons, their patients, and the patient's families are left to work out the details of each potential ethical dilemma—in each case this is most effectively done by collaboratively delineating reasonable and appropriate goals for care, focusing on both what is achievable and what is in alignment with the patient's own wishes for self-determination. Neurosurgeons must not be afraid to admit when information is not clear or complete, and they must also share the responsibility for decision making in a real way with the patient or surrogate decision maker, so that what is truly in the "patient's best interest"[2-4] is likely to be achieved.

# References

1. Amadio JP. Neurosurgery ethics: perspectives from the field, circa 2015. *Virtual Mentor*. 2015;17:3.
2. Code of Ethics. [cited 2017 January 3, 2017]; ABNS Code of Ethics; 2017. Available from: http://www.abns.org/en/About%20ABNS/Governance/Code%20of%20Ethics. aspx/.
3. AANS Code of Ethics. [cited 2016 November 15, 2016]; from AANS website – Code of Ethics – revised 2014; 2014. Available from: https://www.aans.org/en/About%20AANS/~/media/Files/About%20AANS/Governance%20and%20Leadership/aanscodeofethics. ashx.
4. Umansky F, Black PL, DiRocco C, et al. Statement of Ethics in Neurosurgery of the World Federation of Neurosurgical Societies. *World Neurosurg*. 2011;76(3–4):239–247.
5. Girdano J, A preparatory neuroethical approach to assessing developments in neurotechnology. *Virtual Mentor*. 2015;17(1):6.
6. Esplin BM, Andre G, Ford PJ, Beasley K. Applying guidelines to individual patients: deep brain stimulation for early-stage Parkinson disease. *Virtual Mentor*. 2015;17(1):10.
7. Lipsman NL, Andres M. Cosmetic neurosurgery, ethics, and enhancement. *Lancet Psychiatry*. 2015;2:2.
8. Beauchamp TLC, James F, *Principles of Biomedical Ethics*. 4th ed. New York, NY: Oxford University Press; 1994:546.
9. 21 Ohio Rev. Code. 2108.40; 2008.

10. A definition of irreversible coma. Report of the Ad Hoc Committee of the Harvard Medical School to examine the definition of brain death. *JAMA.* 1968;205(6):4.

11. Backlund EO. Death with dignity—on the withdrawal of life-sustaining measures. *Neurosurgery and Medical Ethics. Acta Neurochirurgica Supplement.* 1999:4.

12. Abram MB. Defining Death: Medical, Legal and Ethical Issues in the Determination of Death. A Report of the President's Commission for the Study of Ethical Problems in Medicine and Biomedical and Behavioral Research. 1981:166.

13. Backlund EO. Brain death in practice—a retrospective review. *Neurosurgery and Medical Ethics. Acta Neurochirurgica Supplement.* 1999:4.

# 14 Ethics in Congenital Heart Surgery

Steven Bibevski, MD, PhD
Roman Yusupov, MD
Edward L. Bove, MD

PROLOGUE ▶ Although there had been repair of aortic coarctation and ligation of patent ductus, the field of pediatric cardiac surgery may be said to have begun at a particular time and place, namely, at the Johns Hopkins Hospital on November 29, 1944. Dr Alfred Blalock operated and Mr Vivien Thomas stood behind him, the only person in the room to make directive and critical comments. The resident assistant was Dr William P. Longmire. Dr Blalock created an anastomosis between the subclavian artery and pulmonary artery, greatly increasing the flow in the pulmonary circuit. The so-called "blue baby" operation took the world by storm. A new era had begun.

An important figure is missing from the above scenario. Dr Helen Taussig was still actively teaching medical students when I (Lloyd A. Jacobs, MD) matriculated at the Johns Hopkins School of Medicine in 1965. I remember her distinctly: she was small and spoke very softly but had a commanding presence. She inspired. Historians relate that she also inspired Blalock by suggesting the rerouting of blood from the systemic circuit into the pulmonary circuit and that Blalock worked with Vivien Thomas to perfect the procedure in the laboratory. It is a matter of historical record that she was in the operating room on November 29.

Thus was born an entire field, which has experienced astonishing progress. Concomitant with this progress, however, was the encounter of pioneers in this field with many new ethical dilemmas.

Dr Edward L. Bove is the Helen and Marvin Kirsh Professor of Cardiac Surgery and Chair of the Department of Cardiac Surgery at the University of Michigan in Ann Arbor, Michigan.

Dr Steven Bibevski is a surgeon in pediatric and congenital cardiac surgery at Joe DiMaggio Children's Hospital in Hollywood, Florida.

Dr Roman Yusupov is a clinical geneticist in the division of pediatric genetics at Joe DiMaggio Children's Hospital in Hollywood, Florida.

A discussion on ethics in any medical field or specialty is heavily dependent on the complete circumstances surrounding the patient. Indeed, it is seemingly impossible to cover all scenarios related to a particular case discussion because of the high degree of variability in every case. For example, surgical repair of tetralogy of Fallot in an asymptomatic patient with no other abnormalities would generate very little ethical discussion in our current society. We perform the operation while the patient is asymptomatic to avoid complications and improve quality of life in the future. What if, however, we consider repair of tetralogy of Fallot in an asymptomatic patient who has a comorbidity that would shorten life expectancy? What if the comorbidity would result in death before the patient would be likely to develop the complications of tetralogy of Fallot? In this scenario, one might ask, would the quality of life be improved with operation? Would medical expenses be reduced by offering the operation? What if we do not know the answers to these questions? Does everyone get treated equally according to protocol or do we weigh all factors that affect the patient? Do we place a value on human life in terms of functionality and ability to interact with society? Should this change depending on the society where the patient lives if resources are scarce? Who makes these decisions? This variability and situational dependence is the very essence for the need of an ethical discussion in congenital heart disease (CHD).

The importance of an ethics discussion in congenital heart surgery extends well beyond clinical scenarios in this cutting-edge specialty. We might also consider nonclinical scenarios. In a highly complex field such as congenital cardiac surgery where experience and skill matter, do we allow trainees to perform the surgery under supervision or do we have the most experienced person perform the surgery? Should the person performing the operation be disclosed to the family? When there is no standard therapy, what kind of disclosure is necessary before proceeding with treatment that has an unknown outcome? 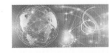 Nowhere are these questions more poignant and timely than in congenital heart surgery, and we will attempt to address some of these questions in this chapter by using examples to guide the discussion.

## Can We Versus Should We

The American health care system has enjoyed an extended period of time in an environment that has supported clinical and ethical decision making largely independent of economic considerations. Decision making has therefore rested on medical indications, family preferences, and the limits of medical knowledge. Medical reform is, however, a major topic of discussion in American health care at the time of this writing and has been a major point of discussion in other economies for some time. With greater scrutiny of the costs of various preventive and therapeutic interventions, there is an increased need to be cognizant of the implications of our decision making in both the short and long term. This is likely to raise considerable ethical debate spanning prenatal screening of CHD, to offering postnatal intervention and beyond, into the spectrum of adult CHD. For example, the results of the Helsinki prenatal ultrasonography screening trial, conducted from the perspective of the national economy, concluded that the implementation of a one-stage ultrasonography screening program for detection of fetal anomalies was advantageous from a cost-effectiveness perspective.[1] The results of the randomized 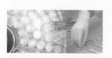 study showed significantly lower perinatal mortality in the screened group, most likely attributed to better early detection of major malformation and subsequent induced abortions. It very quickly becomes difficult to draw a line between malformations for which it would be cost-effective to terminate the pregnancy and those for which it would not. In the realm of CHD, prenatal screening is clearly associated with improved survival and reduced costs for some diagnoses. The ability to prepare a family for the pending medical and surgical plan has also been demonstrated to provide significant benefit to families.[2] Aside from the immediate and extended economic impact,[3] there is a significant impact on the social aspect of families who have a child with CHD.[4]

## Social Stress on a Family With a Child Who Has Undergone Palliative Cardiac Surgery in a Complex Medical Background

A topic that the authors believe does not get adequate attention when counseling families is the impact on the family when the child goes home. In a complex medical background where a child has neurologic deficits, feeding difficulty requiring a gastric tube, frequent medical visits, and overall dependency for many years, what is the impact on the family? Are these families adequately aware of the impact that correcting an otherwise fatal cardiac anomaly will have on their family? Will the other children in the family get less attention and parental time because the sibling requires constant medical care? The impact of a child's chronic disease on the family is defined as a concept integrating an individual's subjective perception of the effects of the child's ongoing health condition on various aspects of family life.[5] This includes changes in the work situation or financial status of the family, in the quality and quantity of interactions with family members and friends, in recreational activities, and in personal consequences for future living. These questions were addressed in a paper by Werner et al.[4] The main findings of this study were that parents of children with CHD are particularly affected in the personal aspects of their lives and that lower levels of perceived social support predicted a greater perceived disease impact on the family. The significance of parenting stress in families with pediatric health conditions is well covered in the comprehensive review by Golfenshtein et al.[6] We strongly recommend including a social assessment of the family when making recommendations for families with children with CHD and emphatically so in a child with an underlying genetic background.

## Navigating the Ethical Decision-Making Process in Congenital Heart Disease

A discussion of all the possible scenarios in CHD is impossible, given the wide variety of congenital heart defects and the possible comorbidities. How then do we assess a case for possible ethical issues and resolve any controversies that may arise? This is particularly important when considering that CHD represents the group of anomalies with the highest incidence at birth and is responsible for 50% of the infant mortality from congenital anomalies. In addition, CHD is frequently associated with chromosomal and/or extracardiac anomalies; the incidence of chromosomal and or extracardiac anomalies may be double that of the general population.[7]

The foundations of any ethical dilemma reside in the key principles and we will discuss each below as part of the process of navigating a particular case.

## Respect for Autonomy

We have an obligation to respect the autonomy of other persons. Essentially, this means that we should respect the decisions made by other people concerning their own lives even if those decisions are different from our own. This is obviously not directly applicable to infants and children for whom the burden typically falls on the parents. In this circumstance, the parents become the intermediary for the discussion.

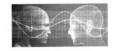

Respect for autonomy requires us to empower others for whom we are responsible, in this case, empowering the family to make decisions on behalf of their child. This concept is highly complicated when families look to the physicians for guidance. It is often stated that "the family wants everything done" but how well and honestly has the family been counseled? How much have our own beliefs and preferences tainted the discussion? How much do they comprehend? Is it possible to predict what the social stressors will be in this particular family?

Perhaps this is the reason why these difficult discussions for patients with CHD often fall to an ethics committee, where a multidisciplinary team is present to give differing perspectives in the discussion. By providing information from varying viewpoints, including nursing, clergy, palliative care, other medical specialists, and perhaps laypeople on the team, a more rounded perspective may be had, and families can feel more supported in their decision making. Unfortunately, difficulties can and often do arise even in the setting of such a committee.[8,9]

How then do we deal with a case in which the family wants everything done, but the scientific data suggest a nonviable outcome? This is especially important in congenital heart surgery where resources can be scarce, treatment is expensive, and a child who survives a previously fatal condition may now consume many more resources. It is easy to state that the physician or ethics team should be stewards with a responsibility to the health care system as a whole and may choose to withhold care; however, this is now being done on an individual basis rather than lumping all patients in a single category.[10]

## The Principle of Beneficence

The core principal of beneficence, viz, the obligation to bring about good in all our actions, seems simple in concept but can be complex. What if there 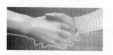 are 2 treatment options available, one with good results and decreased costs in the short term, but with suboptimal long-term outcomes, and another with a higher risk for death or complications in the short term but that has much better long-term outcomes? What if your center is experienced with option A, but option B is available only at a competing medical center?

The belief that by offering treatment we are imparting beneficence seems obvious; however, questions arise such as "What is the best treatment for this patient, in this situation, with the current resources, and the family's wishes?" Is it enough that we take positive steps to prevent harm, or does beneficence require the provision of the optimal treatment to achieve the best results?

Discussion of the following case serves as a useful exercise. When corrected early in life, patients born with transposition of the great vessels survive into late adulthood without significant impediments. Untreated, however, the outcome is very poor. Do we put the child through an operation believing that we can overcome the expected complications and provide a more predictable course, or do we observe the child, anticipating that the outcome is not likely to be optimal?

This brings us to the principle of nonmaleficence. We have an obligation not to harm others: "First, do no harm." The corollary is, where harm cannot be avoided, we are obligated to minimize the harm we do. Therefore, in the example mentioned earlier, if we expect the outcome of operation to be salutary, then should we proceed with the operation, understanding that there are risks involved and understanding that not proceeding may do more harm than good. Ultimately, each action must produce more good than harm.

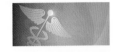

## The Principle of Justice

We have an obligation to provide others with whatever they are owed or deserve. We have an obligation to treat all people equally, fairly, and impartially. The difficulty in this principle lies within the variability of severe genetic syndromes with only moderate predictability of outcomes. Trisomy 13 and trisomy 18, unlike trisomy 21, have long been associated with exceedingly poor quality of life, very shortened life expectancy, and demands for extensive health care and social resources. In this setting, are we doing more harm to families, the patient, and society by providing a lifesaving operation, only to be left with a child who has unknown mental awareness and is dependent for all daily essentials such as feeding, toileting, and hygiene? Cases such as this have generated extensive discussion recently, whereas, in the past, there was little ethical dilemma; operation was generally withheld. Recently, however, reports are emerging where these patients are being offered operation and are surviving beyond a year of life.[11] During the preparation of this manuscript, a prenatal diagnosis of complex CHD was made in a fetus with trisomy 18. The parents requested that the genetic diagnosis be excluded from all medical and surgical decision making and that all life-prolonging therapies be made available to the infant. There was conflict among the medical team, and the case was resolved when a term echocardiogram showed fetal demise. Nonetheless, the case highlights the principles of ethics in surgery and the lack of consensus that may exist among a medical team.

## The Ethics of Training in Congenital Heart Surgery

The discipline of congenital heart surgery requires unique skills and education that are not currently provided in a standard thoracic surgery residency. Furthermore, many postresidency congenital cardiac surgery fellowships lack uniformity and quality control. In the United States today, the path to becoming a congenital cardiac surgeon is a long one. Following 4 years of medical school, a general surgery residency must be completed (although an American Board of Surgery certification is no longer required) before a standard cardiothoracic residency is undertaken. An additional 1 or 2 years is then spent learning the intricacies of the specialty of congenital heart surgery. The entire process can take 15 or 16 years. It might be argued that much of that preparation is unnecessary and, indeed, efforts are under way to establish new 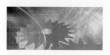 paradigms for training today's cardiothoracic surgeon. Nevertheless, the majority of today's residents will follow training programs based on the traditional pathway to certification. Many factors influence the quality of the finished product. These include institutional case volume, case mix and severity, the academic and hospital environment within which the resident functions, interpersonal commitment, and the ever-increasing conflict between educational and service demands. Furthermore, these issues must be considered in light of the increasing difficulties of training in today's environment. The demands of patients and payers have created a "microscopic" atmosphere in which every outcome is examined, critiqued, and even made public. Perhaps no specialty is more under this microscope than cardiac surgery, and pediatric cardiac surgery, in particular. Today's sophisticated echocardiograms reveal every outcome in detail, often before the surgeon has the opportunity to close the incision. For the trainee in congenital heart surgery, the shift to early repair and the impact of interventional cardiology have resulted in fewer straightforward cases for the resident to begin his or her experience. Work-hour restrictions have further affected the resident's ability to see as many cases as possible, leading many programs to consider lengthening their residency programs even further. Finally, it might be argued that a resident entering a cardiothoracic residency today is less well prepared to perform major cardiovascular cases because of the profound reduction of their exposure to open vascular operations during their general surgery experience.

How does the senior, responsible surgeon for any given congenital heart operation teach her or his resident to do the procedure? Could it not be argued that the result is likely to be better if the most experienced surgeon at the table does the case? Given the difficult visualization of the operative field when operating on very small babies through limited exposure, it can be a challenge for both the surgeon and the first assistant to see the anatomy at the same time. This issue always represents a challenge in any teaching program but must be faced if an accredited congenital heart residency program is to certify that its trainees are qualified to enter independent practice. Even a seemingly minor error in technique may result in a serious complication in the small heart of a newborn baby. Clearly there is no simple answer to this question, but those who take on the responsibility of educating tomorrow's surgeons must be committed to providing the appropriate environment for learning. The above argument that the "best" results will be achieved only at the hands of the senior surgeon can be countered by the argument that sending an improperly trained surgeon out into the world is equally worrisome, if not more so.

Defining the competent surgeon has become more difficult in today's environment. The number of skills required has increased. The cardiac surgical trainee must be prepared to handle open as well as endovascular procedures, understand complex and sophisticated imaging techniques, be knowledgeable in critical care medicine, be comfortable with immunology and transplantation, and learn to live in a world where specialists from many varied backgrounds all play a role in the management of the patient. The time has come where a prescribed number of years of training coupled with the personal observations of the faculty and program director are insufficient to provide the seal of approval for a resident to enter practice. Residency programs should separate practice from performance, much the same as athletes and musicians do. A structured curriculum with mandatory standards and a skills coach should be provided. Computer-based and virtual reality teaching tools should be utilized to their fullest extent. Competency to enter practice should be assessed by the ability of the candidate to master the necessary knowledge and skill sets, not by a predetermined number of years of training.

## The Ethics of Decision Making: Doing Things Right Is Not the Same as Doing the Right Thing

It is not uncommon for surgeons in congenital heart centers to be referred patients with complex CHD who have undergone a prior palliative operation, sometimes more than 1. Unfortunately, in some of these cases, the palliative operation, even though it may have been performed properly, makes the definitive repair more complex and riskier than it needs to be. Thus, the adage: *Doing Things Right Is Not the Same as Doing the Right Thing.* Although there may be many reasons why this is the case, the explanation may lie in selfishness and hubris. The unwillingness to "lose the case" to another center, or perhaps to admit that the definitive repair is beyond the ability of the referring surgeon or center to perform, too often prevails when making these decisions. Furthermore, the ultimate repair may require dismantling the connections made at the prior procedure, adding further risk to the operation.

Similar dilemmas are often encountered when more than 1 option for correction is possible. Should a complex, higher-risk operation be done when a "simpler" lower-risk procedure could be performed, even if the simpler operation has a worse long-term outcome? This scenario generally arises in children where their complex anatomy indicates that a decision between a palliative, single-ventricle approach and a complicated two-ventricle repair must be selected. Usually, the single-ventricle approach can be done at 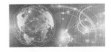 a lower early risk, but these patients will ultimately have difficulties at some point in life because their physiology is incompatible with a good-quality long-term existence. At that point, options may be limited, if they exist at all.

## Innovation Versus Regulation

The field of congenital cardiac surgery is a relatively new one. Many of the advances made in the past were the result of innovative approaches to problems that were uniformly lethal. When a family was faced with certain death or a risky, untested procedure, many opted for the untested procedure. This early environment fostered an era of unprecedented progress. Today's environment is, however, dramatically different. Success of surgical procedures today is measured in fractions of a percent, and there are many eyes on results of individual programs and individual surgeons. How then do we make progress and innovate in this restrictive environment? Should decisions about trying something new and potentially better lay in the individual surgeon's hands, or should anything being "tested" be done as part of a formal research study with the institutional review board review and formalization? How significant a deviation from the standard care would warrant such review? Moreover, in the field of congenital heart surgery what *is* the standard?

On the one hand, if an open, free-for-all on innovation is fostered, many new and better approaches to problems may be discovered. On the other 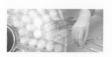 hand, individual enthusiasm for an approach or a device may cloud a person's judgment to the point where harmful procedures may be done. Even with the extensive scientific training, well-intentioned "experimental" treatments may in fact be harmful until enough data are generated to demonstrate the detrimental effect.

Because the field of congenital cardiac surgery is a relatively young one, many of the interventions we offer have been developed in a colloquial fashion, and approaches to certain defects can be remarkably different. For example, the conduction of a Norwood operation is typically done under deep hypothermic circulatory arrest. This mandates that the operation be performed in an expeditious manner, as time is of the essence. More recently, surgeons who were uncomfortable with deep hypothermic circulatory arrest developed an approach, which uses low-flow antegrade cerebral perfusion, obviating the need to stop the circulation completely. This provides the ability to perform the surgery at warmer temperatures and, in theory, eliminates the time pressure. Unfortunately, it will take decades to determine if the results are equally good, and patients are not always informed that there are 2 approaches to brain preservation.

## Genetic Case Examples for Discussion

In the era of persistent and steady increase of health care costs in the United States, one of the main components of daily physician practice is deciding what interventions are clinically appropriate. Physicians are constantly being urged to be financially prudent and to exercise judicious and economical practices. There is hermeneutical or factual evidence regarding benefits that an intervention will have, and then there is an ethical dilemma to whom and how to distribute those benefits.

Physicians, including surgeons, do not have an obligation to offer treatment that they think will not benefit patients. Medical futility refers to an intervention that is not likely to produce any significant benefit for the patient. The best known example is cardiopulmonary resuscitation. By providing futile interventions, physicians may increase the patient's discomfort and pain. Such interventions may give parents and family members false hope. Finally, they misuse finite medical resources that may benefit other patients.

Medical futility does not fly in the face of respect for patient autonomy. Although a patient or a parent has a right to choose and ask for a particular medical treatment option, it does not entitle him/her to receive such treatment at any cost. Physicians have an obligation of offering treatments that comply with professional standards of care, one of which is a clear benefit to the patient. These professional standards are based on scientific data that are extrapolated from basic or clinical research, case reports, and other published information. In fact, many medical associations develop disease-specific guidelines based on such scientific data with the ultimate aim of proving whether a particular intervention is futile or not.

As long as a physician openly communicates his/her view with the patient or family members regarding futile medical intervention supported by valid scientific information, it should preclude any further ethical dilemmas. As long as this concept is upheld, all clinical team members would ideally reach a consensus. Futile medical or surgical intervention contradicts the main pillar of medicine, the one of "do no harm." Of course, a family has an option of going to another medical center for a second opinion or requesting a meeting of a medical ethics committee.

Experimental procedures should not be called medically futile until there is solid empirical clinical evidence documenting that outcome in a group of patients. That, however, does not mean that a physician is obligated to perform an experimental procedure and cannot be held liable if he/she does not do so.

Medical futility is not the same as medical rationing. Medical rationing refers to the allocation or distribution of procedures based on some guidelines that potentially withhold beneficial treatment for some individuals. With scarce resources and enlarging health care populations, there is an inevitability of medical care rationing. Resources, including health care, are 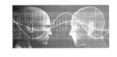 finite although the need for such resources appears to be limitless. Rationing is irrelevant only in a utopian society, which is not the case with the American society at the present time.

If there is to be any health care rationing, it should focus on the quality of life, not on social status, inability to pay, age, or sex. Thus, performing corrective heart surgery on an otherwise healthy patient at the expense of the patient with multiple congenital anomalies due to trisomy 18 should not be called rationing.

## Deciding Whether to Perform Complex Cardiac Surgery on a Patient With Multiple Congenital Anomalies Due to a Genetic Abnormality That Predisposes to High Morbidity/Mortality

A newborn baby boy with complex CHD is to be considered for operation. He has a prenatal diagnosis of trisomy 18, which is associated with significant mental retardation. The baby has other congenital anomalies, including intra-uterine growth retardation, cleft lip/cleft palate, micrognathia, and very small kidneys. The clinical geneticist informs the family that survival beyond the first birthday is about 10% to 15%.

A recent registry-based study in 16 European countries revealed that about 80% of babies with trisomy 18 had a cardiac anomaly, with 20% of them with a severe cardiac anomaly. Among babies with trisomy 13, about 57% had a cardiac anomaly and 17% of them had a severe cardiac anomaly.[12]

Unfortunately, sometimes congenital heart defects occur with other structural defects that would fall under the concept of "lethal anomalies." Such conditions have been associated with in utero demise or in the newborn period, despite medical treatment. Trisomies 13 and 18 are classic examples. That trisomy 13 and trisomy 18 are lethal conditions can be further advanced by acknowledging the fact that at least half of fetuses do not survive through birth. Overall, the risk of spontaneous fetal loss for trisomy 13 ranges from 49% to 66% and for trisomy 18 the range is from 72% to 87%. In addition to that, a prenatal diagnosis may lead to termination of pregnancy, but some women choose to continue their pregnancy.[13,14]

The median survival for a newborn with trisomy 18 is approximately 14 days and for a newborn with trisomy 13 is approximately 10 days.[15]

Survival rates beyond the first year of life in children with trisomy 13 and trisomy 18 have risen in the past decade from about 6% and 12%, respectively, to 12.6% and 19.8%, respectively, during the past few years.[16,17]

Despite the enthusiasm and apparent improvement in survival rates, 1 key fact remains the same: children with trisomy 13 and trisomy 18 have significant lifelong irreversible neurodevelopmental disabilities and congenital 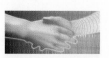 birth defects that are frequently not compatible with life or long-term survival. Would a life-sustaining cardiac operation only prolong the inevitable outcome of early death or still result in an incapacitated patient who is not able to perform daily functions and properly communicate with an outside world? In many instances the surgical risk alone is exceedingly high.

Parents of children with trisomy 13 and trisomy 18 very frequently request full intervention, including surgical procedures. Based on studies using parental questionnaires, 25% to 30% of patients chose a plan of full intervention.[18,19] This number is more likely to rise because of increasing modes of communication between parents and higher reported rates of survival. In the era of social networking, many parents whose children have trisomy 13 or 18 communicate with each other via support groups or "Google" the desired information. A majority of caretakers who participate in online support groups and social networking report a positive outlook on family life and the quality of life of their child with trisomy 13 or 18. Learning about a positive outcome 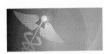 in another child with the same condition empowers parents and makes them believe that their child may have the same outcome.

Unfortunately, there are a lot of variables that may intervene and preclude achieving the same success story. Most of these variables can be overlooked by parents because information about them may not be shared or only reported in nonmedical media. For example, when describing their child's congenital heart defect to other parents online, most parents are likely to use general language with less technical terminology. Not many will post their child's echocardiogram or cardiac magnetic resonance imaging (MRI) results with detailed measurements. The same goes for brain MRI, electroencephalogram, child's growth parameters, respiratory support parameters, and other imaging or functional tests. This by itself may create a bias and lead to unwarranted expectations.

Parents frequently believe that their interpretation of the quality of life of their disabled children contrasts with that of their providers. Understandably, most parents view the lives of such children as valuable and we as physicians ought to support this view. However, at the same time, it is very important to properly educate parents by providing them with recent medical information. It is also important to note that many parents also report significant financial sacrifices, which may increase with each survival year.

There is a lot of debate whether children with trisomies 13 and 18 have a meaningful life. It is an important debate and it must continue. However, the debate should not supersede the objectivity of science, the main pillar on which medicine is based. Science does not yield meaning; it deals with facts, not emotions. The same holds true for the economy, of which health care is a major part. That is why there are increasing calls to avoid unnecessary testing and procedures that contribute to excessive health care costs with limited health care outcomes.

The 2010 American Heart Association guidelines recommend against resuscitation for children with trisomies 13 and 18 on the basis of "unacceptably high morbidity."[20]

Many clinicians believe that medical and surgical interventions do not clearly demonstrate improved survival in patients with trisomy 18, they do not improve significant neurocognitive disabilities, and they are "clearly associated with significant morbidity, resource allocation, and cost."[21]

Recently a questionnaire was administered to Canadian pediatric cardiologists regarding management of patients with trisomy 18. The following are the 3 options: not offering operation, offering palliative operation, and offering complete intracardiac repair. Most (67%) supported comfort care for affected patients with a heart lesion. None supported palliative surgery for those with complex heart lesions. This study shows that Canadian pediatric cardiologists support comfort care and medical treatment but not surgical treatment for trisomy 18 patients with cardiac lesions.[22]

There are those who argue that the burdens of 3 cardiac operations, along with the guarded prognosis for survival, justify withholding surgery for infants with hypoplastic left heart syndrome.[23]

## Same Condition, Different Severity

Three years ago, a baby girl was born at your hospital with hypoplastic left heart syndrome, mild dysmorphic features, small growth parameters, feeding issues, and 2 to 3 toe syndactyly. A cardiac operation is performed successfully. Over time, the baby is diagnosed with Smith-Lemli-Opitz syndrome, a rare autosomal recessive disorder of cholesterol metabolism. Of note, cholesterol and 7-dehydrocholesterol levels are only moderately normal. The baby is thought to have only mild manifestations of this condition.

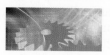

Now, the same parents, who are very observant Catholics, gave birth to a baby boy who also has hypoplastic left heart syndrome, along with significant growth retardation, cleft palate, ambiguous genitalia, polydactyly with 2 to 3 toe syndactyly. The clinical geneticist once again confirms the diagnosis of Smith-Lemli-Opitz syndrome on biochemical testing and notes that this time cholesterol level is very low. He informs the cardiac surgeon that this is a more severe presentation of the same condition, with a higher risk of early death. The parents would like to have lifesaving cardiac surgery performed on this baby also.

Over time, clinicians may encounter patients with the same underlying etiology, sometimes from the same family. However, the clinical manifestations of that etiology may differ from one family member to another. When deciding on a treatment plan for patients with multiple congenital anomalies due to the same etiology, it is very important to first understand the cause of that etiology and to assess the severity of the manifestations of the genetic defect.

The same genetic condition, involving a congenital heart defect, may have variable phenotypes. The congenital heart defect by itself may be the same, but associated noncardiac features may be better or worse. The clinical vignette described above is just one of the many possible examples of the wide spectrum of presentation within a particular condition. Smith-Lemli-Opitz syndrome, a relatively rare autosomal recessive disorder of cholesterol metabolism, usually results in multiple congenital anomalies. The most common ones are prenatal and postnatal growth retardation, microcephaly, moderate to severe intellectual disability, cleft palate, cardiac defects in up to 50% of cases (with a strong predominance of endocardial cushion defects and hypoplastic left heart syndrome), genital anomalies, and postaxial poly-dactyly.[24] The clinical spectrum is wide, and individuals have been described with normal development and only minor malformations. However, most patients have decreased cognitive function, ranging from borderline intellectual capability to severe intellectual disability. There exists an inverse correlation between serum concentration of cholesterol and the clinical severity, with high mortality in patients with the lowest cholesterol concentrations.[25]

It is relatively easy to convince oneself to perform corrective heart surgery on a patient with a milder phenotype. Real ethical dilemmas arise when a patient presents with a more severe phenotype, especially if he/she is a family member of someone previously treated by the same clinical team. That it may be a rare condition that has not been encountered before by the treating physician makes it even more challenging. The first step would be to understand the pathophysiology of the condition. Objectively assessing the patient at hand and comparing the patient not with a family member but with a cohort of patients reported in the medical literature is imperative. An appropriate treatment team should be assembled for a multidisciplinary approach and for a more collective experience. The first, milder, case that occurred in the family may be an exception to the rule and cannot be taken as a standard, nor should medical and surgical management of such a case be the standard in guiding management of subsequent patients with the same condition.

## Genetic Cause Is Unknown Despite Extensive Testing

A newborn baby girl is transferred from a nearby small hospital shortly after birth. She is already known to have multiple congenital anomalies, including tetralogy of Fallot, craniosynostosis, microcephaly with periventricular leukomalacia and intraventricular hemorrhage on brain MRI, seizures, profound hypotonia, and dysmorphic facial features. Parents are first-degree cousins emigrating from the Middle East. Extensive genetic testing does not reveal the underlying diagnosis.

Very frequently, physicians have to deal with rare clinical presentations, which they have never seen before. This happens with particular frequency in the field of clinical genetics. In many instances, the genetic mechanism of disease is never elucidated, despite extensive genetic testing. In such cases, physicians must make a clinical diagnosis based on available data. Based on that decision, a treatment plan for surgical intervention is formulated 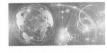 by a group of specialists. In this particular case, despite corrective cardiac repair and surgical treatment of craniosynostosis, the patient died shortly after 1 year of age. This patient never developed meaningful social skills, had global developmental delays, and required continuous monitoring and frequent interventions, with almost weekly doctor appointments and frequent hospitalizations. The overall cost to keep this child alive for about 1 year was more than $1 million. Was this amount of money well spent or could it have been better used for other purposes? Would appropriate palliative care without cardiac surgery have been a better option? In retrospect, most physicians treating this child thought that way.

Of note, close to $5000 was spent on this patient just for genetic testing that did not reveal the underlying diagnosis. And, although this is just a very tiny portion of overall expense that was incurred for the care of this patient, when more such patients are genetically tested, the overall amount of money may reach staggering proportions.

With the rapid advances in the field of genetics and genomics as well as the rapid expansion and availability of next-generation sequencing, more and more clinicians will rely on genetic testing to establish a diagnosis. There are multiple genes that have been clearly linked to various forms of cardiomyopathy, cardiac conduction defects, and structural and congenital heart defects. As the number of patients being tested increases, so does our understanding of genotype and phenotype correlations. These are some of the reasons why physicians use genetic testing as part of their decision making. Despite decreasing cost, genetic testing is still quite expensive. It may run from several hundred dollars for a routine karyotype to a few thousand 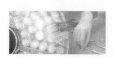 dollars for a sequencing panel, which rises even further for comprehensive whole exome sequencing, and the price may increase to about $10 000 for expedited results (usually within a week or 2). In most instances, when inpatient genetic testing is sent to an outside laboratory, the hospital covers the cost of such testing. In a busy tertiary care facility, with daily inpatient genetic consults, the annual cost of genetic testing may accumulate in the range of $500 000 to $1 million. In the era of fiscal responsibility, is this money well spent or could it have been better used for other resources, including surgical procedures?

## Genetic Testing Cannot Be Performed Because of Insurance Noncoverage and Financial Issues

A 2-year-old boy who recently came to the United States with his family from a Caribbean island is found to have large ventricular septal defect and atrial septal defect on the echocardiogram. The child is also known to have profound hypotonia with weakness, poor weight gain, global developmental delays, and respiratory failure requiring tracheostomy. The child needs a lifesaving cardiac operation. The clinical geneticist suspects a neuromuscular disorder. Basic genetic testing rules out common neuromuscular problems. More comprehensive genetic testing is not covered by the child's insurance and his parents cannot pay out of pocket. Without genetic testing and exact diagnosis, it is very difficult to predict the severity of the condition and life span for this patient.

On one hand, it would not be ethical to wait for genetic test results, which may take weeks; if cardiac surgery is to be performed, it should be done as soon as possible. On the other hand, understanding the full pathology may lead to a better long-term strategy and outcome. Other system dysfunctions may exacerbate the clinical presentation and cause a more severe phenotype. One of the jobs of the treatment team is to identify which system dysfunction is primary and which ones are secondary. In this particular case a neuromuscular problem appears to be the primary issue that is important not only in short-term but also in long-term management. The child's congenital heart defect appears to be secondary, which is likely to affect only short-term management. An important question to consider is the following: If the primary issue, namely, neuromuscular disorder, is not compatible with life in the long term, how important is it to pursue short-term management in the form of congenital heart defect repair? Even if the exact pathogenesis of the neuromuscular disorder cannot be elucidated at the time, the severity of the presentation at hand should guide physicians regarding long-term prospects. Ideally, a consensus should be reached regarding the potential outcome of the neuromuscular disorder by itself, before cardiac intervention is attempted.

## Overall Guideline

The following 3 factors are proposed as key decision factors when withholding surgical therapy from a child with a congenital heart defect is being considered:

1. Congenital structural cardiac defect that would require 2 or more operations for palliation.
   Combined with at least 1 of the following:
2. Another major congenital anomaly, neurologic impairment, or intrauterine growth retardation of unknown or unclear etiology.
3. A well-described chromosomal abnormality or genetic condition with proven predisposition to poor neurocognitive abilities, global developmental delay/mental retardation, seizures, or epilepsy.

If factors (1) and (2) are present, a medical ethics panel with parents and medical/surgical team should be convened to help decide whether to pursue surgical intervention.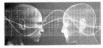

If factors (1) and (3) are present, withholding the cardiac operation because of an overall poor quality of life is suggested with palliative care only.

# References

1. Leivo T, Tuominen R, Saari-Kemppainen A, Ylöstalo P, Karjalainen O, Heinonen OP. Cost-effectiveness of one-stage ultrasound screening in pregnancy: a report from the Helsinki ultrasound trial. *Ultrasound Obstet Gynecol.* May 1996;7(5):309–314.
2. Bratt EL, Järvholm S, Ekman-Joelsson BM, Mattson LÅ, Mellander M. Parent's experiences of counselling and their need for support following a prenatal diagnosis of congenital heart disease—a qualitative study in a Swedish context. *BMC Pregnancy Childbirth.* August 15, 2015;15:171.
3. Raj M, Paul M, Sudhakar A, et al. Micro-economic impact of congenital heart surgery: results of a prospective study from a limited-resource setting. *PLoS One.* June 25, 2015;10(6):e0131348.
4. Werner H, Latal B, Valsangiacomo BE, et al. The impact of an infant's severe congenital heart disease on the family: a prospective cohort study. *Congenit Heart Dis.* May–June 2014;9(3):203–210.
5. Stein RE, Jessop DJ. The impact on family scale revisited: further psychometric data. *J Dev Behav Pediatr.* February 2003;24(1):9–16.
6. Golfenshtein N, Srulovici E, Medoff-Cooper B. Investigating parenting stress across pediatric health conditions—a systematic review. *Issues Compr Pediatr Nurs.* September 14, 2015:1–49.
7. Baker K, Sanchez-de-Toledo J, Munoz R, et al. Critical congenital heart disease–utility of routine screening for chromosomal and other extracardiac malformations. *Congenit Heart Dis.* March–April 2012;7(2):145–150.
8. Yates AR, Hoffman TM, Shepherd E, Boettner B, McBride KL. Pediatric sub-specialist controversies in the treatment of congenital heart disease in trisomy 13 or 18. *J Genet Couns.* October 2011;20(5):495–509.
9. Mavroudis CD, Mavroudis C, Jacobs JP. The elephant in the room: ethical issues associated with rare and expensive medical conditions. *Cardiol Young.* December 2015;25(8):1621–1625.
10. Janvier A, Farlow B, Barrington K. Cardiac surgery for children with trisomies 13 and 18: where are we now? *Semin Perinatol.* June 2016;40(4):254–260.
11. Boss RD, Holmes KW, Althaus J, et al. Trisomy 18 and complex genital heart disease: seeking the threshold benefit. *Pediatrics.* July 2013;132(1):161–165.
12. Springett A, Wellesley D, Greenlees R, et al. Congenital anomalies associated with trisomy 18 or trisomy 13: a registry-based study in 16 European countries, 2000–2011. *Am J Med Genet A.* December 2015;167A(12):3062–3069.
13. Morris JK, Savva GM. The risk of fetal loss following a prenatal diagnosis of trisomy 13 or trisomy 18. *Am J Med Genet A.* 2008; 146(7):827–832.
14. Houlihan OA, O'Donoghue K. The natural history of pregnancies with a diagnosis of trisomy 18 or trisomy 13; a retrospective case series. *BMC Pregnancy Childbirth.* 2013;13:209.
15. Wu J, Springett A, Morris JK. Survival of trisomy 18 (Edwards syndrome) and trisomy 13 (Patau syndrome) in England and Wales: 2004–2011. *Am J Med Genet A.* 2013;161:2512–2518.
16. Nelson KE, Rosella LC, Mahant S, Guttmann A. Survival and surgical interventions for children with trisomy 13 and 18. *JAMA.* 2016;316(4):420–428.
17. Meyer Liu G, Gilboa SM, Ethen MK, et al. National Birth Defects Prevention Network. Survival of children with trisomy 13 and trisomy 18: a multi-state population-based study. *Am J Med Genet A.* April 2016;170A(4):825–837.

18. Janvier A, Farlow B, Wilfond BS. The experience of families with children with trisomy 13 and 18 in social networks. *Pediatrics*. August 2012;130(2):293–298.
19. Guon J, Wilfond BS, Farlow B, Brazg T, Janvier A. Our children are not a diagnosis: the experience of parents who continue their pregnancy after a prenatal diagnosis of trisomy 13 or 18. *Am J Med Genet A*. February 2014;164A(2):308–318.
20. Morrison LJ, Kierzek G, Diekema DS, et al. 2010 American Heart Association guidelines for cardiopulmonary resuscitation and emergency cardiovascular care: part 3, ethics. *Circulation*. 2010;122(18 suppl 3):S665–S675.
21. Graham EM. Infants with trisomy 18 and complex congenital heart defects should not undergo open heart surgery. *J Law Med Ethics*. 2016;44(2):286–291.
22. Young AA, Simpson C, Warren AE. Practices and attitudes of Canadian cardiologists caring for patients with trisomy 18. *Can J Cardiol*. April 2017;33(4):548–551.
23. Kon AA. Healthcare providers must offer palliative treatment to parents of neonates with hypoplastic left heart syndrome. *Arch Pediatr Adolesc Med*. 2008;162(9):844–848.
24. Kelley RI, Hennekam RC. The Smith-Lemli-Opitz syndrome. *J Med Genet*. 2000;37:321–335.
25. Cunniff C, Kratz LE, Moser A, Natowicz MR, Kelley RI. Clinical and biochemical spectrum of patients with RSH/Smith-Lemli-Opitz syndrome and abnormal cholesterol metabolism. *Am J Med Genet*. 1997;68:263–269.

# 15 The Spectrum of Pediatric Surgical Ethics

Matthew Ziegler, MD
Moritz M. Ziegler, MD, MS
(Honorary), BS

PROLOGUE ▶ In addition to the obvious issues related to the size of anatomic structures and the great complexity of many congenital anomalies, the most vexing issue faced by the pediatric surgeon is the question of surrogacy. For the pediatric surgeon, the parents of the patient are themselves patients, needing cognitive and spiritual care, sometimes more urgently than the putative patient. The injunction to benevolence toward these is as binding as is the familiar "do no harm."

In instances where the parent's surrogacy cannot be taken at face value, where there may be conflict between parents, or when ulterior motivations are suspected, ethical decisions are particularly difficult. When surrogates are unavailable physically or emotionally, the surgeon's obligation may become blurred. Careful attention to the Zieglers' exemplars will be helpful.

Matthew Ziegler and Moritz M. Ziegler are a father-son team that brings the twin attributes of long experience and excellent training and current expertise. Their illustrative topics will be helpful to all surgeons.

Dr Matthew Ziegler is a surgeon in the division of colorectal surgery at William Beaumont Hospital and an assistant professor at Oakland University School of Medicine in Royal Oak, Michigan.

Dr Moritz M. Ziegler is a retired surgeon-in-chief at Children's Hospital Colorado and the University of Colorado School of Medicine.

*"With no language but a cry..."*
*Willis Potts, MD*
The Surgeon and the Child

## Introduction

Medical ethics are applied to patients of all ages, but a particularly challenging subgroup is encountered in the range from newborn to adolescent. Numerous unique questions and conundrums are the challenges within this population, and many age-old controversies persist to the present day. Can children provide consent for treatment? If not, who is the rightful responsible party? 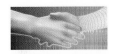 Can surgical innovation be tested in infants and children? If so, how can the young patient be protected from adverse outcomes? If not, how can surgical innovation for this vulnerable population be advanced and perfected? Other difficult problems facing modern medical ethics include, but are not limited to, the following: the appropriate age for gender assignment in newborns with ambiguous genitalia and other disorders of sexual development (DSDs); children born with a devastating chromosomal abnormality who present with a life-threatening surgical emergency; and children who require a blood transfusion but whose parents object to this intervention on religious grounds. The purpose of this chapter is to define these and similar issues and offer a general approach that might be applied to individual circumstances, with the goal of preserving the young patient's safety and autonomy while providing support to the parent/guardian as well as to the surgical innovator.

## Surgical Ethics Defined

"Surgical ethics" is a broad subject, and its application is paramount to the success of the complex relationship among the surgeon, patient, and family.[1] Certain moral virtues that may play a vital role here include trustworthiness, equanimity, compassion, advocacy, courage, humility, and hope. These principles may be particularly challenging to enact during the process of informed consent for young patients, where many rules, definitions, and observed practices exist. Indeed, many physiologic, moral, and socioeconomic factors have to be considered within the context of this special population.

Surgical ethics has evolved into the principles of respect for persons, beneficence, and justice.[2] It follows, then, that a process of informed, voluntary, and confirmed consent is mandatory before any surgical procedure. This includes a description of the scope and nature of a risk/benefit assessment as well as the details of the operation. In the setting of research, a description of subject selection and its associated consent process is also mandatory. This bioethical conversation is based on conservatism and reflects a direct counter to past abuses; the principles therein must be balanced against the drive to rigorously apply medical advances.[3]

## Brief Historical Overview of Pediatric Surgical Ethics

The origin of surgical ethics is often attributed to Hammurabi, the ruler of the first dynasty of Babylon. In 1750 BC he declared that a patient who was

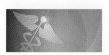 harmed by a surgeon would be best served by amputation of the surgeon's hands.[3] An equally compelling but less punitive declaration was made by Hippocrates in 400 BC when he devised the concept of *"Primum Non Nocere."*[4]
Translated, "First, do no harm," this simple phrase has become the cornerstone of modern medical ethics, and its message is ingrained into the minds of medical students from the very beginning of their education.

Much later, a significant development in the field of human subject clinical research took root in the early 20th century when a Boston surgeon named Ernest Codman called for unencumbered transparency of surgical outcomes. Codman suggested that surgeons track and record their operative results and follow their patients longitudinally to improve on current practices.[5] These measures are standard today, but at the time they were rejected by the surgical elite, Codman ultimately was forced out of Boston. He returned several years later to establish the "End Result Hospital," and he is now generally acknowledged to be the father of surgical outcomes for his vision and groundbreaking scientific methodology.[6] Codman's efforts more than a century ago with no doubt laid the foundation for 2 important surgical outcomes research projects under the auspices of the American College of Surgeons—the National Surgical Quality Improvement Program (NSQIP) and NSQIP-Pediatric.[7,8]

Following Codman's brave foray into surgical ethics, the next major challenge within this field was brought to light in Nuremberg, Germany, following World War II. The Nuremberg war crime trials exposed the many atrocities perpetrated by the Nazis against their human subjects, who were adult and child victims of grotesque experimentation, obviously in the absence of consent. The subsequent Helsinki Declaration, devised in 1964, put forth that "the human subject holds precedence over both science as well as society."[9] Although this important document sought to preserve patient autonomy, transgressions persisted. In 1966, Beecher reported a series of published human subject research articles whose authors failed to obtain, or at the very least document, patient permission for participation in the studies.[10] In response to such reports, the Belmont Commission was established in the 1970s and charged with the task of investigating and defining the principles of ethical research for human subjects.[11] The commission determined that "clinical practice" would enhance patient well-being with a reasonable likelihood of success. In contrast, "research" would test a hypothesis, permit conclusions to be drawn, and contribute to generalizable knowledge. Included in the commission's report was a statement of basic ethical principles involving respect for persons, beneficence, and application to the conduct of research. The American College of Surgeons continued its pledge to honor surgical ethics when it formed the Committee on Emerging Surgical Technology and Education in 1995 to monitor the application of "new technology" to patient care.[12]

## Ethical Boundaries: Patient Care or Innovative Surgical Research

As ethical principles in surgery evolved with time, the blurred boundaries between patient care and clinical research required evaluation and clarification. Many surgical innovations are incremental and technical and may occur spontaneously in the intraoperative setting. However, not all departures from standard practice connote research, and the fact that a procedure is experimental also does not make it research. However, any new procedure or technique should become a subject for formal research to provide evidence-based validation data. This approach, in essence, helps to assure efficacy and patient safety before a widespread application of novel technology.[13]

A study by Reitsma and Moreno identified 59 journal articles that provided evidence of surgical innovation. Of 21 respondents to further inquiry from the authors, only 14 described their work as research. Of the 14, only 6 sought institutional review board (IRB) approval.[14] A number of respondents believed that governmental regulations were not appropriate when considering a potential application for innovations in surgery. Another study investigated the obstacles confronted by comparative trials in surgery and identified 4 significant barriers:

1. The use of a placebo or sham surgery for comparison may not be ethically justified.
2. It is nearly impossible to "blind" the investigating surgeon.
3. The timing of the surgeon's innovation in the context of their expertise and position on the learning curve.
4. The incrementalism in surgical research and the speed of change it might produce.[15]

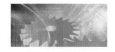

Indeed, 2 fundamental needs within this realm of medical ethics are the protection of the patient and the progression of research. Unfortunately, the aforementioned obstacles have played a role in stifling trials of various innovations in pediatric surgery, which might otherwise demonstrate superior efficacy and value in certain patient subgroups. Examples include the arterial switch performed for transposition of the great arteries; the Norwood procedure for hypoplastic left heart syndrome; and various in utero fetal procedures such as diaphragmatic hernia repair, relief of genitourinary obstruction, and hydrocephalus repair.[13]

## The Physician-Pediatric Patient Relationship

In the arena of pediatric surgery, a unique relationship exists among the patient, parent/guardian, and surgeon. The patient and his/her family must be placed at the center of all decision-making processes, and the surgeon must promote goodness and act with beneficence.[15] The ultimate success of this interaction depends on communication, choice, competence, compassion, continuity, and the absence of a conflict of interest.[16] The child's surgeon must uniquely behave in this discussion, with an emphasis on beneficence, as a source of information that should not impose on the infant and family his/her own ethical dogma, although a complete and open explanation is in order. Rather, the practice of beneficence offers to the family a spectrum of choices that even include the withdrawal or withholding of a therapy for the baby,[17] culminating in infant death.

Such a situation might be better understood when a putatively fatal pathophysiology afflicts the infant. Such complications represent a large spectrum: a genetic or chromosomal anomaly; the effect of profound prematurity; an acquired entity such as a midgut volvulus complicating the structural anomaly of malrotation of the colon that potentially could result in massive to complete small intestinal loss; a baby born with severe pulmonary hypoplasia complicating a congenital diaphragmatic hernia that during a course of neonatal extracorporeal membrane oxygenation therapy, the baby's physiologic parameters demonstrate clinical futility; and perhaps most frequent and devastating is the premature baby who acquires necrotizing enterocolitis, an infectious inflammatory enteritis that occurs in a compromised host (a profoundly premature neonate is the most susceptible), that results in sepsis along with focal to massive bowel death.[18] The intestinal necrosis is of major importance and magnitude because it is the most significant determinant of the eventual nutritional rehabilitation of the patient. Necrotizing enterocolitis is an entity with significant morbidity that eventually may be complicated by multisystem organ failure that includes the complication of cerebral hemorrhage. A devastated child might be afflicted with severe intestinal failure, complicating pulmonary insufficiency, all in the face of a moderate to severe mental/motor deficit.

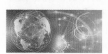

It is in the face of such reality that neonatal intensive care units are often the center of ethical debate, for example, the standard of practice when one examines the mortality following full support versus the mortalities when therapy is either withheld or limited and then withdrawn. One report stated 72% of deaths were in the not started or withdrawn category versus 28% of the mortality following full therapy.[19] The care effort is directed to salvage the good outcome baby no matter their associated health or family history instead of using limited intensive care unit resources on that neonate who will have an irreversible profound morbidity, producing a personal, family, and societal challenge to simply stay alive.[20] It is exactly this situation that might find the parents, family members, neonatal specialist, and pediatric surgeon to be not all on the same page in determining the continuation or withdrawal of support for such a critically ill neonate. Today the likely mechanism to handle such a complex challenge is to keep the patient and family at the center of the debate while simultaneously recruiting an independent third party to represent the baby's interest or ask for a formal ethics committee consultation to weigh in on the final disposition of the infant.

## Informed Consent

The origin of informed consent for surgery is often attributed to the 1767 case of Slater v. Baker and Stapleton, when 2 surgeons, in an effort to improve fracture alignment, refractured a patient's leg while changing a bandage. The patient in this case argued that the surgeons did not obtain permission to perform this procedure.[16] In the 1905 case of Mohr v. Williams, the principle of informed consent was again brought to light after a wrong-site ear surgery was performed. This case also helped specify that a surgeon could not perform an alternate operation without the patient's consent. The process of informed consent evolved throughout the 20th century as the incidence of malpractice claims steadily increased. In general, this process requires that competent persons or their designated surrogate has both a right and legal responsibility to decide which course of treatment is preferred.[17] In 1992, the bioethicist Ezekiel Emanuel defined the 4 required components of informed consent:

1. The provision of understandable information, including a description of the processes, risks, benefits, potential outcomes, and alternatives.
2. The physician's assessment of the patient's ability to understand the information.
3. The physician's assessment of the patient's competence to make an informed decision.
4. The ability of the patient to make such decisions free of coercion.[21]

Our society has granted legal and ethical rights to parents to make decisions for their children, and children are considered legally incompetent until the age of 18 or 21 years, depending on the state of residence. Exceptions to these rules include pregnancy and cases of sexually transmitted diseases, among others. The concept of a "mature minor," able to make his/her own end-of-life support decisions, has also been called into question. Furthermore, the principle of "patient assent" has been applied to adolescent populations. This is a process that requires the physician to involve the adolescent in the exchange of information about his/her health care and to assess whether he/she understands the details of the proposed diagnostic and treatment interventions. The ideal physician/patient/parent-guardian relationship in these scenarios involves a process of informed consent based on an open, thorough dialogue with understandable language that addresses the concerns of all involved parties.

In addition to outlining the appropriate components of informed consent, Emanuel also argued that a physician may persuade a patient to accept an alternate set of health values that would impact a treatment decision if it was in the patient's best interest. This practice of steering an individual toward a specific medical decision, often known as "nudging," may blur the line between paternalistic beneficence and respect for autonomy. The consenter must be cautious not to nudge to the point that the decision favors the surgeon and not the patient.[22]

## Exceptions to the Consent Process

In 1971, an infant with trisomy 21 and duodenal atresia was admitted to the neonatal intensive care unit at Johns Hopkins Hospital. The baby's parents requested that neither medical nor surgical procedure be performed that might facilitate feeding or prolong life. The Hopkins' team concurred with the family's decision and placed the baby in the nursery periphery with comfort care and minimal fluid and electrolyte intake; the baby survived for 20 days before succumbing to inanition. The child's hospital course was videotaped and became an important albeit controversial ethical teaching case.

A 1973 report in the *New England Journal of Medicine* by Duff and Campbell vetted the issue of neonatal nonsupport and withdrawal of care at the Yale New Haven Neonatal Intensive Care Unit, where 43 of 299 consecutive deaths (14%) were related to either support withdrawal or lack of initiation.[21,23] Although many of the deaths occurred in high-risk babies, this report was met with a moral outcry from many. Among the more vocal pro-life advocates from this contingent was Dr C. Everett Koop, the surgeon-in-chief at the Children's 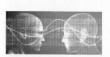 Hospital of Philadelphia. Koop's support of neonatal life was the subject of several publications, and he was dismayed by the Yale report.[24,25] A decade later, the federal government studied a series of "Baby Doe" cases to determine the appropriateness of treatment intervention. These cases included a baby with esophageal atresia, with tracheoesophageal fistula and trisomy 21, and a baby with an open thoracolumbar myelomeningocele. In both cases, the family denied permission for operative treatment; a very public debate followed. In 1984, when Dr Koop was then the surgeon general of the US Public Health Service, the Congress amended the Child Abuse Prevention and Treatment Act for hospitals receiving federal funding. The revision mandated that programs must be in place to respond to examples of medical neglect such that the withholding or withdrawing of surgical or medical therapy from neonates would not occur unless they were comatose or the likelihood of therapeutic success approached zero. This represented a heavy imposition on parents' rights to decide on life-saving treatment while curbing the treatment discretion of the hospital and its medical staff.[25,26]

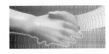

## Religion and the Physician Authority for Health Care Delivery

In the United States, most religious beliefs are congruent with standard physician recommendations and modern medical care. However, in cases of life and death, certain therapies may conflict with religious practice. A prime example of this is the need for a blood transfusion in the child of a Jehovah Witness parent or guardian. This belief stems from Genesis 9:3-4, which states, "Only flesh with its soul—its blood—you must not eat." Based on these biblical verses, a Jehovah's Witness will typically not accept the administration of whole blood, packed red blood cells, plasma, platelets, white blood cells, and even autotransfusion. Component factors such as albumin, clotting factors, and immune globulins may be individualized. Most hospitals will continue to administer these blood products to Jehovah Witness children if deemed medically necessary, often under a court order.[26]

## Disorders of Sexual Development (DSDs)

DSDs occur at an incidence of 1 in 4500 live births. The generic definition of a DSD is a disorder in which the chromosomal, gonadal, or anatomic sex is atypical.[28] The timing of the diagnosis is variable and may occur in the neonatal period, at the time of puberty onset, or even in adulthood. The scope of the deformity also varies from a normal external appearance to a visible anomaly involving multiple organs. The heterogeneity of these conditions can pose a challenge in counseling parents on how to raise and educate their children in the setting of a given DSD; in general, parents are best served by teaching in a manner that parallels the child's chronologic and conceptual growth. Milestones, then, become quite important—such as the time of a diagnosis, surgical procedure, or start of a major developmental stage. It is important to note that most of these children will be heterosexual. It is also important for the surgeon to recognize the value in delaying elective surgery until the child is mature enough to participate in the decision-making process.[27,28]

One significant controversy on the topic of DSDs is the surgical approach to the rare and complicated multiorgan cloacal exstrophy deformity. This condition consists of an omphalocele, open and separated bladder halves, a separated anterior pelvic rim, often a myelomeningocele, and bifid external genitalia. As recently as the 1980s, the general consensus was that surgery for this condition was too complex and the outcomes were too poor to warrant aggressive intervention in the neonatal period. Over time, a single-stage operation was adopted, which involved reconstruction of the external genitalia. It became evident that a bifid micropenis in a genetic male could not be reconstructed to provide normal function, and many of these babies were converted to a female phenotype in the neonatal period. However, these "female" babies often acted in a similar manner to their male counterparts with normal genitalia; indeed, it became evident that sex imprinting occurs very early in development.[28] A more contemporary approach to these children was soon devised—one in which gender is not surgically assigned until an age when both the child and his/her parents can participate in the decision-making process.

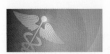

Another important issue for this patient population is medication compliance. This is often seen in the noncompliant peak of 6 to 8 years old and again in early to midadolescence—ages typically associated with strong peer group conformity. A further challenge involves conveying information to the child regarding his/her projected genital function, fertility, and sexual satisfaction. Children deserve an accurate assessment of their particular anatomy and physiology, and this discussion should be conducted at an age-appropriate time.

## Ethical Introduction of Pediatric Surgical Innovation

The introduction of surgical innovation presents a unique challenge to maintain ethical standards in the care of children. Fortunately, several strategies have been proposed to this end. Strasberg and Ludbrook identified "significant innovations" as those that require retraining and/or recredentialing of the provider, and they categorized these innovations as either diagnostic or therapeutic. They examined whether a healthy patient who was exposed to a given innovation would be placed at increased risk, and they defined a patient protection process that emphasized autonomy and the use of patient registries to enable the detection of adverse outcomes.[29]

A second strategy for the ethical introduction of surgical innovation might be termed the "surgical oversight paradigm."[30] Under this model, the chief of surgery assumes an authoritarian role and is responsible for issues such as credentialing and privileging the surgical staff, publishing the operating room schedule, leading the operating room team, being responsible for a surgical safety and quality outcomes audit, leading the morbidity and mortality conference, and taking part in additional professional and public reporting. Here, the surgeon fulfills a moral obligation to improve surgical quality.

A third strategy is represented by a statement from the Society of University Surgeons.[31] The Society has defined a formalized statement akin to the "surgical oversight paradigm" in which the surgeon-in-chief is assigned additional authority for supervising and monitoring surgical innovation. The Society has also rejected the Morbidity and Mortality Conference as a suitable forum in which to consider such proposals. The position statement also attempts to carefully distinguish whether the innovation represents a variation on a standard procedure (a minor modification that does not require specific disclosure), a unique departure from accepted standards (a modification or innovation of potential patient significance that does require disclosure), or rather an initial stage of what will become a formal research project (as an investigation designed to contribute to the generalizable knowledge). There is no patient age discrimination in this statement that suggests it would be easily applicable to the pediatric age group.

Still another method for introducing surgical innovation specifically in the pediatric age group was proposed by the American Academy of Pediatrics (AAP) in a policy statement published in 2017, although no data are available to test its efficacy as of the writing of this chapter.[32] This statement outlines a process that includes a history, physical examination, and detailed description of the proposed therapy. The risks and benefits are defined, and the projected efficacy of the application is compared with the expected outcomes from alternative therapies. In addition, the skills of the surgeon and entire treatment team are assessed, and any special preparatory work considered necessary or helpful to the novel technique is evaluated. The application and consent process includes any conflicts of interest, and the hospital's IRB is consulted if the innovation might be considered "research" under a formalized protocol. When the consenting surgeon appears to be affected by an "optimism bias," the presence of an objective third party during the consenting process may be helpful. Once the 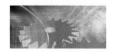 definition of innovative therapy is met, an oversight and adjudication process is required to assure patient protection, maintain the public's confidence and trust, and promote an innovation that would provide new and substantial benefits to patients. In the event of an urgent or emergent situation, the aforementioned process may be abandoned in favor of a rapid approval initiative that includes the patient and his/her family, the clinical team and other experts, and often a member of the hospital ethics team.

A fifth strategy approaches innovation as an institutional and not an IRB issue.[3] This paradigm represents a mixed integration, rather than a fusion, of research and innovation. It requires an open discussion and ongoing dialogue of ethical concerns, regulatory requirements, the informed consent process, documentation, the amount and definition of the source to guide resource provision and allocation, and a designated individual or group charged with providing project oversight.[33] Boundaries and approaches under this strategy must be set and defined. Strict oversight may be needed when the innovation produces a significant risk increase compared with alternative approaches, when the procedure is so novel that the risks and benefits remain uncertain, and when the procedure itself raises resource allocation concerns. If this "combination paradigm" becomes the care standard, an enhanced informed consent and peer review process will be mandatory.

As a real-life example, this latter strategy was adopted by the Department of Surgery at the Boston Children's Hospital from 1998 to 2002. Once established, it promoted accountability, improved provider and patient protection, supported innovation that led to ongoing clinical trials and the development of a patient registry, and promoted a culture of collaboration between the surgical and regulatory communities with a shared responsibility and decision-making process.[34] A simple methodology was used to introduce the new paradigm, which first required the investigator to submit a proposal (including a description and rationale for the procedure) to the surgeon-in-chief for review. Two faculty members who were not involved with the project were
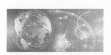
assigned as reviewers and submitted an opinion either supporting or rejecting the proposal. If the proposed innovation was accepted, a written informed consent document was developed with the help of the IRB and hospital legal staff and then submitted to the patient and/or parents/guardian. When appropriate, an assent document was included. Under this system, the IRB served as a record keeper, and the records were subject to periodic review. The investigator was required to limit application of the innovation to 3 patients before a formal IRB presentation became mandatory.

Although a successful outcome was achieved with this approach, several limitations and challenges were encountered. It quickly became evident that a change in culture favoring greater accountability for the surgeon-patient relationship was required. The concept that all components of this new system were mandatory and would be uniformly applied to all new surgical innovations, without exception, took time to establish. Perhaps the largest infraction was the repeated use of this interim oversight paradigm to bypass the IRB in favor of a peer-activated shortened approval process.

## Use of Medical Devices in Children

The use of medical or surgical devices in pediatric patients does not fall under the same guidelines and methods for approval and use as those applied to the adult population.[35] In adults, these devices fall under the Federal Food, Drug, and Cosmetic Act, and they are assigned to 1 of 3 risk categories. The higher the risk assessment of the procedure, the more rigorous the approval requirements for the use of the device will be. New high-risk devices typically require a Premarket Approval Application, which mandates that all outcomes data from animal and clinical trials (although not necessarily in the pediatric age group) have demonstrated efficacy, safety, and value. Devices for adults are approved for application by the Food and Drug Administration (FDA), whereas devices for children are developed and used under an "off-label" or "physician-directed" application. In pediatrics, when device use is proposed for rare conditions (less than 4000 cases annually), the FDA may opt to implement the Humanitarian Device Exemption when data demonstrate "reasonable safety and probable benefit."[36] The law then requires that these cases be reviewed and approved by the IRB. Similarly, the frequent application of adult devices to the pediatric age group falls under the "off-label and physician-directed" rubric. Such off-label use is legal and is not regulated by the FDA, which views these cases as simply the practice of medicine.[37] The recent policy statement from the AAP, written largely by members of its surgical section, strongly supports this system.[32] In 2007, the AAP also helped pass the Pediatric Medical Device Safety and Improvement Act, which provided necessary regulatory reforms for device approval, incentives and funding for new device development, and advocacy efforts to encourage public and private health care payers to approve payments for such off-label uses. Finally, in 2009, the FDA Office of Orphan Products formed a Pediatric Device Consortia Grant to fund pediatric device development. This program has seen steady growth and currently has 5 consortia focused specifically on this goal.

## Conclusion

We have summarized a brief overview of surgical ethics as applied to the newborn and young child. We have specifically not focused this discussion on any number of details for a single subject, but rather we have attempted to describe the scope of "pediatric surgical" ethics and the unique challenges that are a result of dealing with a prepubertal constituency. For those readers interested in working or even serving in this field, it goes without saying that both the challenges and rewards are great.

## References

1. Britannica.com.
2. McGrath MH, Risucci DA, Schwab A. *Ethical Issues in Clinical Surgery: For Residents.* Chicago, IL: American College of Surgeons; 2007.
3. Krummel T, Ziegler M. IPEG panel on challenges of medical innovation: introduction. *J Laparoendosc Adv Surg Tech A.* 2006;16:634–638.
4. Kantarjian H, Steensma D. Relevance of the Hippocratic Oath in the 21st century. *ASCO Post.* 2014.
5. Howell J, Ayanian J. Ernest Codman and the end result system: a pioneer of health outcomes revisited. *J Health Serv Res Policy.* 2016;2:274–277.
6. Dervishes O, Wright K, Saber A, Pappas P. Ernest Codman and the end-result system. *Am Surg.* 2015;81:12–15.

7. Khuri S. The NSQIP: a new frontier in surgery. *Surgery.* 2005;138:837–843.
8. Raval M, Dillon P, Bruny J, et al. Pediatric American College of Surgeons National Surgical Quality Improvement Program: feasibility of a novel prospective assessment of surgical outcomes. *J Pediatr Surg.* 2011;46:115–121.
9. Wendler D, Rid A. In defense of a social value requirement for clinical research. *Bioethics.* 2017;31:77–86.
10. Beecher H. Ethics and clinical research. *N Engl J Med.* 1966;274:1354–1360.
11. Protection of human subjects; Belmont Report: notice of report for public comment. *Fed Regist.* 1979;44:23191–23197.
12. Peregrine T. Emerging trends in lifelong learning: new directions for ACS surgical education programs. *Bull ACS.* 2013;98:9–17.
13. Leclercq W, Keslors B, Schettinga M, et al. A review of surgical informed consent: past, present and future. A quest to help patients make better decisions. *World J Surg.* 2010;34:1406–1415.
14. Reitsma A, Moreno J. Ethics of innovative surgery: US surgeons' definitions, knowledge, and attitudes. *J Am Coll Surg.* 2005;200:103–110.
15. Angelos P. The ethics of introducing new surgical technology into clinical practice. *JAMA Surg.* 2016;151:405–406.
16. Hazebrock F, Tibboel D, Wijnen R. Ethical aspects of care in the newborn surgical patient. *Semin Pediatr Surg.* 2014;23:309–313.
17. Axelrod D, Goold S. Maintaining trust in the surgeon patient relationship: challenges for the new millennium. *Arch Surg.* 2000;135:55–61.
18. Singh J, Lantos J, Meadow W. End-of-life after birth: death and dying in a neonatal intensive care unit. *Pediatrics.* 2004;114:1620–1626.
19. Barton L, Hodgman JE. The contribution of withholding or withdrawing care to newborn mortality. *Pediatrics.* 2005;116:1487–1491.
20. Petty JK, Ziegler MM. Operative strategies for necrotizing enterocolitis: the prevention and treatment of short-bowel syndrome. *Semin Pediatr Surg.* 2005;14:191–198.
21. Emanuel E, Emanuel L. Four models of the physician-patient relationship. *JAMA.* 1992;267:2221–2226.
22. Cohen S. Nudging and informed consent. *Am J Bioeth.* 2013;13:3–11.
23. Duff R, Campbell A. Moral and ethical dilemmas in the special-care nursery. *N Engl J Med.* 1973:289–290.
24. Koop CE. *The Slide to Auschwitz.* Deerfield, NJ: IA Palmer; 1976.
25. Schaeffer F, Koop CE. *Whatever Happened to the Human Race.* Old Tappan, NJ: Fleming H. Revell Company; 1979.
26. Caniano D. Ethical considerations in pediatric surgery. In: Ziegler M, Azizkahn R, Weber T, vonAllmen D. eds. *Operative Pediatric Surgery.* New York: McGraw Hill; 2014:16–21.
27. Fallat M, Hertweek P, Ralston S. Surgical and ethical challenges in the disorders of sexual development. *Adv Pediatr.* 2012;59:283–302.
28. Howell C, Caldamone A, Snyder H, et al. Optimal management of cloacal exstrophy. *J Pediatr Surg.* 1983;18:365–369.
29. Strasberg S, Ludbrook P. Who overseas innovative practice? Is there a structure that meets the monitoring needs of new techniques. *J Am Coll Surg.* 2003;196:938–948.
30. McKneally MF, Daar AS. Introducing new technologies: protecting subjects of surgical innovative research. *World J Surg.* 2003;27:930–934.
31. Biffl W, Spain D, Reitsma A, et al. Responsible development and application of surgical innovation: a position statement of the Society of University Surgeons. *J Am Coll Surg.* 2008;206:1204–1209.

32. Section on Surgery, American Academy of Pediatrics. Responsible innovation in children's surgical care, Policy Statement. *Pediatrics.* 2017;139:87–94.
33. Krummel TM, Azizkhzn R, Holcomb GW, et al. IPEG panel on challenges of medical innovation: case one. *J Laparoendosc Adv Surg Tech A.* 2007;17:64–66.
34. Javid P, Kim HB, Duggan C, Jaksic T. Serial transverse enteroplasty is associated with successful short-term outcomes in infants with short bowel syndrome. *J Pediatr Surg.* 2005;40:1019–1023.
35. Section on Cardiology and Cardiac Surgery, Section on Orthopedics, American Academy of Pediatrics. Off-label use of medical devices in children, Policy Statement. *Pediatrics.* 2017;139:83–86.
36. Available from: www.fda.gov/Forindustry/DevelopingproductsforrareDiseases Conditions/DesignatingHumanitarianUseDevicesHUDS/Legislation RelatingtoHUDsHDEs/ucm283517.htm.
37. Frattarelli D, Galinkin J, Green T, et al. American Academy of Pediatrics Committee on Drugs. Off-label use of drugs in children. *Pediatrics.* 2014;133:563–567.

# 16

# Clinical Research: Conflict of Personal and Systemic Ethics

Robert H. Bartlett, MD

PROLOGUE ▶ Several chapters in this book focus on the dilemma of agency versus utilitarianism. The standard phraseology of utilitarianism is "the greatest good for the greatest number." The notion of agency avers that the surgeon is bound to the individual patient, to act only and always in the patient's best interest and as he/she would have chosen.

Dr Bartlett points out, correctly I believe, that this conflict is sharply focused in the design of clinical trials in which the end point is death. The undertaking of such clinical trials is good "for the greatest number" but so was, potentially at least, the knowledge gained at Tuscaloosa regarding syphilis. Moreover, there may exist a conflict within the surgeon regarding the question of to whom the fruits of his/her beneficence is owed.

The ancient and venerable discipline of surgery has almost always been deeply committed to the individual patient with whom the covenant has been made. The relatively new doctrine of utilitarianism, now widely subscribed to, presents many conflicts to the surgeon's adherence to the ancient ethics of the craft, and as is so frequently the case the surgeon is left to his/her own inner resources to deal with this conflict. The tending to inner strengths continues to be imperative to the surgeon's resilience.

Dr Bartlett is a renaissance man, who has concerned himself with these issues throughout his long career as a clinical innovator, a scientific investigator, and a consummate surgeon. He weighs carefully the arguments in that agenda and offers a solution that minimizes the conflict of interest in conducting clinical research. Dr Bartlett's long  participation in clinical research concerning the efficacy of extracorporeal membrane oxygenation (ECMO) and his thoughtful compassion for patients make his discussion to be of great value.

Dr Robert H. Bartlett is professor emeritus of surgery at the University of Michigan Medical School.

Surgeons are often involved in clinical research to determine if one operation, drug, device, or other intervention is better than another. A common research question is whether a new approach is better than the current standard of care. Surgeons may be the focal point of the investigation (minimally invasive vs open colectomy) or a participant (antibiotic A is better than antibiotic B) or simply using trial data in their practice (the timing of resuscitation measures in shock).

The ethical issues are both systemic and personal. The systemic ethical issues revolve around the question: How can we compare treatment A with treatment B when some patients will inevitably be assigned to what proves to be the inferior treatment? The answer to this question hinges on the notion of "equipoise." We all assume that we do clinical trials only when we do not know if treatment A is better than treatment B. "We" means the overall clinical community. Comparing 2 methods of repairing a direct inguinal hernia is a good example. We design trials to define entry criteria, details of the operation, side effects, and endpoints. We can explain the study to patients, assign a patient to one approach or the other, and interpret the results. Clinical equipoise exists as a presupposition.

The personal ethical issues are more difficult. The individual investigator may perceive clinical equipoise but often does not have personal equipoise. An investigator comparing new versus conventional care must have a personal opinion that the new treatment will be better, otherwise why study it? The only way that studies of new approaches can be done is that clinical equipoise trumps personal equipoise.

Clinical trials of life support in acute fatal illness in which the end point is death bring all these ethical and study design issues into sharp focus. The problem is the control group. How can we assign patients to a control group that will ultimately result in death? And is there a better way to conduct the research that does not arbitrarily assign patients to a treatment that will ultimately have the worse outcome? A classic example is the use of ECMO in the treatment of severe respiratory failure. There have been 10 clinical trials comparing ECMO support to a conventional care group. This discussion is a recapitulation and review of those trials published in the *Journal of Intensive Care Medicine.*[1]

There have been 10 published clinical trials of ECMO in acute, potentially fatal, respiratory failure in which treated patients were compared with controls receiving conventional care.[2–12] The end point of these trials was death. The study designs of these trials were reviewed with particular attention to logistics, ethics, consent, statistical analysis, and the ultimate value of the trial to medical practice.

There are 5 prospective randomized controlled trials (RCTs),[2–6] 3 in adult respiratory failure and 2 in neonatal respiratory failure. There are

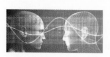

2 prospective RCTs using adaptive designs,[7,8] both in neonatal respiratory failure. There is 1 sequential controlled trial in neonatal respiratory failure.[9,10] There are 2 matched-pair controlled trials, 1 in pediatric respiratory failure[11] and 1 in adult respiratory failure caused by H1N1 influenza virus.[12] The first 2 prospective randomized trials in adult respiratory failure were conducted decades ago.[2,3] Neither of these trials showed a difference between ECMO and the control groups. The next 8 trials all showed a major survival benefit to ECMO compared with conventional care controls.

## Study Design and Ethical Considerations

The key question posed by the analysis of these studies is as follows: Is there a better way to study life support than a prospective controlled randomized design? RCTs are considered to be the gold standard, but in this case the end point is death, so the ethical issues are critical.

Clinical research on life support techniques in acute fatal illness poses unique problems for the investigator. These problems are personalized when the research investigator is also a treating physician. The physicians are responsible for their patients primarily and for doing clinical research secondarily. It is commonly said that the investigators in controlled clinical trials should be neutral regarding the intervention—that there is no bias that one treatment or the other might be better (equipoise). However, the investigators in these trials, at least this investigator, knew that ECMO could sustain life in the absence of any lung function and were strongly biased toward the belief that survival with the technology would be better than dying without it. The investigators realized that controlled comparative studies were necessary, so the studies were conducted with good scientific intent and methodology but without neutrality on the part of the investigators. Does the axiom of beneficence apply to an individual patient more than the population? Each investigator had to answer this question for each patient.

Is equipoise an important requirement for a clinical trial? In many simple trials, the physician-investigator can honestly claim the lack of bias and personal equipoise.[13] Even if he/she believes that treatment A will be better than treatment B, the greater good is served by the trial's clinical equipoise.[14] The current view is that clinical equipoise predominates. Personal bias is inevitable in any prospective controlled trial, but participating in a trial is believed to be ethical if the practicing community believes the question requires a clinical trial.[14] What does this mean? Johnson reported that a randomized trial is unethical if more than 70% of the practicing community considers the question answered.[15] Avins proposed some alternative designs intended to make randomized trials more fair and more ethical, if ethical dilemmas can be quantitated.[16] All of this discussion is amplified in trials of life support in acute fatal illness.[17] After the first 2 poorly designed trials of ECMO, the investigators in the ECMO trials dealt with the ethical dilemma by using adaptive designs or separating the conventional caregiver from the ECMO center caregiver. These approaches minimized but did not eliminate the ethical dilemma of the physician-investigator.

The neonatal ECMO trials have generated extensive discussion about ethics and clinical research, probably because the ethical, emotional, and scientific issues are magnified in studies in newborn infants. Ethicists and pediatricians John Lantos, MD, and Joel Frader, MD, examined all the issues based on the 2 adaptive design trials.[18] They identified 6 features that made the neonatal ECMO trials particularly difficult. They concluded that "the investigators did as well as they could, given the complexity of the clinical and ethical issues." They observed that neonatal ECMO had become the standard of care by 1990, based partly on the trials and partly on common sense in neonatal practice. Others disagreed, mostly critical of the adaptive study designs rather than the ethics involved.[19–22] In 1997, Malcontent (a pseudonym) argued that only a prospective randomized trial could answer the scientific question.[23] He/she implied that the practice of ECMO, routine in the United States by that time, was motivated by the desire of physicians to make money. What is more unethical, the postulate or the unsubstantiated accusation? Malcontent cited the recent randomized trial of neonatal ECMO conducted in the United Kingdom, claiming that the ethical dilemma of assigning a patient to the control group was justified by the greater good of more scientific proof. In an invited response, Lantos argued 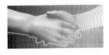 that the UK randomized trial was unethical because the adaptive trials and worldwide experience showed a clear benefit to ECMO when the study was conducted in 1993 to 1995.[24] Addressing both the scientific and the ethical issues, Lantos wrote "there were 24 excess deaths in the conventional arm. I'm not sure how I would feel if I was one of the parents whose baby received conventional care and died."

Using the adaptive neonatal ECMO trials as an example, V. Mike, PhD, a biostatistician from Cornell, proposed a concept she called "ethics of evidence."[25] This concept is an exposition of the dilemma of balancing the best evidence from clinical trials against the inevitable uncertainty of clinical medicine. Mike pointed out that the adaptive design trials, although statistically valid, did not convince most practitioners because they were not accustomed to unique study designs. She speculated on how neonatal ECMO should have been studied in early randomized trials and how clinicians should have better communication and understanding with statisticians. The best expert to address these issues, she asserted, would be a clinician-statistician-ethicist.

An eloquent and thoughtful discussion of clinical trials in acute fatal illness was published by Truog, MD, in 1992.[26] This discourse was based on the 2 randomized adaptive design trials of ECMO in neonatal respiratory failure. He had a unique perspective on the issues because he was a critical care pediatrician, an ethicist, and a clinical researcher and he had firsthand experience with the trials. His description of the problems and his analysis of the solutions hold true today, 22 years and 6 more ECMO clinical trials later. His comments specifically addressed clinical trials of life support in acute fatal illness. In that context, Truog pointed out that (1) there is a deep and fundamental 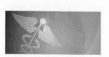 conflict in the role of physician-investigator because as a physician the individual is responsible for his/her patients but as an investigator the individual is responsible for the quality of the research; (2) although clinical equipoise provides a theoretical justification for the ethics of the trial design, it does not resolve the psychological angst of the physician-investigator, entailed in withholding treatments that this individual physician believes to be lifesaving; and (3) prospective randomized trials of potentially life-sustaining therapies are therefore always problematic, and alternatives should be strongly considered. He concluded that "the ideal study design would both preserve the essence of the traditional patient-physician relationship and provide results that are reflective of up-to-date modifications in both experimental and standard therapies. For these reasons, an RCT would fail on both counts."

Are RCTs the gold standard? In life support trials? In any clinical trials? Vincent argued that randomized trials should be abandoned in intensive care.[27] Three different studies examined the value of observational trials compared with RCTs. All showed essentially no difference between the outcomes of these study designs.[28-30] Freeman et al identified 3 RCTs in which the mortality was much higher in the treatment group, a fact that could have been identified by observational studies before patients were arbitrarily assigned to a fatal treatment.[31] A poorly designed RCT can impede clinical research and practice for decades (eg, as demonstrated by the first 2 ECMO trials). Conversely, Albert[32] argued that randomized trials may provide different conclusions than observational trials. He assumed that the conclusions of the randomized trials in his examples were correct and those of the observational trials were not. Based on personal experience with some of these examples, I do not agree with his premise. However, we interpret his analysis: the observational trials he cites were comparing a cohort of patients managed with treatment A with that of patients managed with treatment B, with no attempt to compare similar patients as in a sequential study or a matched-pair design. It is this controversy that has led both clinicians[27] and ethicists[15] to seek alternatives to RCT in critical care.[33]

If RCTs are untenable, if not unethical in acute fatal illness, there are 2 alternatives: adaptive designs and matching designs. Nonrandomized adaptive designs are well suited to simple questions in which the end point is a clinical result and there is no need to blind the randomization.[34] Blinded randomization is necessary in trials of life support. The 2 ECMO trials using adaptive designs required that the treating physicians did not know the assignment of treatment before entering the patient in the trial. This was called "randomized play-the-winner" rule. In retrospect, this was an unfortunate choice of words implying that chance was a major part of the statistical design. Using the randomized play-the-winner or similar technique for these studies of life support in acute fatal illness minimized but by no means eliminated the ethical dilemma of the investigators. These studies were praised by statisticians for addressing the ethical and logistical dilemmas while still reaching statistical significance based on a small number of patients.[35] However, because of the disparity between the numbers in the treatment and control groups, clinicians simply did not believe these trials.[19-22] These 2 trials are the only trials of randomized adaptive designs in acute fatal illness. Although both were statistically and clinically successful,[36] it is unlikely that any further randomized adaptive design trials will be undertaken in life support trials because, as Mike described,[23] clinicians have been taught that RCTs are the gold standard. However, the dilemma is very well addressed by matching designs.

Of the ECMO trials, 3 used matching designs. The sequential Netherlands trial of neonatal ECMO compared 3 cohorts of patients based on diagnosis. Individual patients were not matched. Both the pediatric study by Green and the H1N1 study by Noah[12] matched individual ECMO patients to patients in the contemporary database, then compared the outcome between the 2 groups. In the study by Green, a preliminary regression analysis identified ECMO as a significant factor in outcome,[37] then the ECMO patients were individually matched to similar patients in the database and the 2 groups were compared. In the study by Noah, referral to an ECMO center was the primary variable, and patients were matched to patients from a non-ECMO center. Three methods of matching were used and compared individual matching,[38] propensity score matching,[39] and "GenMatch," which combines both.[40] Each method produced essentially the same results. A landmark example of a matched-pair design related to ECMO was the Food and Drug Administration (FDA)-qualifying trial of the Berlin Heart pediatric ventricular assist device.[41] The Berlin Heart company wanted to do a FDA-qualifying trial to sell their device to pediatric patients with profound heart failure leading to heart transplant. Two hundred cases had already been

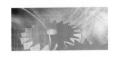

conducted as Investigational Device Exemption and most survived. Assigning children to a control group where all would die seemed unethical, but the FDA required data demonstrating efficacy. In an unprecedented move, the FDA suggested conducting a matched-pair trial, comparing study patients with similar patients in the Extracorporeal Life Support Organization database of children with heart failure managed with ECMO bridging to heart transplant. The study was conducted in 48 patients, matched 1:2 to patients in the Extracorporeal Life Support Organization database. The successful recovery rate was 90% with the Berlin Heart compared with 70% with ECMO alone. The device was approved by FDA. This matched-pair approach will serve as the mechanism for qualifying all ventricular assist devices in the Intermacs database.[42]

## Consent

Consent policies evolved during the 40 years were covered in this review. In the early trials, detailed informed consent was sought and given for the ECMO group but not for conventional care. This was based on the idea that the patient has already given consent for conventional treatment and further consent for the control arm is not necessary.[43] Discussion of this topic, stimulated in part by the ECMO studies, led to the policy that consent should be sought and given for any clinical trial itself, including the treatment and data collection in both arms.[44] This was the policy for the UK randomized trials. In those trials, randomization to ECMO required transport to an ECMO center, compared with staying in the home intensive care unit. Few families refused consent. The matched-pair trials were not subject to consent based on the argument that consent is not required for the analysis of deidentified data.

## Economics

Of these studies, 4 were not only outcome but also cost-benefit studies. The 2 randomized trials in the United Kingdom were supported by the National Health Service based on the justification that the cost per survivor could be 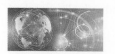 determined, and the cost could be converted to quality-adjusted life-years. The study of early versus late ECMO was designed to determine the outcome and cost of 2 starting points for ECMO. The Netherlands sequential trial included the determination of cost per survivor, which was an important factor in deciding whether ECMO would be reimbursed by the national health system.

## Best Design for Studies of Life Support

From the review of these 10 studies, we conclude that the best study design is a matched-pair approach. The goals of a life support study are simple; is survival significantly better compared with conventional care, and what is the cost in time, effort, and money? With a matched-pair design, these questions can be answered with the smallest number of cases, with the best comparison of patients in the 2 groups, at the least expense. The logistical and ethical issues are minimal. The control group can be drawn from a large number of cases managed by the best conventional care. These cases can be in the study center only or a larger database if optimal conventional care is assumed and documented. The variations in care between the groups can be included in the matching categories. There are several methods of matching the patient groups, from sequential analysis, as in the Netherlands trial, to developing a detailed propensity score. The study can be done retrospectively or prospectively. Matching can be done 1:1 or more. The Netherlands study in which all were neonates matched only for diagnosis. The pediatric study began with a large database and then used logistic regression to identify the significant variables. The ECMO patients could then be matched to control patients with these categories. The H1N1 study had many categories of matching, so that 5 of the ECMO patients could not be matched from the large database.

## Conclusions From the Analysis of the ECMO Trials

Clinical research to evaluate the effectiveness of life support systems in acute fatal illness has unique problems of logistics and ethics and consent. There have been 10 prospective comparative trials of ECMO in acute fatal respiratory failure, using different study designs. The matched-pair method is the best study design for evaluation of life support systems in acute fatal illness.

## Conclusions

Surgeons often have a role in clinical research; therefore, they must understand the types of study designs and the logistical and ethical issues involved with clinical research (human experimentation). The ECMO studies are good examples because the practical and ethical issues are brought into sharp focus. Each surgeon investigator must decide if clinical equipoise overrides personal equipoise to ethically participate.

## References

1. Bartlett RH. Clinical research in acute fatal illness: lessons from extracorporeal membrane oxygenation. *J Intensive Care Med.* 2016;31:456–465.
2. Zapol WM, Snider MT, Hill JD, et al. Extracorporeal membrane oxygenation in severe acute respiratory failure: a randomized prospective study. *JAMA.* 1979;242:2193–2196.
3. Morris AH, Wallace CJ, Menlove RL, et al. Randomized clinical trial of pressure-controlled inverse ratio ventilation and extracorporeal $CO_2$ removal for adult respiratory distress syndrome. *Am J Respir Crit Care Med.* 1994;149:295–305.
4. UK Collaborative EMCO Trial Group. UK collaborative randomized trial of neonatal extracorporeal membrane oxygenation. *Lancet.* 1996;348:75–82.

5. Peek GJ, Mugford M, Tiruvoipati R, et al. Efficacy and economic assessment of conventional ventilatory support versus extracorporeal membrane oxygenation for severe adult respiratory failure (CESAR): a multicentre randomized controlled trial. *Lancet.* 2009;374:1351–1363.

6. Schumacher RE, Roloff DW, Chapman R, Snedecor S, Bartlett RH. Extracorporeal membrane oxygenation in term newborns. A prospective cost-analysis. *ASAIO J.* 1993;39:873–879.

7. Bartlett RH, Roloff DW, Cornell RG, Andrews AF, Dillon PW, Zwischenberger JB. Extracorporeal circulation in neonatal respiratory failure: a prospective randomized study. *Pediatrics.* 1985;76:479–487.

8. O'Rourke PP, Crone RK, Vacanti JP, et al. Extracorporeal membrane oxygenation and conventional medical therapy in neonates with persistent pulmonary hypertension of the newborn: a prospective randomized study. *Pediatrics.* 1989;84:957–963.

9. Geven WA. Comparative trial of ECMO for neonatal respiratory failure in The Netherlands. *Presented to Extracorporeal Life Support Organization.* Dearborn, Michigan; 1995.

10. Poley MJ. *Cost-Effectiveness of Neonatal Surgery: A Matter of Balance* [Thesis]. Rotterdam: Erasmus University. Chapter 5; 2005.

11. Green TP, Timmons OD, Fackler JC, Moler FW, Thompson AE, Sweeney MF. The impact of extracorporeal membrane oxygenation on survival in pediatric patients with acute respiratory failure. Pediatric Critical Care Study Group. *Crit Care Med.* 1996;24:323–329.

12. Noah MA, Peek GJ, Finney SJ, et al. Referral to an extracorporeal membrane oxygenation center and mortality among patients with severe 2009 influenza A (H1N1). *JAMA.* 2011;306:1659–1668.

13. Shafer A. The ethics of the randomized controlled trial. *N Engl J Med.* 1982;307:719–724.

14. Freedman B. Equipoise and the ethics of clinical research. *N Engl J Med.* 1987;317:141–145.

15. Johnson N, Liliford RJ, Brazier W. At what level of collective equipoise does a clinical trial become ethical? *J Med Ethics.* 1991;17:30–34.

16. Avins AL. Can unequal be more fair? Ethics, subject allocation, and randomized clinical trials. *J Med Ethics.* 1998;24:401–408.

17. Gelfand S. Clinical equipoise: actual or hypothetical disagreement? *J Med Philos.* 2013;38:590–604.

18. Lantos JD, Frader J. Extracorporeal membrane oxygenation and the ethics of clinical research in pediatrics. *N Engl J Med.* 1990;323:409–413.

19. Elliott SJ. Neonatal extracorporeal membrane oxygenation: how not to assess novel technologies. *Lancet.* 1991;337:476–478.

20. Editorial. Persistent fetal circulation and extracorporeal membrane oxygenation. *Lancet.* 2;1988:1289–1291.

21. Greenough A, Emery E. ECMO and outcome of mechanical ventilation in infants of birthweight over 2 kg. *Lancet.* 1990;336:760.

22. Soll RF. Neonatal extracorporeal membrane oxygenation-bridging technique. *Lancet.* 1996;348:70–71.

23. Malcontent. Fumes from the spleen. *Paediatr Perinat Epidemiol.* 1997;11:260–264.

24. Lantos JD. Was the UK Collaborative ECMO trial ethical? *Paediatr Perinat Epidemiol.* 1997;11:264–268.

25. Mike V, Krauss AN, Ross GS. Neonatal extracorporeal membrane oxygenation (ECMO): clinical trials and the ethics of evidence. *J Med Ethics.* 1993;19:212–218.
26. Truog RD. Randomized controlled trials: lessons from ECMO. *Clin Res.* 1992;40:519–527.
27. Vincent JL. We should abandon randomized controlled trials in the intensive care unit. *Crit Care Med.* 2010;38:S534–S538.
28. Benson K, Hartz AJ. A comparison of observational studies and randomized controlled trials. *N Engl J Med.* 2000;342:1878–1886.
29. Ioannidis JPA, Haidich AB, Pappa M, et al. Comparison of evidence of treatment effects in randomized and nonrandomized studies. *JAMA.* 2001;286:821–830.
30. Concato J, Shah N, Horwitz RI. Randomized, controlled trials, observational studies, and the hierarchy of research designs. *N Engl J Med.* 2000;342:1887–1909.
31. Freeman BD, Danner RL, Banks SM, Natanson C. Safeguarding patients in clinical trials with high mortality rates. *Am J Respir Crit Care Med.* 2001;164:190–192.
32. Albert RK. "Lies, damned lies…" and observational studies in comparative effectiveness research. *Crit Care Med.* 2013;187:1173–1177.
33. Miller FG, Joffe S. Equipoise and the dilemma of randomized clinical trials. *N Engl J Med.* 2011;364:476–480.
34. Chow SC, Chang M. Adaptive design methods in clinical trials—a review. *Orphanet J Rare Dis.* 2008;3:11.
35. Royall RM. Ethics and statistics in randomized clinical trials. *Stat Sci.* 1991;6:52–88.
36. Chevret S. Bayesian adaptive clinical trials: a dream for statisticians only? *Stat Med.* 2012;31:1002–1013.
37. Timmons OD, Dean JM, Vernon DD. Mortality rates and prognostic variables in children with adult respiratory distress syndrome. *J Pediatr.* 1991;119:896–899.
38. Diamond A, Sekhon JS. Genetic matching for estimating causal effects: a general multivariate matching method for achieving balance in observational studies. *Rev Econ Stat.* 2013;95:932–945.
39. Sekhon JS. Matching: multivariate and propensity score matching with automated balance search. *J Stat Softw.* 2011;42:1–52.
40. Glance LJ, Osler TM, Mukamel DB, Dick AW. Use of a matching algorithm to evaluate hospital coronary artery bypass grafting performance as an alternative to conventional risk adjustment. *Med Care.* 2007;45:292–299.
41. Fraser CD, Jaquiss RD, Rosenthal DN, et al. Prospective trial of a pediatric ventricular assist device. *N Engl J Med.* 2012;367:532–541.
42. Kirklin JK, Naftel DC, Kormos RL, et al. Fifth INTERMACS annual report: risk factors analysis from more than 6,000 mechanical circulatory support patients. *J Heart Lung Transplant.* 2013;32:141–156.
43. Zelen M. A new design for randomized clinical trials. *N Engl J Med.* 1979;300:1242–1245.
44. Zelen M. Randomized consent designs for clinical trials: an update. *Stat Med.* 1990;9:645–665.

# 17 Ethical Considerations on the Trauma Service

Benjamin N. Jacobs, PhD, MD

PROLOGUE ▶ The world's oldest surgical text, the Edwin Smith Papyrus, is of Egyptian origin and dates from about 1600 BC, although it is thought to be a copy of texts perhaps as old as the pyramids. It is a case-oriented textbook of trauma, containing meticulous descriptions of 48 instances of wounds or fractures. Perhaps even more important is that the Smith Papyrus rests on an algorithm that defines alternative decisions, which declare its presupposition to be a freedom of choice and an ethical import to every surgical decision.

The critical decision schema of the Edwin Smith Papyrus, after a clinical description, confronts the surgeon with a triage algorithm of 3 choices: to treat the patient with an expectation of success; to treat the patient even though the outcome is doubtful; and, third, to declare the words "an ailment not to be treated."

The distinction between the first 2 categories emphasizes the power of the expectations of the patient and his/her family and friends. The frank admission of futility implicit in the third pathway, given as it was in about one-half of the cases, has been the subject of speculation as to its motives. Many discussants of the Edwin Smith Papyrus have suggested that the third pathway served the purpose of avoiding injury to the surgeon's reputation. Others, and I am among them, speculate that the admission of futility constitutes the first stirrings of compassion for the dying. The notion recurs among the writers

122

of the Hippocratic Corpus in stressing that one should not inflict harm. The third pathway in the algorithm suggests the notion of a "good death." Trauma and burn surgery often, still today, confronts the surgeon with similar moral choices.

Dr Benjamin N. Jacobs is a fifth-year resident in surgery at the University of Michigan Medical School with an interest in trauma and burn surgery, as well as vascular surgery.

## Introduction

Trauma remains one of the leading causes of mortality in the United States, particularly in the elderly and young people, and the trauma bay is an environment fraught with intensity, emotion, and, particularly, high stakes. As with any high-stakes environment, the possibility for complex ethical questions emerges. Inevitably, after a month on the Trauma Service, the house officer will be able to recollect a number of instances where, returning home in the morning for rest, he/she finds himself/herself ruminating whether the right choice had been made. All practitioners of medicine and, perhaps, with a little hubris, surgeons more than most have an overwhelming desire to preserve life. Indeed, it is this 2-fold goal, the preservation of life and the mitigation of suffering, that drives all members of the surgical profession. In certain circumstances, we find these 2 goals at opposition with one another. Perhaps this is nowhere more true than in the trauma bay.

Thankfully, the *clinical* questions in trauma are often relatively straightforward. Guided by the algorithms of the American College of Surgeons Advanced Trauma Life Support and by the "worst things first" or "life, limb, looks" philosophy—and driven by the importance of acting swiftly in a hemorrhaging patient—many complex clinical and ethical questions can be answered by the simple rejoinder: "I did what I thought best, based on the information we had, and I didn't have time to get any more."

Perhaps it is incorrect to say that the stakes on the Trauma Service are any higher than on, say, the Transplant or Vascular Surgery services. It may be more accurate to say the stakes are different. It is from this difference that many of the ethical questions unique to trauma arise. This is because, in the trauma bay, one, more often than not, sees young, healthy patients—no chronic renal insufficiency, no congestive heart failure—who have every reason to expect long years of continued life when they leave our care.

Consequently, we must ask the question: In what state are we leaving them? May an intervention to preserve life ultimately harm the individual who must live that life? The surgeon has taken an oath to "do no harm"—the principle of non-maleficence—and must ask of every patient and every action whether he/she is harming or helping. We must not simply characterize

our enemy as death alone but must understand that suffering takes many forms. It is this difficulty that makes the stakes in the trauma bay much different than we may find on other services. To quote Shakespeare's *Hamlet*:

> *But that the dread of something after death,*
> *The undiscovered country, from whose bourn*
> *No traveller returns, puzzles the will,*
> *And makes us rather bear those ills we have*
> *Than fly to others that we know not of?*
> *Thus conscience does make cowards of us all*

In the surgeon's case we might modify this: the dread of something *worse* than death.

Do we have the right to decide what is worse than death? Are we able to evaluate such things? These are the questions to be addressed in the following chapter. Hopefully, we will come to at least a few 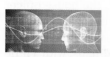 firm conclusions. But like most ethics books, and most chapters in them, we will raise more questions than we can provide answers for. We consequently challenge the reader simply to read, and to reflect, and to dedicate his/her life in surgery to both, with equal ferocity.

## Consent in the Trauma Bay

Most house officers have encountered this situation: a patient arrives in the trauma bay, the seat-belted driver and sole victim of a motor vehicle collision. Proceeding with the primary survey, the patient is found to have a depressed Glasgow Coma Scale and a positive FAST examination. In nearly all situations like this one, the clinical choice is clear: life-saving maneuvers of some kind must be initiated. However, there is no way to obtain consent from the patient for his/her operation.

As was discussed in prior chapters, the pillars of medical ethics—autonomy, nonmaleficence, and beneficence—arose from the reaction of the medical and scientific communities to the atrocities of the early and middle parts of the 20th century. The concept of autonomy tells us that a patient must be allowed to decide the course that is best for him/her, and it is on this concept that informed consent is founded. Informed consent is separate from and more complex than a patient simply saying "sure, okay" to an operation. The requirements of informed consent are that the patient must have (1) the capacity to decide and understand, (2) knowledge and understanding of the risks and benefits of the treatment in question, and (3) been given the opportunity to weigh these risks and benefits and to draw his/her own conclusion about the best course of action.

However, as we know well, many trauma patients are intubated on arrival, or hypotensive, or otherwise in extremis and consequently unable to register, reflect on, and verbalize consent. Indeed, identifying and contacting a representative of a trauma patient in a timely fashion is often necessary and, nearly as often, challenging. One study indicated that 77% of trauma patients were able to provide consent—either directly or via a legally authorized representative—within 30 minutes of arrival to the trauma bay,[1] which really does not seem so bad, except that the same study found that inability to obtain consent within 30 minutes was associated with severe head injury and shock—*precisely* those 2 things that we would be most to likely intervene on within the first 30 minutes of hospital arrival. Another study investigated whether those patients who were able to consent were able to recall the details of the consent process on postoperative day 1.[2] Although 90% of trauma patients were able to name the operation they received, only 22% were able to accurately recall the complications that had been discussed with them.

That said, when faced with a young, otherwise healthy trauma patient presenting needing a significant operation, but one that will allow him/her to return to his/her life, family, and work in relatively short order, it is simple enough to assume how the patient would respond if he/she could. But there are almost always additional layers of complexity.

Consider the following patients, actual examples of "unconsentable" patients that we have encountered:

- 16-year-old female amateur athlete, with an isolated T4 spinal fracture sustained in a fall.
- 31-year-old, healthy female, awake and talking but too confused to consent, with abdominal tenderness and a fluid stripe at the splenic flexure on FAST examination.
- 27-year-old unhelmeted motorcycle pilot polytrauma with a depressed skull fracture, presenting with Glasgow Coma Scale of 3T.
- 57-year-old male with coronary artery disease and chronic obstructive pulmonary disease presenting with 70% total body surface area burns after an oxygen explosion in his home.
- 89-year-old female pedestrian struck by car with subdural hematoma and hip fracture.

Which one of these patients may be easily separated from the others? The 31-year-old female, with a splenic fracture and hypotension—but otherwise healthy—will in all likelihood recover well after an open splenectomy and return to her 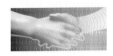 life, work and family. An easy decision is made here, as we can assume no other response, were this patient able to consent than that we should perform the operation.

In each of these other patients, however, there are further issues to consider. In these cases, we must ask questions about what the patient would want, what his/her likelihood of survival or eventual recovery is, what his/her quality of life will be (and whether and how that matters), and what the cost to the health care system in general is (and also whether and how *that* matters). To understand and answer these questions, we return to our core ethical concepts of beneficence, nonmaleficence, and empathy. Surgeons, the best of them, anyhow, are experts at returning to first principles when faced with a challenge.

Considering our hypothetical patients, based on the nature of each patient's injuries, we can expect that their quality of life would be at least changed if not severely diminished, even if a life is saved. We might then worry that by our action we are "dooming" these patients to a life of hardship and suffering. Does this not violate the principle of nonmaleficence? The writings comprising the Hippocratic Corpus, written during the fifth and fourth centuries BC, and from which much of our modern surgical culture flowered, contain the clear admonition against "tormenting the sick unnecessarily."

When we think about that concept of beneficence, which bears some similarity to what has been called the Golden Rule, we must see that the key is not to do unto others what we *ourselves* would want. As an aside, there are 2 competing formulations of this Golden Rule that arose in Palestine around the same time: Jesus of Nazareth's "*Do* unto others" and the Rabbi Hillel's "*Do not* do unto other that which is hateful to you." These inverse formulations live on in some way in our concepts of beneficence and nonmaleficence.

For example, if House Officer Jennifer happened to really enjoy peanuts, she would likely be glad to have House Officer Nicole—who happened to be down in the cafeteria while Jennifer is stuck on call in the intensive care unit (ICU) overnight—stop by the unit to bring her a bag of peanuts. It does *not* follow, though, that because Jennifer really enjoys peanuts while on call, she should therefore bring peanuts to whoever might also be stuck in the hospital. Some people just do not like peanuts; some have severe allergies that preclude even being near them. Obviously, this is meant to be simple and a little goofy. But the point is to illustrate that it does *not* follow from the concept of beneficence that we may simply substitute our own desires or judgment for the unconsentable patient's judgment.

If the doctrine of informed consent requires capacity and understanding on the part of the patient, the requirement placed on the surgeon is that he/she makes a *good faith* effort to understand the patient's desires, culture, and 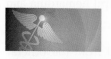 life project. We look then to the concept of *empathy*: in which we see the situation not from our perspective but from the perspective of the patient. Again, it matters not whether we ourselves would never, ever want to be cannulated for extracorporeal membrane oxygenation or undergo a craniectomy for a traumatic brain injury (TBI). It does not matter. What is at issue is would *this patient* want such a thing.

Are we even capable of this? Indeed, physicians consistently rate the quality of life of their patients as worse than the patients themselves do.[3] We may evaluate our hypothetical nonagenarian patient and think "Well, this lady lives in a nursing home, she is in a wheelchair, etc. Her quality of life is bad, and so we should withhold such and such treatment." We may, from our experience in the world and in the hospital, believe that an intervention on a nonagenarian that will likely result in a prolonged ICU stay followed by further months in acute rehab would not be of interest to most nonagenarians. However, it has been shown that patients' ratings of their own quality of life do not necessarily correlate with the desire for life-sustaining treatment or do not resuscitate orders. Often, when we see a patient and characterize 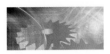 him/her as "languishing" in the ICU, to use a common medical colloquialism, the patient's family would use another word: "fighting."

Furthermore, there remains the clinical difficulty of accurately predicting a long-term neurologic outcome in the TBI patient, although clinical outcomes prediction tools are actively being researched at this time. It is extremely hard to know, by the time we have to act and send the patient off with neurosurgery to do a craniectomy, what that patient's life will be like in 6, 12, or 24 months.

It is important to remember as well that people change; they are flexible. Indeed, we know from our own experience and from the literature that our choices at any given time are highly context dependent. It may be that, waking up from anesthesia, this young girl with the high spinal injury is devastated and states that she would rather have not been resuscitated. At that time the months of rehabilitation, the knowledge that her old life is gone, take all her focus. However, is it possible that after some time, the patient may begin to understand that although life is different, it can still be fulfilling. This has been investigated, and we do know that most people are capable of adjusting to a life of disability in this way.[4,5] One study evaluated whether patients believed, at 3 years after a poor neurologic outcome from TBI, they would have consented to their operation and treatment had they been able to.[6] Out of 13, despite their outcome, 11 agreed that they would have. Indeed, this suggests that adaptation to adverse circumstances is *possible*, and even likely. This is what Honeybul has termed "recalibration."[7]

Do we have the right, though, to say to patients facing a significant detriment in quality of life: "well, we think you'll change your mind."? Even if we speak from our experience: "in my experience, most people learn they can live a fulfilling life after this injury." God forbid we quote the evidence cited above to the patient. This seems very much like "well, we *know* you'll change your mind, and you'll feel better about this." This feels profoundly paternalistic. Consider another scenario in which a "we think you'll change your mind" argument is used: to refuse a tubal ligation for a 20-year-old who wanted one, for instance? The use of this argument seems very wrong indeed.

But when faced with a dying patient we must act quickly. There is a line of thought that seems to lead to opposite conclusions. Blaise Pascal (1623-1662) was a mathematician, a scientist, and a logician. He proposed a thought experiment that has been termed "Pascal's Wager." Pascal's Wager speaks from a theistic viewpoint and proposes that earning a life after death has an upside only. If the belief is true, one attains glory; if the belief is false nothing is lost, restful oblivion awaits. In Pascal's view theistic belief allows one to have all to gain and nothing to lose.

Similar logic is often heard in the surgical clinic or consultation room. "Operation gives you a chance, however, small, to live, which is all; without it, death is inevitable. You have all to gain and nothing to lose." Surgeons tend to almost always evince a strong bias to action and are often complicit helping the patient to wager on an operation, even in the face of inevitable suffering and decrement in quality of life. The challenge of jousting against nearly impossible odds seems often to be justified by Shakespeare's words:

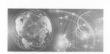

*"Diseases desperate grown by desperate appliance are relieved or not at all."*

Perhaps the most important consideration of all is to avoid this implicit bias. It is not acceptable to be guided by the preservation of life alone. Both the preservation of life and the mitigation of suffering together are the goal, and we must be guided only by the balance of probabilities, analyzed through the lens of the patient's experience and culture. There is no clear answer or algorithm to follow, other than to remember always to return to first principles. The patient rolls into the trauma bay and we stop for a beat and recall our ABCs; we must do the same with our ethical principles—autonomy, beneficence, nonmaleficence, and empathy. When we cease to fear death as the greatest failure, then there is no outcome that is to be really feared—we always have an out.

It is important, here, to recall that there are many who desire aggressive life-saving treatments in situations with a vanishingly small likelihood of a positive outcome. In our hypothetical patient with 90% total body surface area burns, with known compromised cardiac and pulmonary status, is it our right to withhold life-saving treatment in the emergency department? Ethically speaking, there is no difference in withholding and withdrawing treatment. The outcome of the end of life is ethically the same whether we withhold treatment in the emergency department or withdraw treatment in the ICU when the legally authorized representative can be located and spoken to.

The notion that, in some individuals or groups, treatment is futile and should be avoided is still extant and still controversial today. Most house officers have been at some conference at some point where a hospital lawyer and someone from the ethics committee tried to explain futility; nobody leaves those conferences with a clear picture of what futility is, when it matters, or what to do about it. Moreover, a surgeon may avoid futile operations to protect his/her ego, to keep his/her complication rate low, or believing that cost avoidance dictates it.

Surgeons have reacted to situations of futility since antiquity. In about 1862, an Egyptian scroll, written in cuneiform on the pressed pith of the papyrus plant, was purchased from a native dealer at Thebes by one Edwin Smith. The Edwin Smith papyrus remained largely inaccessible until about 1930 when James H. Breasted published a facsimile and a translation of it.[1]

The Edwin Smith papyrus constitutes the oldest surgical text in existence. It contains a "Book on Wounds," which originated perhaps 1500 years BC, but is thought to be based on practices that were already ancient by that time. The most interesting aspect of the papyrus, the aspect that seems also to have interested Breasted, are the verdicts given at the end of each patient presentation. In a sizeable number of instances, the verdict given is "an ailment not to be treated." A closer study of the text shows clearly that the ancient surgeon arrived at his/her judgment believing that treatment was futile. When refusing treatment, the motives of the surgeon (equally among ancient surgeons and us today) are often questioned. It is clear that the ancient surgeons, in their all-too-common refusals, were motivated by reputation building.

Finally, any discussion of the concept of informed consent requires us to address the issue of informed consent in research as well. Given the prevalence of traumatic injury, it is clear that it represents a grave public health problem. Particularly within the Golden Hour, research designed at optimizing our treatment of traumatized patients is key to improving outcomes in these patients and setting standards and guidelines and, indeed, creating trauma systems. However, research—as described in the Declaration of Helsinki and the Belmont Report—can only be conducted in the presence of the informed consent of the participants. How can these challenges be dealt with in the trauma setting?

It has been the case that many of the treatments in the trauma setting have been vetted through many years of experience, trial and error, and inferences from elective general surgery practice. Increasingly, large retrospective databases such as the American College of Surgeons National Trauma Quality Improvement Program have been used to increase our knowledge of best trauma practices. However, these databases have many limitations and the Gold Standard of medical research remains the randomized controlled trial. The Food and Drug Administration has established a policy such that patients requiring emergency surgical treatment can receive experimental treatment *without* prior written informed consent. This is called the Exception from Informed Consent Policy (EFIC).

The EFIC dictates that patients may receive an experimental therapy without consent if all of the following conditions are met: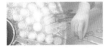

1. Available treatments are unproven or unsatisfactory.
2. The research cannot otherwise be performed to determine whether the therapy is safe and effective.
3. It is not feasible to obtain informed consent from the subject or the subject's legal representative, and there is no reasonable way to identify potential subjects prospectively.
4. Participation in the research holds out the prospect of direct benefit to the subject.

5.  The risks and benefits of the experimental procedure/treatment are reason-
    able compared with those associated with the subject's medical condition
    and standard therapy.
6.  The proposal has been reviewed and approved by an institutional review
    board.

A further requirement is that a legally authorized representative must be con-
tacted at the earliest possible time.

Before engaging in this kind of study, trialists are required to engage in
community consultation. They have to go out and discuss the trial with the
community, publicize it to some extent, and discuss it with community leaders. At this time, however, there is no standardized process by which commu-
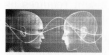nity consultation must proceed.[8] It has been demonstrated
that community members largely do support the idea of
enrollment without consent.[9] Perhaps this is due to an
understanding within the community of the importance
of research and its possibility of improving the safety, health, and welfare
of community members. Interestingly, this same study found that patients,
although willing to support the concepts underlying the EFIC for their own
care, were reluctant to support it fully when thinking about the care others
may receive.

## Conclusion

Surgeons are guided by overwhelming desire to preserve life and to mitigate
suffering. It is when we find ourselves between this Scylla and this Charybdis
that we are challenged concerning what to do. Perhaps nowhere else in the
hospital is this more common than in the trauma bay. As we consider these
questions, we must not simply characterize our enemy as death alone but
must understand that suffering takes many forms. It seems important to me
to make note of a notion that is very commonly neglected by the modern surgeon: the idea of the "good death."

What is perhaps the earliest description of the "good death" may be found
in the book of Job (5:26). Being at peace is put forward as an ingredient, and
although pain and dread are not mentioned explicitly, their absence is clearly
part of that peace. One's offspring are spoken of; modern patients are often
desperately worried about their children. The good death is never the premature death: "Thou shalt come to thy grave in a full age...." These aspects of
a good death are all still relevant, and it is after all true that futile operations
mitigate against the likelihood of the good death.

There are many testimonials to this idea. Alfred Rethel (1816-1859) created
a drawing entitled "Death as a Friend." William Osler called pneumonia "the
old man's friend." Drew Gilpin Faust, now president of Harvard University,

has written of the idea of the good death in relation to the American Civil War. The complete surgeon recognizes that the good death is a part of the good life. However, the fact remains that we cannot know, and yet we must act. This means that we must live with our uncertainty, and that we *must own* our mistakes and miscalculations. Perhaps not unlike an elective operation on a patient with many comorbidities in whom we know there is a good likelihood of complications; when it goes wrong we accept that we have miscalculated and strive to learn from our mistake and use that knowledge in the future to be better, to help move.

Indeed, it is likely while stationed on the Trauma Service that we all perform our private ethics morbidity and mortality conference on Thursday mornings as we try to sleep with daylight streaming through the windows before we return to the hospital for our next call. It is perhaps enough to say that we are thinking about it. To not consider, to not learn, to fail to live in and thrive in uncertainty is a capital mistake for the surgeon. Remember: Socrates is wise, because he knows he is not wise.

# References

1. Sava J, Ciesla D, Williams M, Street J III, White P, Wang D. Is informed consent in trauma a lost cause? A prospective evaluation of acutely injured patients' ability to give consent. *J Am Coll Surg.* 2007;205(3):405–408.
2. Bhangu A, Hood E, Datta A, Mangaleshkar S. Is informed consent effective in trauma patients? *J Med Ethics.* 2008;34(11):780–782.
3. Uhlmann RF, Pearlman RA. Perceived quality of life and preferences for life-sustaining treatment in older adults. *Arch Intern Med.* 1991;151(3):495–497.
4. Honeybul S, Gillett G, Ho K, Lind C. Ethical considerations for performing decompressive craniectomy as a life-saving intervention for severe traumatic brain injury. *J Med Ethics.* 2012;38(11):657–661.
5. Ditto PH, Jacobson JA, Smucker WD, Danks JH, Fagerlin A. Context changes choices: a prospective study of the effects of hospitalization on life-sustaining treatment preferences. *Med Decis Making.* 2006;26(4):313–322.
6. Honeybul S, Gillett GR, Ho KM, Janzen C, Kruger K. Long-term survival with unfavourable outcome: a qualitative and ethical analysis. *J Med Ethics.* 2015;41(12):963–969.
7. Honeybul S, Janzen C, Kruger K, Ho KM. Decompressive craniectomy for severe traumatic brain injury: is life worth living? *J Neurosurg.* 2013;119(6):1566–1575.
8. Maher Z, Grill EK, Smith BP, Sims CA. Does proximity to violence negatively influence attitudes toward exception from informed consent in emergency research? *J Trauma Acute Care Surg.* 2015;79(3):364–371.
9. Sims CA, Isserman JA, Holena D, et al. Exception from informed consent for emergency research: consulting the trauma community. *J Trauma Acute Care Surg.* 2013;74(1):157–165; discussion 165–156.

# 18 Ethical Decision Making in Vascular Surgery

Anthony J. Comerota, MD
Susan M. Shafii, MD

PROLOGUE ▶ The consequences of vascular disease and the complications of operations to palliate its effects are protean. Moral decisions are particularly difficult against the background of an inexorable systemic disease that, almost certainly, will ultimately take the life of the patient. In this circumstance, it would seem to be appropriate to incur great risk for even a small chance of a small extension of life. Such is not the case however.

The end manifestations of vascular disease may constitute, if those of any disease do so, fates worse than death. A major stroke with aphasia or significant paralysis, end-stage renal disease, or bilateral lower extremity amputations exemplify such fates. Any analogy to Pascal's famous wager, which advocates that any risk be taken, does not apply in instances where these states or surgical complications may ensue. Nowhere else does the natural course of the disease, or the complications of operations that may produce precisely the same consequences, present such daunting moral choices.

Dr Anthony J. Comerota is an adjunct professor of surgery at the University of Michigan Medical School.

Dr Susan M. Shafii is an assistant professor of surgery at the University of Minnesota Medical School.

*"I will remember that there is art to medicine as well as science, and that warmth, sympathy, and understanding may outweigh the surgeon's knife or the chemist's drug."*

*Hippocratic Oath*

## Introduction

The practice of medicine and surgery is rapidly changing. Medical education, financial reimbursement, technologic advances, and provider specialization are examples of how fast our profession has morphed. With all of the external stressors, physicians can lose their compassion to care for patients with the same dignity and professionalism that existed when the decision to become physicians and surgeons was made. Vascular surgery in particular has an 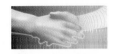 aspect of ethical challenges that frequently arise, which are left solely in the hands of vascular surgeons to handle, as society has chosen not to address those challenges. Two scenarios are presented and discussed.

The first scenario involves a family requesting maximal medical and surgical efforts for an apparently futile clinical condition in a patient with a limited life span even if all efforts are successful. Furthermore, the family's wishes appear to conflict with the patient's wishes.

The second scenario is poignantly opposite. The family withdraws care, which likely would have preserved a young patient's life, without requesting his wishes because his condition would adversely affect his quality of life.

In the first scenario, the medical event was, in all likelihood, an end-of-life event despite maximal care. In the second scenario, the event was not likely an end-of-life event if maximal care was offered. Hopefully, the discussions of these real-world cases and the algorithm provided will assist with future decision making when scenarios such as these arise.

## Clinical Scenario 1

### Elderly Male With High-Risk, Ruptured Abdominal Aortic Aneurysm

An 86-year-old, somewhat frail, gentleman is referred because of his 7.5 cm abdominal aortic aneurysm (AAA), which was identified by the patient. He told his cardiologist that he felt a "heartbeat" in his stomach. He is a retired architect, still performs some consulting work, and is a popular member of his assisted living community.

A computed tomography (CT) scan obtained by his cardiologist shows the 7.5 cm AAA, which has a short (7 mm) neck that is markedly angulated (90°). His iliac arteries are tortuous and calcified; therefore, open repair is his only option.

His cardiologist has given you a thorough summary of his medical problems, which include coronary artery disease (prior myocardial infarction), congestive heart failure (EF: 32%), diabetes controlled on long-acting insulin, chronic renal failure (creatinine: 2.4), chronic  obstructive pulmonary disease (FEV-1: 30%), and hypertension controlled with 2 agents. He is being treated for depression since his wife passed away 8 months ago. He states that his life has lost its meaning, and during the last 8 months, he has lost 24 pounds.

On examination you find a right cervical bruit, an easily palpable AAA that is not tender, and no left popliteal or distal pulse, and the remaining vascular examination is normal.

You recognize that the patient is at prohibitive risk for his needed open repair and enter into a discussion with the patient who fully comprehends his associated risks. He states that he is not afraid of the procedure but does not want prolonged life support and does not accept potential dialysis. He enjoys his relatively independent lifestyle and refuses to consider living in a full-service nursing facility. He recognizes his increased risk of rupture but accepts that risk, as both you and he agree that forgoing elective repair is the proper decision.

Four months later the patient presents to the emergency department tachycardic, hypotensive with abdominal and back pain, and a distended abdomen. The patient is not coherent. A CT scan confirms everyone's suspicion of a ruptured AAA with a large retroperitoneal hematoma. His hemoglobin level is 8.5 and his blood type is AB negative. There are 4 units of AB negative blood in the hospital, 2 of which have been crossmatched for a 12-year-old hemophiliac.

The patient's son and daughter have accompanied him to the hospital. Although they have no official power of attorney, they insist that "everything be done" to save their father. You explain to them your opinion regarding his chances of survival. You also relay your prolonged discussion with him 4 months earlier, his desires to avoid prolonged life support and dialysis, and his emphasis on quality of life. Their response is that "we can cross that bridge when we get to it."

## Ethical Questions

1. What is the proper course of action for the vascular surgeon?
2. Does the vascular surgeon have an ethical responsibility to the patient or is it now to the patient's children?

3. How does the vascular surgeon balance the patient's wishes with the family's wishes?
4. Is it justifiable to consume enormous health care resources when the anticipated outcome appears futile?

## Discussion

In situations similar to this, it is always uncomfortable, and most vascular surgeons acquiesce to the family's wishes and perform the required operative procedure. We all know the subsequent scenario. Many patients survive the operative procedure, which is followed by a prolonged stay in the intensive care unit, prolonged intubation, intense invasive monitoring, watching carefully for bowel (colon) ischemia, maintaining marginal renal function, and, often, dialysis. After the family members have endured 4, 5, or more days, they observe the ongoing required respiratory support, the need for dialysis (which they often decline), and the need for hyperalimentation in the face of progressive deterioration. The family then decides to terminate life support and offer comfort care. It is unclear how much the patient has suffered during this time, but what is clear is that the enormous resources have been expended without a reasonable chance for patient benefit.

How can vascular surgeons avoid this repetitive scenario in patients at prohibitive risks for elective repair of their AAA, if they subsequently rupture?

One simple solution is to have a prepared document detailing the high risk of elective repair and the patient's and family's acceptance of the risk of potential rupture. If rupture occurs, the futility of intervention is recognized and comfort care is agreed on by all. We have not yet witnessed such planning, although are about to implement this in our practice following discussions with our ethics committee and legal department.

Because such a document does not exist, what should the vascular surgeon do when major life-prolonging procedures and care are requested, if not demanded by the family despite the vascular surgeon recognizing the futility of such an approach?

It is interesting that decisions to limit such life-prolonging care seem to be made more easily by the patient and family members during discussions surrounding elective procedures; however, attitudes often change when rupture occurs and death is imminent, yet the futility of care has increased exponentially.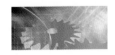

Winkler et al[1,2] have suggested an approach that integrates both medical expertise and value judgments in navigating these difficult waters (Figure 18.1). We will draw on their set of criteria to assist vascular surgeons in responding to families' request for what appears to be inappropriate treatment.

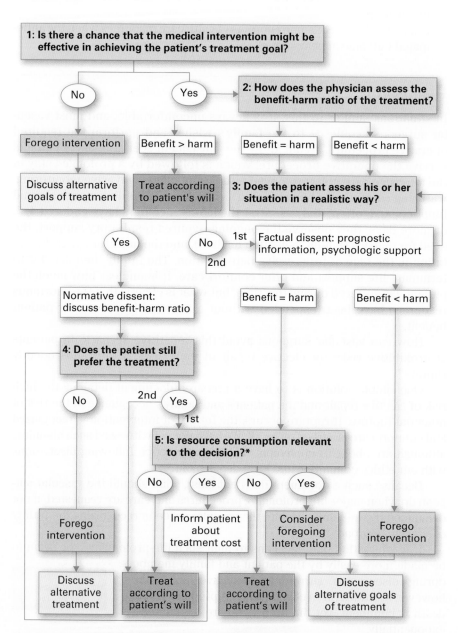

**FIGURE 18.1 Algorithm to guide patient care decision making.** (Reprinted with permission from Winkler EC, Hiddemann W, Marckmann G. Evaluating a patient's request for life-prolonging treatment: an ethical framework. *J Med Ethics*. 2012;38(11):647.)

There are 4 major elements to guide decision making in this scenario:

1. *Is the intervention requested effective?* Elective repair of AAAs is highly effective. However, in this patient's situation, the potential for extreme morbidity, which accompanies the open procedure, was recognized and was the deciding factor to decline elective operation. The logical extension to the observation that elective repair is prohibitive would be that emergent repair should not be considered because of the compounding of comorbidities.
2. *Is there a clear understanding of the benefit-to-harm ratio?* In this situation, the physician and patient agreed that elective repair was associated with much greater harm than potential benefit. Does this ratio change when the patient presents with a ruptured aneurysm? It has been stated that, at least in theory, the benefit-to-harm ratio is a continuous variable. In this case, it is the vascular surgeon's judgment that the harms of this procedure would far outweigh the potential benefits based on the patient's expressed desires to avoid prolonged life support and avoid dialysis and poor quality of life—in other words, a high degree of medical futility.[3]
3. *Has the patient assessed his medical condition in a realistic fashion?* The patient enjoyed his relatively independent lifestyle and was not willing to be cared for in a full-care nursing facility. It was apparent to the vascular surgeon that the patient approached the management of his AAA in an objective and a realistic manner. He recognized that in all likelihood if he survived the procedure, his quality of life would be completely unacceptable. His children did not consider their father's expressed opinion to the vascular surgeon.
4. *Should resource consumption play a role in decision making?* Our health care system faces increasing demands while budgets cannot keep pace. If one assumes that at the same time, limits on spending are inevitable and rule-based consensus rationing of health care is preferred to case-based rationing at the bedside. This is where society's responsibility becomes crucial.

If aggressive treatment is chosen in this case, the question of whether to transfuse with his blood type or for him to receive O positive appears easy. The AB negative blood should be reserved for the younger patient and others who would clearly benefit. However, is the blood bank 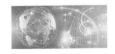 technologist capable of making that decision in an emergency? Most likely they are not!

The patient had a realistic understanding of his management options and put them into proper perspective with his choices for how he wanted to live his life. His decision fit well with proper use of resource consumption because the realistic assessment of his outcome appeared poor if operative intervention was chosen.

On the other hand, the family's request for "everything to be done" mandates enormous consumption of resources (most or none of which they will pay). Furthermore, the treatment is associated with a poor benefit-to-harm ratio. This case would consume enormous resources, but outcomes were unlikely to be beneficial to the patient and run counter to the patient's expressed desires. As physicians become increasingly involved in resource usage, a more explicit process developed by a broad consensus is required as physicians (especially in the United States) are uncomfortable about making resource-sensitive decisions at the bedside. Considering all of the issues involved, there may be justification for a unilateral decision to be made by the vascular surgeon to withhold operative repair of this patient's ruptured AAA.

---

## Clinical Scenario 2

## Young Male With Acute Mesenteric Ischemia in the Setting of Active Ulcerative Colitis

A 49-year-old gentleman with a 9-year history of ulcerative colitis who developed an acute flare-up 2 weeks ago presents with a 2-day history of worsening abdominal pain. He was discharged to home from the hospital 3 days earlier after being treated with aggressive immunotherapy. A CT scan at the time of initial hospitalization demonstrated an edematous colon. He now returns with worsening abdominal pain and a leukocytosis of 30 000. A repeat CT scan was obtained and demonstrated edematous colitis. Surgical consultation was obtained, and the patient was taken for exploratory laparotomy and colectomy.

On entering the abdomen, it was noted that approximately 100 cm of small bowel was frankly necrotic. The small bowel was stapled off and resected. The remaining small bowel had marginal perfusion with patchy areas of necrosis. There was no pulse in the superior mesenteric artery (SMA). Discussion between the family and the colorectal surgeon focused on the intraoperative findings and potential transfer to a hospital with vascular services, if mesen-

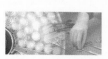

teric revascularization was to be performed. The family requested transfer and revascularization. The abdomen was packed and temporarily closed, and the patient was airlifted to a tertiary referral center. CT angiography of the aorta was obtained immediately on arrival, which demonstrated an occluded SMA and a large aortic thrombus in the proximal descending thoracic aorta.

The patient was taken to the operating room for an SMA thromboembolectomy and evaluation of the remaining bowel. On entering the abdomen, there was extension of the necrosis, which now involved the entire small bowel. No perforation identified. Discussion with the family by the general surgeon ensued while the vascular surgeon proceeded with the revascularization procedure. After successful revascularization of the SMA, the general surgeon returned after his lengthy discussion with the family. It was the opinion of the general surgeon that the patient would not have been a candidate for small bowel transplant and would require lifelong total parenteral nutrition (TPN). The patient's wife indicated that her husband would not want to be TPN dependent or have multiple additional surgical procedures. The abdomen was then closed without resection of the necrotic bowel. The following morning 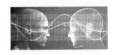 the family chose to proceed with terminal extubation and hospice care. Given the patient's young age, he was somewhat alert and appropriately responsive after extubation. He lived for 2 days before ultimately expiring.

## Ethical Questions

1. Because the vascular surgeon and general surgeon at the tertiary care institution never met the patient to understand his wishes, how should they have approached this problem given the patient's young age?
2. The patient underwent the original operation with the understanding that he would have a colectomy. The ultimate outcome and findings were never discussed with him. Should the surgeon have resected the remaining necrotic bowel and let the patient decide his own fate given the change in diagnosis?
3. Should the vascular surgeon have proceeded with thromboembolectomy before the family members reaching their decision regarding his ultimate care?
4. The patient was hemodynamically stable throughout. Was it wrong for the physicians and caretakers to follow the wife's wishes rather than discussing with the patient?

## Discussion

This is a difficult case from many aspects. There does not appear to be a reason to not take the wife's word as an extension of the patient's wishes. In addition, proper proxy and decision-making policies were followed. However, because he was young without significant cardiac, renal, or pulmonary comorbidities and was hemodynamically stable during the surgical perioperative period, it was expected that he would survive the terminal extubation if his necrotic bowel was removed. Should the patient have been given the option to decide his own fate?

One solution could have been to resect the remaining bowel that was frankly necrotic and planned to move forward with discussion with the patient after he awakens from surgery. The problem with this route is that as we all know the perioperative complication rate after an emergency vascular surgery procedure is high, and the potential for this discussion with the patient is unknown. By the time the discussion could have occurred, the remaining small bowel would have had to been completely removed and the continuity, restored. He would have then been on the path to lifelong TPN.

In young patients with chronic medical conditions, such as ulcerative colitis, and other medical conditions that wax and wane, should we press our colleagues to have clear guidelines on obtaining patient's wishes and develop 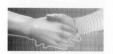 advance directives to guide us in emergency situations? The intraoperative findings in this case potentially justify either of the 2 disparate decisions. In some cases, patients are willing to accept lifelong TPN with all the accompanying comorbidities. The ultimate decision, though, is how the patient would view his/her life with all of its new constraints.

Jones and McCullough[4,5] described the previously accepted futility concept put forth by Tomlinson and Brody[5,6] that sets limitations on medical therapy and helps guide clinicians through an algorithm. There are 4 categories that comprise the algorithm: physiologic futility, clinical or overall futility, imminent demise futility, and quality-of-life futility.

"Physiologic futility" is described when the physiologically desired outcome is not expected, such as an extended cardiac resuscitation with no return of cardiac activity. The second category is "overall or clinical futility," in which the proposed intervention would not restore the patient's ability to proceed with human development and interact with the outside environment. An example of this is a vegetative state, and some would categorize TPN in this category as well. The third category is the "imminent demise futility," in which the patient will almost definitely die before discharge from the hospital and likely not recover interactive capacity before expiration. The elderly high-risk patient with the ruptured AAA fits this category. The final category, "quality-of-life futility," is when the projected condition will result in an intolerable inability to engage in valued life tasks or to derive sufficient pleasure from doing so, from the patient's perspective.

This case will not end in physiologic futility in the immediate timeframe, nor is it considered overall clinical futility, as the patient would likely have recovered from the bowel resection and had meaningful interpersonal interactions with the individuals and the surrounding environment. The 2 types of futility that are encountered in this case are the "imminent demise futility" during the surgical case and the long-term aspect of "quality-of-life futility" for the remaining portion of the patient's life. In regard to "imminent demise futility," if the remaining small bowel was not resected, then the patient would reliably die before hospital discharge from abdominal sepsis and bowel perforation. The decision to not resect the remaining necrotic bowel after revascularization, however, was made by the wife's understanding of the patient's long-term view of "quality-of-life futility." His desire to not be TPN dependent was not relayed by anyone but his wife. Are we obligated to accept her understanding of his end-of-life decision if we have an opportunity to obtain it from the patient? This scenario can also be equated to the decision of initiating emergent dialysis in a young chronic kidney disease patient who may not be a candidate for a kidney transplant.[4] Both scenarios pose single end-organ damage, in which we have the medical technology to sustain life but with consequences on "quality of life" and medical expense. Hemodialysis is a more acceptable alteration in life given the high prevalence of end-stage renal disease and federal funding. Both scenarios in surviving patients require central venous access, include risks of potential bloodstream infections, and require reliance on artificial life support. Comprehensive understanding of the futility algorithms and discussions with colleagues and families will help guide expectations and appropriate decision making.

## Acknowledgment

The authors recognize the expert editorial assistance of Shakela Watkins, MA, in the preparation of this manuscript.

## References

1. Winkler EC, Hiddemann W, Marckmann G. Evaluating a patient's request for life-prolonging treatment: an ethical framework. *J Med Ethics.* 2012;38(11):647.
2. Winkler EC, Hiddemann W, Marckmann G. Ethical assessment of life-prolonging treatment. *Lancet Oncol.* 2011;12(8):720–722.
3. Council on Ethical and Judician Affairs, American Medical Association. Medical futility in end-of-life care: report of the council on ethical and judicial affairs. *JAMA.* 1999;281(10):937–941.
4. Jones JW, McCullough LB. Extending life or prolonging death: when is enough actually too much? *J Vasc Surg.* 2014;60:521–522.
5. McCullough LB, Jones JW. Postoperative futility: a clinical algorithm for setting limits. *Br J Surg.* 2001;88:1153–1154.
6. Tomlinson T, Brody H. Ethics and communication in do-not-resuscitate orders. *N Engl J Med.* 1988;318:43–46.

# 19 Ethics of Surgery in the Elderly

Christopher S. Chiodo Ortiz, BS
Jorge Ortiz, MD

PROLOGUE ▶ Modern health care and, more particularly, modern public health commitments to clean water and segregated sewers have extended the life of humans measurably. In almost every specialty of surgery, and for almost every specific operation, a historical pattern may be discerned. An operation or operative approach is introduced, which is followed by application first to younger patients and then to septuagenarians, octogenarians, and occasionally ultimately to nonagenarians. An operative approach or a specific operation is successfully applied more and more frequently to the frail elderly patient.

Modern decision analysis, when applied to decisions about the appropriateness of an operation in a specific patient, leans heavily on estimates of risk. Such data are increasingly available and are always of value for decision making in addition to the clarification of patients' values.

Mr Christopher S. Chiodo Ortiz is a 2016 graduate of Bucknell University with a Bachelor of Science degree in biology. He is currently applying to postbaccalaureate programs and plans to begin the medical school application process in the near future.

Dr Jorge Ortiz is an associate professor and chief of surgical transplant at The University of Toledo College of Medicine.

Tremendous advances in the field of surgery occurred simultaneously with increased life spans in the United States. In 2009, there were 40 million people aged 65 years and older. By 2030, this is estimated to grow over 72 million and by 2050, it is expected to be 89 million.[1] Therefore, more elderly will receive surgical evaluations. Because age is associated with higher postoperative morbidity and mortality, as well as differing patterns of surgical illnesses and significant complications, operative therapy may not be appropriate for every patient at every age.

The additional comorbidities, greater use of medication, and threat of poor outcome[2] have strained health care, and many ethical conundrums exist. Recent advancements in medical science make operations technically possible for older individuals, but it must determine if performing operations in patient groups with poorer associated outcomes is appropriate.[3]

Elderly patients are more likely to experience general surgical conditions. Mortality following emergency surgery increases with age. Patients older than 75 years exhibit a notable increase in mortality rates.[4] For example, in acute appendicitis, older patients suffer a 7-fold increase in postoperative mortality.[5]

Cardiac surgery is offered to an expanding range of patients. Superior outcomes are noted as techniques improve and evolve.[6] Several studies show that outcomes in the elderly may not be inferior.[6] Yet it is clear that postoperative complications are far more likely to occur, thus driving up costs and labor.

Approximately 20% of the elderly present with vascular disease. In patients above the age of 75 years, complications are poorly tolerated in open vascular procedures. However, advancements in endovascular techniques have improved outcomes in the elderly. Morbidity and mortality are not significantly different between elderly individuals in good health and younger patients. Accordingly, demands on vascular surgeons, as well as other surgical specialists, and caseloads will increase.[7]

A significant proportion of complications in the elderly are associated with mental status deterioration. Delirium is a hospital-acquired altered state of mind characterized by agitation, delusions, incoherent speech and thought. About 80% of elderly patients in the intensive care unit experience it. Additionally, about 10% will remain delirious at discharge.[8-13] It is correlated with poor short- and long-term outcomes. Patients who experience delirium are likely to remain in the hospital longer, have lower subsequent 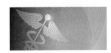 quality of life, and are 3 to 10 times more likely to die in the hospital or shortly thereafter.

The Confusion Assessment Method allows doctors to recognize delirium.[8-13] Medications such as benzodiazepines should be administered carefully. Measures to normalize the environment may also reduce risk.[8–13] It is critical that physicians contemplating the option of operation test for delirium. If a patient is unable to comprehend the procedure needed, it may not be ethical to continue, especially if the patient is exhibiting other indicators of poor outcomes.

Like delirium, dementia may render the patient unable to reach a rational decision about their health care and potential procedures. In patients presenting with either of these conditions, physicians should consult the family and advanced care directives. In deteriorating patients, it may not be prudent to operate if they are unlikely to survive. The physician must guide the family by providing as much information as possible and sharing realistic outcomes. Ensuring the patient is comfortable may well be the best alternative.

Postoperative cognitive dysfunction is a subtler deterioration in mental status than delirium and dementia. In a study of 331 geriatric patients, it was observed in about 10% during the 3 months following a major operation.[14] In procedures where cognitive dysfunction is a recognized risk, physicians must contemplate the ethics of proceeding if it may precipitate mental deterioration.[14]

Frailty is a recently developed metric used to prognosticate surgical outcomes.[15] It affects the ability to endure any physiologic situation and inhibits reclamation of functional utility after the ailment or injury. Negative postsurgical outcomes are correlated with increasing scores on the Rockwood frailty index. In a study of 220 patients, 37% were deemed frail. Seventy-seven experienced postoperative problems, 42 of which were considered major complications. Seven frail patients died. Frailty, not chronologic age, was the major predictor of negative postoperative outcomes, including complications and duration of hospital stay.[15]

Other frailty scales exist, such as the Edmonton Frail Scale. This evaluates functional performance, health, attitude, medications, independence, and support from family and friends. In the Up and Go test,[16,17] the physician asks patients to stand, walk about 3 m, and then return to their seat. If the duration of the test is longer than 12 seconds, there is a high likelihood that this patient may be frail.[18,19]

Ethical concerns must be considered throughout the evaluation. This will allow physicians to improve outcomes as well as prevent ineffectual care, which improperly allocates funding, resources, and time in futile pur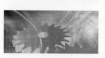suits. These frailty tests provide an objective metric to evaluate at-risk patients. Frailty scores provide an objective "language" shared between disciplines. Even though a person may want or need an operation, frailty can hinder the outcome of the operation and patient recovery, so it may not be ethical nor in the patient's best interest to proceed. It is therefore important to assess not only the impact of age but also the impact of issues associated with age in geriatric surgery.

In the past 15 years, male life expectancy has increased by 2.3 years, and female life expectancy has increased by 2.9 years. However, this figure only applies to those in the top 5% of monetary income in the United States. The life expectancy of the bottom 5% of citizens in terms of income has only increased by 0.32 and 0.04 years for males and females.[20] The health disparity gap between socioeconomic classes, including in terms of longevity, is widening, and this burdens society. The average health care cost for a person 65 years or older is currently 5 times more than the cost for an individual below 65 years of age.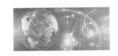

Medicare guarantees elderly Americans, regardless of economic status, access to the US health system. Medicare part A covers the professional portion of surgery, hospitalizations, laboratory tests, and home care. Medicaid provides services to the destitute. Unfortunately, there are still gaps in coverage. Issues with co-pay, travel expenses, and long-term health care are sometimes underappreciated in the underserved. There are deductibles and co-pays that may burden the elderly individual.[21] This stresses not only the index patient but also the family and support system, who may need to cover the additional costs.

Socialized medicine delivers care through a universal health care system. A centralized agency determines the efficacy of care for all by using tax resources. Care is delivered to the individual regardless of their ability to pay. Supporters posit that government oversight in health care would decrease expenses due to the removal of profit margins and administrative overhead linked to private insurance. Additionally, the government's ability to aggregate expenditures on the national level would decrease costs for individual hospitals and patients. Those who do not support a socialized medicine model argue that the universality of health care would cause its quality to deteriorate. In this scenario, care is still burdened by monetary issues, and the government may demand to assess the utility of surgery in the elderly. For example, it may be determined that an elderly individual displays too much risk associated with surgical outcomes to undergo a procedure. Such a determination should be the responsibility of the surgeon, not the payer.

Balancing the needs of the individual with the needs of society is complex. Different schools of ethical thought may provide solutions. Virtue ethicists base decisions on their own moral perception of right and wrong. For example, it may not be virtuous to operate on an elderly patient whose predicted outcomes and postoperative quality of life are poor. It may be virtuous though for the physician to prolong the quality life of an elderly patient in any way possible.

Utilitarian ethics propounds the greatest good for the greatest number. Because elderly patients are associated with higher costs and use of more resources, it may not be deemed appropriate to allocate excessive hospital funding to the elderly. Theoretically, this money could be distributed to 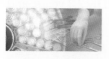 a larger surgical patient group and potentially benefit more people. With more equal allocation of funding, it is possible that patient outcomes would improve in the general population.

In a free market model, where liberty is supreme, individual desires outweigh ethical concerns, as well as concern for the majority. Some would argue that if elderly patients desire an operation and have the economic means to afford it, they should be granted that procedure. If surgeons were to operate on every individual who has means of payment, this could decrease the proportion of positive outcomes. From the surgeon's standpoint, the fee-for-service model would dictate that surgeons provide services when they want, for whatever price the market will bear. If surgeons were salaried, it could be argued, they may not be incentivized to provide extra care to the elderly patient.

In the purest forms of Christianity, Islam, and Judaism, finances would never be a deciding factor in determining the appropriateness of surgery. As a matter of fact, one of the Five Pillars of Islam is to provide for the poor. If individuals require an operation to save life, it would be granted to them. Sanctity of life mandates that all possible procedures would be used to extend survival. These religions view life as holy and sacred, so any medical route that would preserve life would be encouraged. Any that would prematurely end it would be discouraged. Because of this, the patient's "right to die" would not be valued. The patients or their family would be reluctant to decline life-prolonging treatment.

Contrarily, Hinduism accepts the "right to die" as long as the person has no further responsibilities or obligations in their life. Nonviolent forms of suicide such as starvation are accepted. Therefore, from a Hindu standpoint, life-prolonging measures in the elderly may not be acceptable if they are not what the person desires.

The elderly are not a homogenous group. They comprise a multiplicity of religious spheres, economic backgrounds, racial and ethnic enclaves, and cultural upbringings. Each of these life experiences affects their assessment of the risk and benefit in surgery. In some cultures, the elderly are revered for their wisdom. In others, the elderly may not fully participate in decisions regarding their care. Cultural competence among physicians is therefore paramount. If there is a language barrier, it is the physician's responsibility to employ a translator, rather than a family member, to ensure elderly candidates receive all the information concerning their health and their options. At times, an elderly patient may be incapacitated and unable to decide on a health care course. In this case, it is extremely important that the health care team probe the family to determine what the patient would have wanted, not necessarily what the family members wish.

Shared decision making is a strategy in which physicians discuss existing evidence with patients, who then consider the information presented to them and determine their preferences.[22] At the center of shared decision making is the appreciation of the patients' ability to preserve their own health. It is not generally used on a widespread basis at this time.[23] In elderly surgery patients, shared decision making may be a valuable model for determining the appropriateness of a procedure. If a patient is incapacitated or unconscious, a shared decision-making process should proceed with the family. It is crucial that they and the physician review advanced care directives to determine what the patient would have wanted. Prolonging life through "any means necessary" may have been expressed. However, this is not always the best option when considering quality of life and postoperative recovery. For example, a deteriorating geriatric patient with a heart condition may desire any operation that has a chance to save his/her life, but this bias toward self-preservation may affect his/her ability to weigh all the factors. Challenges to shared decision making include lack of health literacy, as well as cultural barriers to the idea of self-directed decisions.

The ethics of surgery in the elderly is a multifaceted issue that health care professionals, as well as the families and patients themselves, must confront. People above the age of 65 years may struggle to handle their expanding health care costs, and this should be considered when determining if an operation is the appropriate route. Significant expenditures can be expected because the elderly population is associated with distinct complications and outcomes after surgery. Elderly patients may be incapacitated and therefore unable to make judgments for themselves. It is critical that the physician inform the patient of every issue regarding their health. Different religions and cultures may view elderly care differently, and different schools of ethical thought may offer differing conclusions regarding the efficacy of surgery. The physician must assess the patient in terms of physiologic age rather than chronologic age. This includes accounting for risk indicators such as dementia, delirium, and frailty because they are associated with worse outcomes. As patients age, it may become difficult for family members to accept the inevitable. It is the responsibility of the physician to improve 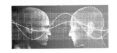 knowledge and respect judgment. The patient, the family, and the physician must consider quality of life, longevity, and all postoperative outcomes and complications.

The surgeon also needs to consider the appropriateness of interventions vis-à-vis society as a whole. Surgery may not always be the most practical alternative in an elderly patient. As health care professionals, it is our job to guide and inform all parties, so the appropriate course of action can be pursued.

# References

1. Kinsella K, He W. *An Aging World: 2008, U.S. Census Bureau, International Population Reports P95/09-1.* Washington, DC: U.S. Government Printing Office; 2009.

2. Desserud KF, Veen T, Søreide K. Emergency general surgery in the geriatric patient. *Br J Surg.* 2016;103(2):e52–e61.

3. Torjuul K, Nordam A, Sørlie V. Action ethical dilemmas in surgery: an interview study of practicing surgeons. *BMC Med Ethics.* 2005;6:E7.

4. Hashmi A, Ibrahim-Zada I, Rhee P, et al. Predictors of mortality in geriatric trauma patients: a systematic review and meta-analysis. *J Trauma Acute Care Surg.* 2014;76:894–901.

5. Andersson RE. Short and long-term mortality after appendectomy in Sweden 1987 to 2006. Influence of appendectomy diagnosis, sex, age, co-morbidity, surgical method, hospital volume, and time period. A national population-based cohort study. *World J Surg.* 2013;37:974–981.

6. Unsworth-White J. Cardiac surgery for the elderly: a surgeon's perspective. *Heart.* 1999;82(2):125.

7. O'Brien G, Martin Z, Haider N, et al. An analysis of vascular surgery in elderly patients to determine whether age affects treatment strategy *Ir J Med Sci.* 2012;181(1):73–76.

8. Balas MC, Happ MB, Yang W, Chelluri L, Richmond T. Outcomes associated with delirium in older patients in surgical ICUs. *Chest.* 2009;135(1):18–25.

9. Barr J, Fraser GL, Puntillo K. Clinical practice guidelines for the management of pain, agitation, and delirium in adult patients in the intensive care unit. *Crit Care Med.* 2013;41(1):263–306.

10. Puntillo K. Pain in the older adult intensive care unit. *Crit Care Clin.* 2003;19(4):749–770.

11. Peitz GJ, Balas MC, Olsen KM, Pun BT, Ely EW. Top 10 myths regarding sedation and delirium in the ICU. *Crit Care Med.* 2013;19(4):749–770.

12. Reade MC, Finfer S. Sedation and delirium in the intensive care unit. *N Engl J Med.* 2014;370(5):444–454.

13. Vaurio LE, Sands LP, Wang Y, Mullen EA, Leung JM. Postoperative delirium: the importance of pain and pain management. *Anesth Analg.* 2006;102(4):1267–1273.

14. Abildstrom H, Rasmussen LS, Rentowl P, et al. Cognitive dysfunction 1-2 years after non-cardiac surgery in the elderly. *Acta Anaesthesiol Scand.* 2000;44(10):1246–1251.

15. Joseph B, Zangbar B, Pandit V, et al. Emergency general surgery in the elderly: too old or too frail? *J Am Coll Surg.* 2016;222(5):805–813.

16. Rockwood K, Song X, MacKnight C, et al. A global clinical measure of fitness and frailty in elderly people. *CMAJ.* 2005;173(5):489–495.

17. Escobedo LV, Habboushe J, Kaafarani H, Velmahos G, Shah K, Lee J. Traumatic brain injury: a case-based review. *World J Emerg Med.* 2013;4(4):252–259.

18. Robinson TN, Zenilman M. Preoperative assessment of the elderly patient: frailty. In: Cameron JL, Cameron AM, eds. *Current Surgical Therapy.* 10th ed. Philadelphia, PA: Elsevier Saunders; 2011:1065–1069.

19. Dasgupta M, Rlfson DB, Stolee P, Borrie MJ, Speechley M. Frailty is associated with postoperative complications in older adults with medical problems. *Arch Gerontol Geriatr.* 2009;48(1):78–83.

20. Dizikes | MIT News Office, Peter. New study shows rich, poor have huge mortality gap in U.S. *MIT News*; April 11, 2016.

21. Rowland D, Lyons B. Medicare, medicaid, and the elderly poor. *Health Care Financ Rev*. 1996;18.

22. Elwyn G, Coulter A, Laitner S, Walker E, Watson P, Thomson R. Implementing shared decision making in the NHS. *BMJ*. 2010;341.

23. Zikmund-Fisher BJ, Couper MP, Singer E, et al. The DECISIONS study: a nationwide survey of United States adults regarding 9 common medical decisions. *Med Decis Making*. 2010;30(suppl 5):20S–34S.

# 20 The Frail Elderly Surgical Candidate

Matthew A. Corriere, MD, MS
Jonathan R. Thompson, MD

PROLOGUE ▶ Modern decision analysis is a derivative of the utilitarianism of Jeremy Bentham and J.S. Mill and has generally used objective verifiable data. There are those who believe decisions should be made only on such an evidentiary base. This approach to the making of decisions is currently supported by an ever-increasing array of databases, an exemplar of which is the American College of Surgeon's National Surgery Quality Improvement Project (NSQIP) risk calculator. The availability of such data greatly facilitates surgical decision making of the highest caliber.

Careful research in social and psychologic determinants of human choice has made clear, however, that human values may vary widely and that most life decisions are based heavily on so-called "human factors," which have heretofore been unmeasurable. There are those who believe that the integration of such factors into decision analysis is not possible. Surgeons have long recognized, however, that it is inadequate to hand the statistical data to the patient and say, "You decide." Fortunately, there is currently developing recognition of this deficiency of decision analysis, and high-quality research is being conducted to bring these "human factors" into health care decisions.

Dr Matthew A. Corriere is doing pioneering work in this area. He is a Frankel Professor of Cardiovascular Surgery and associate professor in the Department of Surgery, Section of Vascular Surgery at the University of Michigan Medical School in Ann Arbor, Michigan.

Dr Jonathan R. Thompson is a vascular surgery fellow in the Department of Surgery, Section of Vascular Surgery, at the University of Michigan Medical School in Ann Arbor, Michigan.

## Introduction

The frail elderly surgical candidate is encountered with increasing regularity as the population ages. Decision making related to surgery on frail elderly patients is complex and requires consideration of the patient's risk and risk tolerance, the implications of nonoperative management, and downstream scenarios that might arise as a consequence of the choice. The surgeon must accurately identify the frail elderly surgical candidate as such, so that treatment can be considered within this context. "Frail" and "elderly" are not mutually inclusive concepts, and ruling out frailty can therefore be as helpful for decision making as identifying this trait, particularly in the very elderly.

Over the past 2 decades, frailty has rapidly advanced from a novel concept to a booming field of clinical research where geriatric medicine, perioperative medicine, and surgery intersect. This chapter will review accepted definitions of frailty, approaches to identifying and quantifying frailty, and associations between frailty and clinical outcomes. With this background information in mind, the frail elderly surgical candidate will then be considered from an ethical perspective.

## Conceptual Framework and Definitions

*Frailty* is a characteristic that many surgeons recognize in patients they treat but may find challenging to define or quantify. Geriatricians commonly define frailty as "…a biologic syndrome of decreased reserve and resistance to stressors, resulting from cumulative declines across multiple physiologic symptoms, and causing adverse outcomes."[1] Frailty is an indicator of decreased physiologic reserve and increased vulnerability. Frailty is associated with mortality, disability, dependent functional status, falls, and need for long-term care among elderly adults.[1] As a unified manifestation with multiple 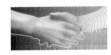 underlying causes, frailty is sometimes referred to as an overarching *geriatric syndrome*.[2,3] Other geriatric syndromes (including falls, incontinence, pressure ulcers, and delirium) are often present in frail elderly patients, but not all patients with a geriatric syndrome are frail.

Frailty, comorbidity, and disability are often simultaneously present in the same patient but are not mutually inclusive concepts (Figure 20.1).

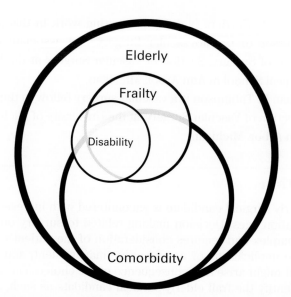

FIGURE 20.1 **Relationships between comorbidity, frailty, and disability among the elderly.** The majority of elderly people have comorbidity but are not frail. Both frailty and disability commonly exist in the same person, but neither affects all elderly patients with comorbidity.

*Comorbidities* are distinct diagnoses or diseases with unrelated causes.[4] Comorbidity is often used to define frailty and considered to be present if a patient has 2 or more diseases that have been diagnosed using established, widely recognized criteria.[5] Because chronic conditions are more prevalent with increasing age, so is comorbidity. Comorbidity is associated with health care utilization and increases the disability and mortality beyond the individual diseases. This implies a synergistic effect, which also may exist when concurrent impairments (such as in strength, balance, or cognition) are present. Patients whose frailty characteristics result from single comorbidity (such as stroke, dementia, or Parkinson disease) are distinguished from patients whose frailty characteristics are the result of multiple (sometimes unknown) causes and are not necessarily considered frail.[1]

*Disabilities* are impairments, activity limitations, or participation restrictions.[6] Both frailty and disability may occur as consequences of diseases (comorbidity) and physiologic changes that occur with aging or are caused by disease. Disability is therefore an effect that may have both frailty and comorbidity as causes. Like comorbidity and frailty, disability is associated with increased health care expenditures in the elderly.[7] Conversely, disability may result in more severe manifestations of frailty or comorbidities even though it does not cause these conditions. Because of these complexities, it is unusual for focused management of a single comorbidity to dramatically improve either frailty or disability. Medical optimization of one comorbidity may antagonize another, sometimes with unanticipated negative consequences.

# Identifying and Quantifying Frailty

Selecting a frailty assessment approach requires consideration of the outcome(s) of interest, level of desired predictive accuracy, goals of the analysis (including whether the unit of analysis is an individual or group of patients), and the available resources for measurement (including both data and personnel). Selected variables used for frailty assessment, along with associated approaches, are listed in Table 20.1. There are 2 general approaches to frailty assessment: frailty as a phenotype and frailty as an accumulation of deficits. These approaches are considered complementary and may be combined into hybrid methods, blending elements of both.[8,9]

Frailty *phenotype* assessments rely on observation or measurement of predefined signs and symptoms.[7,8] Characteristics used to define the frailty phenotype include wasting (which may consist of weight loss, shrinking, or decreased muscle mass), weakness, poor endurance (often measured based on walking

TABLE 20.1 ▶ VARIABLES USED FOR FRAILTY ASSESSMENT

| Category | Variables |
|---|---|
| Weakness | Grip strength<br>Isokinetic measurement |
| Poor endurance | Exhaustion |
| Physical activity and function | Walking time or speed<br>Kilocalories per week<br>"Get Up and Go" test |
| Wasting | Weight, height |
| Sarcopenia | Total psoas area<br>Muscle mass<br>Leg circumference |
| Comorbidity | Dementia, cognitive dysfunction, or delirium<br>Diabetes<br>Hypertension<br>Pulmonary disease<br>Heart disease<br>Depression<br>Cancer<br>Charlson Comorbidity Index<br>Elixhauser Comorbidity Score |
| Disability | Functional dependence<br>Exhaustion<br>Falls<br>Impaired memory<br>Impaired mobility<br>Incontinence<br>Problems with activities of daily living |
| Laboratory data | Low albumin<br>Anemia |
| Social support | Available assistance when help is needed |

speed), and low activity. Within the definition popularized by Fried et al, patients are designated as frail if they meet 3 or more criteria and intermediate (or "pre-frail") if only 1 or 2 are present.[7] Among a wide array of variables used to define the frail phenotype, slow gait speed has been identified as a key indicator highly correlated with results of nonphenotype approaches.[10] Grip strength has been the most commonly used approach for identifying weakness as a component of the frailty phenotype.[1,10] Phenotype assessments usually require prospective measurement and data collection but do not require clinical assessment and are relatively easy to score and interpret. Accordingly, these approaches are often practical for clinical implementation, provided that the necessary personnel and equipment (such as a hand grip dynamometer or a stopwatch and space for measuring walking speed) are available. Because many phenotype approaches use measures that are seldom documented within the scope of routine clinical care, they are less useful for retrospective study designs or secondary data analyses.

*Accumulated deficits* frailty models originated from variables included in the comprehensive geriatric assessment (CGA), which includes medical data in addition to assessment of cognitive, physical, and functional elements.[9,11] Because accumulated deficits approaches are based, at least in part, on data collected through clinical care, regardless of whether frailty assessment was deliberately included as part of the clinical interaction, they are useful for analysis of retrospective, administrative, or registry data where direct observation and measurement of participants is not possible. The CGA provides an extensive amount of information across multiple domains that can be used for frailty assessment but must be performed by a geriatrics specialist and is time- and labor-intensive to obtain; with approximately 70 items, it may take an hour or more to collect. The Clinical Frailty Scale, developed through the Canadian Study of Health and Aging, is based on a subset of variables obtained during the CGA. This scale places patients into 1 of 7 categories based on an interview and medical records review, can be performed by a nonspecialist, and was one of the first accumulated deficits approaches described.[11] This approach reliably approximates more formal frailty assessments and has been demonstrated to correlate highly with more comprehensive assessments that are less practical for routine clinical use. The Edmonton Frail Scale is another example of a shorter accumulated deficits 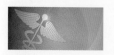 assessment tool that can be used by people without specialized geriatrics training. It is also based on selected elements of the CGA, including cognition, general health, functional status, social support, medication, nutrition, continence, and functional performance.[12] Even more abbreviated accumulated deficits models have been developed for use with registry data (such as the American College of Surgeons NSQIP Data File), including laboratory data.[13]

Direct comparisons between phenotype and accumulated deficits approaches to frailty assessment suggest that phenotype approaches are clinically useful and easily reproducible and provide a relatively broad risk assessment. Phenotype approaches have been criticized, however, for omission of cognitive and psychologic factors that may have significant impacts on frailty.[14,15] It is also important to remember that phenotype approaches provide a "snapshot" of frailty status at a single point in time and therefore may not reflect the dynamic changes in frailty status that occur as patients frequently move between states.[16] By comparison, accumulated deficits assessments use data from the medical record entered over an extended interval of time, perhaps making them less sensitive to short-term fluctuation. Accumulated deficits approaches also allow greater precision and clinical inference but require collection, analysis, and translation of clinical data.[3,15]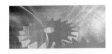

Hybrid approaches blend phenotype variables such as problems with toileting, getting dressed, bathing, and cooking with comorbidity variables, many of which are included in both the Charlson and Elixhauser comorbidity scales, to build a frailty index.[17] Other measures have been developed that rely primarily on clinical judgment.[18] Given these considerations, it may be that awareness and attention to frailty as a potentially important concern may be more important than the specific assessment approach used.

## Frailty and Surgical Outcomes

Interest in frailty as a risk factor originated in the field of geriatric medicine, where associations between frailty and adverse outcomes, including falls, impaired mobility, disability, hospitalization, and death, have affected clinical decision making and management.[1] Although the utility of frailty for predicting death, morbidity, and hospitalization is well documented in the general elderly population, frailty identification may have even greater importance within elderly patients being considered for surgical procedures. Because surgical procedures subject patients to a discrete (and sometimes elective) physiologic challenge, the frail elderly surgical patient faces a different risk:benefit ratio that might affect either the decision to operate or the surgical approach chosen.

A growing body of evidence supports the importance of frailty as an indicator of decreased physiologic reserve, which can translate into increased vulnerability to adverse perioperative events. Adverse outcomes associated with frailty include mortality, delirium, and nonhome discharge.[17] Frailty is also associated with readmission and increased length of hospital stay. Risk associated with frailty has been observed consistently across study cohorts defined by surgeon specialty, diagnosis, or procedure type.[19-21] Robinson et al studied frailty among patients requiring intensive care unit admission following general surgery, thoracic, vascular, or urology operations.[17] These authors found that functional dependence was the strongest predictor of mortality at 6 months among other frailty indicators that included cognitive impairment, low albumin, low hematocrit, falls within the previous 6 months, and comorbidity. Others have also observed associations between frailty and albumin levels, as well as low and low-normal hemoglobin levels.[22-24] Arya et al have described associations between the Modified Frailty Index and risk of perioperative complications, mortality, and nonhome discharge following vascular procedures using the American College of Surgeons NSQIP Data File.[25,26]

*Sarcopenia* refers to age-related decreases in skeletal muscle and related functional consequences.[27] This multifactorial process may be affected by gender, genetics, health risk behavior, diet and nutrition, and lifestyle factors.[28,29] Sarcopenia has a prevalence of nearly 60% among elderly Americans, is asso-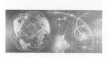ciated with functional impairment (especially for severe sarcopenia among older women),[27] and is often used as a standalone phenotypic frailty indicator. Cross-sectional abdominal images, which are frequently available in surgical candidates, can be used to identify sarcopenia. Total psoas area, measured from cross-sectional images, has been used as a surrogate measure of sarcopenia and demonstrated to predict mortality following abdominal aortic aneurysm repair and liver transplantation.[21,30]

Consistent and pervasive associations observed between frailty and surgical risk have prompted calls for more active screening to facilitate tailored management. Identification of frailty might prompt consideration of nonoperative management, a specific operative approach, or individualized testing to further inform risk and counseling.[17] Whether frailty itself is a modifiable risk factor, however, remains unclear. Interventions that might affect frailty include reorientation for cognitive impairment, strength and balance training, nutrition, and mobilization. Positive impacts of exercise training on functional performance have been observed among elderly nursing home residents, but the improvement occurred without correlative changes in muscle strength, bodyweight, or body fat.[31] These results suggest the possibility that improved performance resulting from exercise programs may derive from improvements in balance and coordination rather than recovery of muscle mass or weight. Nonetheless, these functional improvements still have potential to positively affect risk of falls and other adverse events. Malnutrition is another potentially modifiable risk factor that is included as a part of the CGA, but evidence to support preoperative nutritional interventions to improve surgical outcomes among frail patients is lacking.[32] Specific management approaches for frail elderly patients have been proposed for cancer, cardiovascular disease, and other diagnoses.[33] Severe frailty without treatable contributing factors may warrant a consideration of palliative management strategies and avoidance of physiologic challenges.

## Ethical Considerations for the Frail Elderly Surgical Candidate

Perhaps the most basic ethical consideration for the frail elderly surgical candidate is whether they are still considered an operative candidate once identified as frail. The surgeon evaluating a frail elderly patient therefore should consider whether the treatment is likely to result in more benefit than harm and whether the patient is just as likely, or even more likely, to die of complications of the operation as from the disease being treated.

The decision to proceed with an elective or emergent operation on a frail elderly patient requires that the surgeon, the patient, and/or any surrogate decision makers, such as family or other designated advocates, accept proceeding despite increased risk. In the era of outcomes reporting transparency and links to reimbursement, there is increasing scrutiny on procedures that are categorized as either high risk or low value. Accordingly, surgeons may be incentivized against operations where the risk of adverse events is high, even when the alternatives are unpleasant and may be limited to death. Patients' risk tolerance sometimes increases as odds of success diminish, particularly with emergency surgery. For example, a patient who would not be considered a candidate for elective operation might be willing to accept a prohibitive level of perioperative adverse events or death if the alternative outcome is significantly morbid and certain to occur otherwise. In these circumstances, it is important to establish shared goals of care and expectations, particularly when a return to baseline functional status is unlikely, the gains are short term, and the operation is risky or significantly invasive.

As mentioned previously, frailty is not necessarily a modifiable risk factor. Although interventions may affect specific markers of frailty such as function, cognition, and laboratory parameters of nutrition and anemia, decisions related to surgery on frail patients may not allow adequate time for interventions to reduce operative risk. This is particularly true if the indication for surgery is time-sensitive in terms of outcomes or risk associated with delaying operation.

## Example Case Scenarios

The scenarios listed below are based on frail elderly surgical candidates. For each, consider the following questions related to decision making in frail elderly surgical candidates. In addition to potential clinical outcomes, also think about the ethical concepts of autonomy, nonmaleficence, fairness, and justice.

- What benefit would the patient receive from a successful operation?
- What risks are the patient and surgeon accepting by operating versus not?
- What are the prospects for a "normal" life with and without surgery?
- Does the patient have decision-making capacity?
- Would observation or operation be less likely to result in short-term harm? What about long-term outcomes?
- Does the patient, family, surgeon, or hospital have any real or potential conflicts of interest?
- If the surgeon believes an operation is not a good choice, should it be offered as one of the treatment options?

AD is a 69-year-old woman with hypertension, emphysema, and a type III thoracoabdominal aortic aneurysm. This aneurysm was found incidentally on a computed tomography during a recent admission for a symptomatic pericardial effusion. The aneurysm is 6.2 cm in maximal diameter and meets diameter criteria for elective repair. She is not a candidate for endovascular repair due to aneurysm anatomy. The patient is an active daily smoker, and although she does not use home oxygen or have dyspnea at rest, she is deemed high risk for postoperative respiratory failure and need for tracheostomy by her pulmonologist. The patient wants "everything done" to extend her life.

BK is an 80-year-old man with a history of hypertension, hyperlipidemia, and coronary artery disease, after coronary bypass 10 years ago, who presents with new hemoptysis. The patient is a former smoker (80 pack-years) and quit 10 years ago. He lives at home but requires some help with his activities of daily living, including cooking and cleaning. He is able to bathe himself. 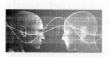 He ambulates with a walker. He is not on any supplemental oxygen. A chest computed tomography scan revealed a mass in his right upper lobe and hilar adenopathy. A subsequent positron emission tomography scan demonstrated metabolic activity in the nodule and in the mediastinum at the hilum. A percutaneous biopsy of the mass demonstrated invasive adenocarcinoma, and the staging endobronchial ultrasonography was negative, although there were enlarged, firm lymph nodes sampled on both sides of the mediastinum during the procedure. The patient's pulmonary function tests suggest that he would tolerate a lobectomy.

JM is a 74-year-old woman with hypertension, chronic obstructive pulmonary disease, end-stage renal disease on dialysis, and rheumatoid arthritis, who presents with an ulcer on her toe. She is severely debilitated from rheumatoid arthritis for which she takes daily prednisone and weekly etanercept injections. She lives alone. She denies claudication but "does not walk much" and only ambulates with a walker. On examination, the toe is malodorous and black with purulent drainage. Noninvasive studies indicate she would not heal from a toe amputation without revascularization. The patient is her own decision maker and wants you to do "whatever is best."

## Conclusion

Frailty is common among elderly surgical candidates, is associated with increased risk of perioperative complications, and warrants consideration during decision making related to operation. Standardized approaches to frailty assessment can allow surgeons to objectively identify and quantify frailty, permitting individualized approaches to both treatment and patient selection. Future research will hopefully identify strategies to improve or reverse frailty, potentially transforming this syndrome from a risk factor into a treatable condition.[34]

# References

1. Fried LP, Tangen CM, Walston J, et al. Frailty in older adults: evidence for a phenotype. *J Gerontol A Biol Sci Med Sci*. 2001;56:M146–M156.
2. Inouye SK, Studenski S, Tinetti ME, Kuchel GA. Geriatric syndromes: clinical, research, and policy implications of a core geriatric concept. *J Am Geriatr Soc*. 2007;55:780–791.
3. Rothman MD, Leo-Summers L, Gill TM. Prognostic significance of potential frailty criteria. *J Am Geriatr Soc*. 2008;56:2211–2216.
4. Iezzoni LI. *Risk Adjustment for Measuring Health Care Outcomes*. Chicago, IL; Arlington, VA: Health Administration Press; AUPHA; 2013.
5. Fried LP, Ferrucci L, Darer J, Williamson JD, Anderson G. Untangling the concepts of disability, frailty, and comorbidity: implications for improved targeting and care. *J Gerontol A Biol Sci Med Sci*. 2004;59:255–263.
6. World Health Organization. *Disabilities*. Available from: http://www.who.int/topics/disabilities/en/. Accessed June 17, 2017.
7. Fried TR, Bradley EH, Williams CS, Tinetti ME. Functional disability and health care expenditures for older persons. *Arch Intern Med*. 2001;161:2602–2607.
8. Cesari M, Gambassi G, van Kan GA, Vellas B. The frailty phenotype and the frailty index: different instruments for different purposes. *Age Ageing*. 2014;43:10–12.
9. Kraiss LW, Beckstrom JL, Brooke BS. Frailty assessment in vascular surgery and its utility in preoperative decision making. *Semin Vasc Surg*. 2015;28:141–147.
10. Hoogendijk EO, van Kan GA, Guyonnet S, Vellas B, Cesari M. Components of the frailty phenotype in relation to the frailty index: results from the Toulouse frailty platform. *J Am Med Dir Assoc*. 2015;16:855–859.
11. Rockwood K, Song X, MacKnight C, et al. A global clinical measure of fitness and frailty in elderly people. *CMAJ*. 2005;173:489–495.
12. Rolfson DB, Majumdar SR, Tsuyuki RT, Tahir A, Rockwood K. Validity and reliability of the Edmonton Frail Scale. *Age Ageing*. 2006;35:526–529.
13. Karam J, Tsiouris A, Shepard A, Velanovich V, Rubinfeld I. Simplified frailty index to predict adverse outcomes and mortality in vascular surgery patients. *Ann Vasc Surg*. 2013;27:904–908.
14. Kulminski AM, Ukraintseva SV, Kulminskaya IV, et al. Cumulative deficits better characterize susceptibility to death in elderly people than phenotypic frailty: lessons from the Cardiovascular Health Study. *J Am Geriatr Soc*. 2008;56:898–903.
15. Rockwood K, Andrew M, Mitnitski A. A comparison of two approaches to measuring frailty in elderly people. *J Gerontol A Biol Sci Med Sci*. 2007;62:738–743.
16. Gill TM, Gahbauer EA, Allore HG, Han L. Transitions between frailty states among community-living older persons. *Arch Intern Med*. 2006;166:418–423.
17. Robinson TN, Eisemen B, Wallace JI, et al. Redefining geriatric preoperative assessment using frailty, disability and co-morbidity. *Ann Surg*. 2009;250:449–455.
18. Studenski S, Hayes RP, Leibowitz RQ, et al. Clinical global impression of change in physical frailty: development of a measure based on clinical judgment. *J Am Geriatr Soc*. 2004;52:1560–1566.
19. Makary MA, Makary MA, Segev DL, et al. Frailty as a predictor of surgical outcomes in older patients. *J Am Coll Surg*. 2010;210:901–908.
20. Robinson TN, Wu DS, Pointer L, et al. Simple frailty score predicts postoperative complications across surgical specialties. *Am J Surg*. 2013;206:544–550.

21. Lee JS, He K, Harbaugh CM, et al. Frailty, core muscle size, and mortality in patients undergoing open abdominal aortic aneurysm repair. *J Vasc Surg.* 2011;53:912–917.

22. Chaves PH, Semba RD, Leng SX, et al. Impact of anemia and cardiovascular disease on frailty status of community-dwelling older women: the Women's Health and Aging Studies I and II. *J Gerontol A Biol Sci Med Sci.* 2005;60:729–735.

23. Slee A, Birch D, Stokoe D. The relationship between malnutrition risk and clinical outcomes in a cohort of frail older hospital patients. *Clin Nutr ESPEN.* 2016;15:57–62.

24. Hazzard WR. Depressed albumin and high-density lipoprotein cholesterol: signposts along the final common pathway of frailty. *J Am Geriatr Soc.* 2001;49:1253–1254.

25. Arya S, Kim SI, Duwayri Y, et al. Frailty increases the risk of 30-day mortality, morbidity, and failure to rescue after elective abdominal aortic aneurysm repair independent of age and comorbidities. *J Vasc Surg.* 2015;61:324–331.

26. Arya S, Long CA, Brahmbhatt R, et al. Preoperative frailty increases risk of non-home discharge after elective vascular surgery in home-dwelling patients. *Ann Vasc Surg.* 2016;35:19–29.

27. Janssen I, Heymsfield SB, Ross R. Low relative skeletal muscle mass (sarcopenia) in older persons is associated with functional impairment and physical disability. *J Am Geriatr Soc.* 2002;50:889–896.

28. Jackson AS, Janssen I, Sui X, Church TS, Blair SN. Longitudinal changes in body composition associated with healthy ageing: men, aged 20–96 years. *Br J Nutr.* 2012;107:1085–1091.

29. Harris T. Muscle mass and strength: relation to function in population studies. *J Nutr.* 1997;127:1004S–1006S.

30. Englesbe MJ, Patel SP, He K, et al. Sarcopenia and mortality after liver transplantation. *J Am Coll Surg.* 2010;211:271–278.

31. Carmeli E, Reznick AZ, Coleman R, Carmeli V. Muscle strength and mass of lower extremities in relation to functional abilities in elderly adults. *Gerontology.* 2000;46:249–257.

32. Fiatarone MA, Fiatarone MA, O'Neill EF, et al. Exercise training and nutritional supplementation for physical frailty in very elderly people. *N Engl J Med.* 1994;330:1769–1775.

33. Singh M, Stewart R, White H. Importance of frailty in patients with cardiovascular disease. *Eur Heart J.* 2014;35:1726–1731.

34. de Labra C, Guimaraes-Pinheiro C, Maseda A, Lorenzo T, Millán-Calenti JC. Effects of physical exercise interventions in frail older adults: a systematic review of randomized controlled trials. *BMC Geriatr.* 2015;15:154.

# 21 Ethical Issues for Global Surgical Engagement: The Case of Obstetric Surgery

Clark T. Johnson, MD, MPH
Timothy R.B. Johnson, MD, AM, FACOG

PROLOGUE ▶ Throughout this book, great emphasis has been placed on individual choices. Indeed, all of ethics ultimately comprises choices; hopefully the choices of each surgeon will give personal meaning to life and simultaneously improve the human situation.

The community of surgeons is increasingly global. The need for an awareness of global disparities is forcefully argued in this essay by a father and son, both experienced obstetrician-gynecologists. Taking cesarean section as a paradigm, disparities are recognized and the need for an individual to make decisions about how one spends one's life is emphasized.

Dr Timothy R.B. Johnson and Dr Clark T. Johnson are both concerned with ethical choices regarding one's participation in global health initiatives.

Dr Clark T. Johnson is an assistant professor in the Department of Gynecology and Obstetrics at Johns Hopkins School of Medicine.

Dr Timothy R.B. Johnson is a professor and the former chairman of the Department of Obstetrics and Gynecology at the University of Michigan Medical School.

For decades, surgeons from wealthy countries in the developed global North have traveled and worked in low-income countries, providing care and increasingly helping to build capacity and infrastructure. Careful consideration must be given to ethical issues, both basic classic clinical ethical precepts of nonmaleficence, beneficence, autonomy, and social justice[1] and also the special situations in low-income countries that require attention to health and professional equity issues, given the marked economic disparities and transcultural, translational, and transnational challenges. A useful categorization of these ethical issues in academic global health engagement has been outlined by the recent "CHARTER for collaboration" between academic institutions and the Ministry of Health in Ghana and the University of Michigan[2]: trust, mutual respect, open communication, accountability, financial transparency, development of servant leadership characteristics, and sustainability. We suggest that such a broadened ethical lens should be directed to global surgical initiatives.

Recent data support the need for surgical services in low-income countries.[3] This important document lays out the evidence and economic basis for ethical choices about disease control and prevention priorities in various surgical domains of global health. For example, for obstetric surgery and specifically cesarean delivery, large populations in low- and middle-income countries do not have fundamental access to universal, safe, indicated cesarean.[4] Policy makers, governments, and donors ask whether or not provision of such service is "cost-effective," whereas many clinical providers probably support these services as fundamental human health rights rather than commodities to be negotiated. In a wide variety of global circumstances, in areas where safe cesarean delivery is not available, its provision is cost-effective in terms of about $200 to $3500 per disability-adjusted life year averted by a combination of both maternal survival and prevention of permanent sequelae, including subsequent obstetric fistulas.[5]

These preventable morbidities make the development of the capacity for obstetric surgery and other lifesaving surgical procedures described by Mock et al[3] a priority and place them within an ethical framework of developmental and individual priorities for global health activism. This knowledge of disparity obliges the surgical community to mobilize solutions to these availability and access problems. In the absence of solutions, there is, in effect, a denial of the daily burden of disease attributed to readily pre- 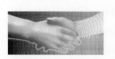 ventable complications of childbirth and common surgical diseases. The ethical imperative to our specialties is ultimately to advocate for patients to help improve health outcomes. This ethical imperative trickles down to individuals, each with the capacity to potentially affect health disparities and poor outcomes globally. Individuals who coordinate their efforts with sustained efforts in effective collaborations committed to ethical principles of engagement can help even more.

In the United States, surgical training is by design done where resources and capacity for the services are provided for a population. In contrast, the needs of global populations may warrant resources be provided in a disparate and isolated geographic area, where the elements of accessible health services that one is trained to expect are not available. Consequently, surgeons interested in authentic global engagement must consider either staying in the place where they have trained or in a similarly resourced setting or providing services where resources might be limited or unavailable. To provide 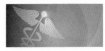 care in a low-resource setting requires firstly ethical considerations for what resources are present, among all the variables that determine where and what a person does for employment. At the population level there will, almost by definition, be disparities in access to health care resources as a result of limited providers. The question remains: What is the ethical consideration of the individual surgeon for the distribution of providers to meet the care of a population. Is this a selfish curiosity of medical tourism[6] or does it represent truly engaged global health aspirations by the individual surgeon?

In the global setting, this consideration of disparities in access to care is complicated by ethical considerations between improvement of areas with greatest need and reinforcement of a current system. Certain areas would benefit greatly by trained providers; however, a circular pattern of "brain drain" prevents retention of trained providers.[7] Natural and structural forces prevent the retention of providers in low-resource settings and aggregate providers to high-resource centers. Comparable forces remain in play in high-income areas, where urban centers retain a disproportionate concentration of surgical specialists, whereas rural areas experience access to care issues similar to low- and middle-income countries. Rural medicine faces many of the challenges in attracting and retaining providers as seen in global medicine.[8]

The autonomy of trained physicians to practice and focus their "work" as desired is paramount, but they must do so following strong ethical principles. Extrinsic factors weigh heavily in this decision, including family factors, the desire to live in specific geographic areas or even in areas where politics or malpractice may affect what type of practice is possible, and so forth. Incentives provided at higher levels have the potential to influence these autonomous decisions[9]—grant repayment programs for working in Federally Qualified Health Centers, for example. Such incentives will likely be attractive to some providers, but not to others, and have their own limitations with disparate global variations.[10]

These influences of government (and potentially some professional societies or nongovernment organizations) can help correct disparity in access but are limited by the motivating efforts in providing the necessary support, financial or otherwise. This is to say these efforts are limited by the will of the people, in the case of government, or by the members of an organization. In the case of government, the effort is further limited by competing goals and priorities of a society. In addition, subsidies to encourage practice in certain areas risk further depletion of workforce capacity where subsidies are not available. Beyond extrinsic factors, engagement in low-resource communities either near home or abroad relies largely on the intrinsic motivation of an individual provider.

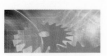

The decision of where to work and what to do for work is largely personal. Extrinsic factors and motivation can influence these decisions, as motivated by policy, but these decisions are ultimately the result of individual behavior. Areas with disparities in health care access rely on the aggregation of these individual decisions to serve the health of a population but with limited tools to help this aggregation.

One of the major challenges of these underserved populations is unawareness of the lack of presumably fundamental health care resources. The challenge of training in a well-resourced setting is nonexposure to limited resourced settings. Some of this is achieved by electives and training experiences that give individuals experience in low-resource settings. For others this can be achieved with interdisciplinary exposure to public health or academic research interests in specific health disparities or underserved populations. For others still, personal experiences and local communities or even religious organizations promote an awareness of those less fortunate. There are surgeons, however, who go through training without a formal exposure to various global health disparities in their discipline. A trainee's exposure to low-resource settings relies largely on individual characteristics or choices made during training.

Globally, there is no shortage of patients with treatable medical and surgical conditions, but there are patients without access to resources for treatment. One would almost expect that creating awareness for these populations is a part of surgical training. With this awareness, an individual can then make an informed decision about how and where to dedicate their work, balancing personal interests with the altruistic interest of improving health outcomes. Although each surgeon must make this decision for himself/herself, the training process should provide the resources for trainees to make informed decisions in this regard. In the absence of awareness or exposure, there is limited motivation to consider practicing independent from what one is familiar with.

The ethical consideration of an individual is to weigh personal experience and preference against the greater health needs of a society. Professional efforts in low- and middle-income countries require a major consideration of economic disparity and social justice not necessarily required in the United States, but the value of health equity as a unifying ethical principle is universal. Each individual will make a different decision about how and how much they contribute, just as each individual must ultimately find comfort in the decision they make. Ultimately, all surgeons are advocates, whether they are aware of it or not. It is incumbent on all surgeons to appreciate their potential role in the larger health system and to contribute ethically as they are able.

# References

1. Jonsen AR, Seigler M, Winslade WJ. *Clinical Ethics: A Practical Approach to Ethical Decisions in Clinical Medicine.* Lange McGraw Hill Education; 2015.
2. Anderson F, Donkor P, de Vries R, et al. Creating a charter of collaboration for international university partnerships: the Elmina Declaration for Human Resources for Health. *Acad Med.* 2014;89(8):1125–1132.
3. Mock CN, Donkor P, Gawande A, et al. Essential surgery: key messages from *Disease Control Priorities*, 3rd edition. *Lancet.* 2015;385(9983):2209–2219.
4. Johnson CT, Adanu RMK, Johnson TRB. Obstetric surgery. In: Debas HT, Donkor P, Gawande A, Jamison DT, Kruk ME, Mock CN, eds. *Essential Surgery: Disease Control Priorities*, 3rd ed. Vol. 1. Washington, DC: World Bank; 2015 [chapter 5].
5. Alkire BC, Vincent JR, Burns CT, Metzler IS, Farmer PE, Meara JG. Obstructed labor and caesarean delivery: the cost and benefit of surgical intervention. *PLoS One.* 2012;7(4):e34595.
6. Anderson FW, Wansom T. Beyond medical tourism: authentic engagement in global health. *Virtual Mentor.* 2009;11(7):506–510.
7. Ahmad OB. Brain drain: the flight of human capital. *Bull World Health Organ.* 2004;82(10):797–798.
8. Strasser R. Rural health around the world: challenges and solutions. *Fam Pract.* 2003;20(4):457–463.
9. Jing L, Liu K, Zhou X, Wang L, Lou J, Sun X. Effectiveness of an incentive policy intervention for rural health-care providers: a longitudinal survey in Shanghai. *Lancet.* 2016;388;(suppl 1):S13.
10. Kruk ME, Johnson JC, Gyakobo M, et al. Rural practice preferences among medical students in Ghana: a discrete choice experiment. *Bull World Health Organ.* 2010;88:333–341.

# 22 Evidence-Based Surgery and Decision Analysis

Thomas A. Schwann, MD, MBA

PROLOGUE ▶ Every choice a surgeon makes is a moral choice. An aphorism from the East states that he/she who alters the natural course of the universe owns forever the well-being of those affected. Therefore it is with the decisions a surgeon makes.

Evidence-based decision analysis stresses that a great many situations in surgery, as in life, which seem at first to be ethical riddles, in fact result from a lack of factual knowledge or a failure to clarify the concepts involved. The surgeon should always, first, endeavor to gather facts and clarify those facts and only afterward declare the situation to represent an ethical dilemma. These should not be considered seriatim, however; knowledge and ethics should proceed hand-in-hand, as they do in appropriate decision analysis.

Dr Thomas A. Schwann is an accomplished cardiac surgeon. In recent years his interests have expanded to include aspects of leadership and decision analysis. He currently, in addition to an active surgical practice, serves as the chief of staff of the University of Toledo Medical Center and is a professor of thoracic and cardiovascular surgery at The University of Toledo College of Medicine.

# Value and Goals of Clinical Practice Guidelines in Health Care

Innovation is the engine that drives human progress and is responsible for our current high standard of living and an unprecedented generation of wealth, with millions of people still existing in abject poverty. In health care, innovation has also contributed to a remarkably increased life expectancy, a reduction (or elimination in the case of small pox) in the scourges of infectious diseases, and insights into the human genome that are predicted to result in revolutionary diagnostic modalities based on biomarkers with the ultimate goal of the development of personalized medicine. Innovation in surgery has transformed the profession from largely a field that focused on amputation and wound care to a discipline dedicated to reversing varied pathologic processes, reconstruction rather than excision, and the development of procedures that extend patients' life expectancy and improve the quality of their lives. Innovation has resulted in a transformation in human knowledge generation and acquisition from a linear to an exponential growth. Buckminster Fuller created the "Knowledge Doubling Curve" (see Figure 22.1) and noted that until the dawn of the 20th century, human knowledge doubled approximately every century. From the 1940s, knowledge was doubling every 25 years. From the 1980s, only 7 years were required to double medical knowledge, and in 2010, that period was reduced to 3.5 years.[1] Today, specific disciplines have been noted to have distinct knowledge doubling times with clinical knowledge doubling every 18 months and general knowledge doubling every 13 months. An analysis from

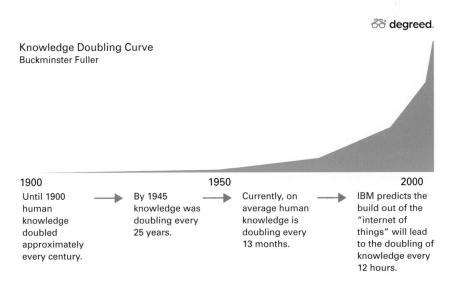

FIGURE 22.1 **Knowledge doubling curve.** (Adapted from Degreed. Courtesy, The Estate of R. Buckminster Fuller.)

International Business Machines (IBM), the birth of the "internet of things" will lead to a staggering rate of knowledge doubling estimated at 12 hours.

Knowledge is expanding faster than our ability to assimilate the information produced, with biologically imposed constraints on our cognitive abilities to constructively and consciously use the emerging data. In health care, how to comprehensively teach the medical students and other learners the basics and the newest emerging advances, what are the most effective techniques for learning this material within the defined time constraints, and, perhaps most importantly, how to successfully manipulate and apply this knowledge avalanche into clinical care to address the myriad of challenges facing health care remain, as of yet, unsolved challenges. The ability to incorporate this information explosion has been further complicated by the remarkable growth in new technology in the treatment of diseases. In such an era of information satiety, clinical practice guidelines (CPGs) have emerged as one method of providing a manageable heuristic tool to guide clinicians in decision making and optimizing care delivery. CPGs are manageable and concise tools that provide clinicians with a summary of the best available evidence-based recommendations, developed by content experts and condensed into practical summaries and directives for optimal management in specific clinical circumstances. In 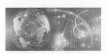 short, these constructs are concise summaries of optimal health care pathways for the average patients. Since their birth in the 1950s, CPGs have exploded in both scope and number paralleling the growth in medical information. Indeed, the Agency for Healthcare Research and Quality has been charged to be the CPG national clearing house (http://www.guidelines.gov).[2] In 1992, the Institute of Medicine opined that CPGs should be "systematically developed statements to assist practitioner and patient decisions about appropriate healthcare for specific clinical circumstances."[3] In addition, to be useful, CPGs must improve the care being delivered by expediting the application of the latest evidence-based effective advances into clinical practice, eliminate waste, and enhance standardization. More recently, CPGs have been used as tools to drive standardization and payment policies, for example, in the U.S. Preventative Services Task Force and for insurance coverage under the Affordable Care Act. Given the increasing importance and reliance on CPGs, the Institute of Medicine recently published standards for developing maximally effective CPGs.[4] There has been an effort to incorporate only level A or level B evidence into CPGs and a view that less robust evidence should be relegated to expert consensus documents or expert opinions/white papers.[5] Given this lower level of evidence behind them, expert consensus opinions should be considered "suggestions" rather than guidelines by the health care community. Despite these specifications for effective clinical support tools, variability exists in the value of these clinical constructs as they span a wide spectrum of formats from CPGs to consensus statements by various expert panels, to position statements, and to white papers. CPGs are only possible where robust comparative data exist to allow a systemic review, which is the sine qua non of CPGs. The dissemination of CPGs via electronic mobile platforms (such as iPhones and the iTunes Store) should ensure ease of availability to the end user and perhaps increase clinician compliance, which is currently relatively low as evidenced by a recent Harris Interactive poll in which only 44% of physicians self-reported that they consistently relay on CPGs in their activities. It has been argued that such skepticism of CPGs contributes to the observation that only about half of health care delivered is appropriate.[6]

Surgical innovation is intended to provide some tangible benefit for the patient by improving outcomes, decreasing costs, or both. In contradistinction to innovation in other health care fields, surgical innovation is rather loosely regulated. Indeed, some would say that it is unregulated and depends only on the creativity and ingenuity of the surgeon. Surgical innovation must be clearly distinguished from surgical research, which is defined as a method of testing a hypothesis so that a scientific conclusion may be drawn.[7] The current lack of regulatory oversight of "standard surgical procedures" may be a reflection of the high degree of variability in the various discreet steps that comprise any given surgical procedure. In the absence of a universally accepted standardized procedure, regulatory oversight is difficult, if not impossible. Even within any given institution, there is variability in the details of a surgical procedure that is surgeon specific and reflects the diversity of the training received by surgeons in their various residency programs. Surgeons make individualized decisions about the size of the incision and how best to perform the multitude of intermediary steps that collectively culminate in the entire successful surgical procedure. Given such variability, macroscopic system-wide quality improvement efforts are difficult because there is no meaningful method of implementing a system-wide change, with alignment of all individual providers to an agreed-on standard. In addition, any system-wide quality improvement effort within the current highly variable surgical practice can be very difficult to measure as it is often impossible to attribute outcomes to a specific version of an operation. This lack of correlation is an impediment to meaningful quality improvement as exemplified by the well-accepted adage from the business world: "if one cannot measure it, one cannot manage it."

The intrinsic variability in surgical procedures, despite their shortcomings, may serve as laboratories for testing the outcomes of these differences in the management of surgical diseases and allows practitioners to use their creativity, imagination, and ingenuity to optimize procedures and processes. Unfortunately, currently there is no infrastructure that is capable of monitoring or systematically measuring the impact of such "experimentation" and frequently we are left only with anecdotal impressions of possible improvements. It is rare, if ever, that data emerge into the public arena on any negative effects of well-intended surgical innovative efforts. Importantly, 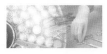 any innovative processes occur at the discretion of the surgeon without the need for external or internal oversight. There are no local, state, or federal regulatory agencies involved in overseeing surgical innovation that does not involve new products or equipment. Notably, no institutional review board approval is required, although ideally this should be part of every significant modification of a surgical procedure. It is also only infrequent that the institutional ethics committee becomes a part of the surgical innovation process. Ultimately it is the responsibility of the medical staff, through their responsibility for quality and oversight of patient safety, delegated from the institutional governing body (the board of trustees), that determines what an appropriate and acceptable level of care is. Input from institutional leadership or departmental chairpersons is useful to ensure that multiple conflicting ethical interests are well adjudicated, and conflict of interests, real or perceived, are resolved. Alternatively, a more structured oversight approach has been proposed in the form of a New Surgical Technology Committee with multiple stakeholders, representing discreet view points and interests, driving the process. Regardless of the degree of oversight, given the Hippocratic dedication to the mantra of "do no harm," it is incumbent principally on each individual surgeon to ensure patient safety and to critically and honestly evaluate any possible deleterious effect of a proposed innovation. How to reconcile the possible but unproven benefits of surgical innovation with patient safety and individual patient benefits versus societal benefits enters the realm of medical ethics. The American College of Surgeons Code of Professional Conduct[7] stipulates that surgeons have a responsibility to be advocates for individual patients as well as be good stewards of societal interests by driving innovation and using resources in a cost-effective manner. Although altruistic and well intended, such dual responsibilities will likely present an ethical conflict for the surgeon. The American Board of Internal Medicine in its Physician Charter on Medical Professionalism in the New Millennium[8] has articulated a guiding Principle of the Primacy of Patient Welfare, which specifies that market forces, societal pressures, and administrative exigencies must not compromise this principle in guiding the clinician's actions. Frequently, surgical innovation is driven through evolutionary incremental modifications to existing techniques as opposed to disruptive transformative new approaches. Exceptions to this represent the development of laparoscopic techniques and, more recently, robotic techniques.

How should surgical innovation be implemented to safeguard patients in an era of increased emphasis on standardization as stipulated in CPGs? In contemporary surgery, significant progress has been made to minimize complications. Thus, more often than not, innovative surgical techniques will have 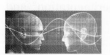 a lower rate of complications than the already low rate associated with the procedure that is being innovated. To assess whether a new approach is superior to the current standard of care, a large number of patients will be required to undergo the procedure, before definitive conclusions about its safety and efficacy can be drawn. In the absence of safety monitoring boards, this can prove challenging and profoundly disturbing for the innovator who is forced to operate in a setting of ambiguity. The ethical issues become particularly pertinent in securing informed consent from patients who may be the first few to undergo a modified procedure. How can one present an informed consent when the perioperative risks or the long-term benefits or outcomes are uncertain? Should the patient be informed that he/she may be one of the first few to undergo this procedure understanding that the learning curve may not yet have been mastered? What is the basis of the belief that the 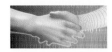 new or innovative procedure will produce the anticipated results, especially in the absence of extensive comparative outcome trials? The innovating surgeon must be cognizant of the potential conflicts of interest between his/her duty to protect patients' interests and other possible motivating factors driving the process such as the desire of the hospital to be viewed as being on the cutting edge and a leader in innovation, especially if the institution has invested heavily in the program and its marketing, be based more on hope of excellent outcomes than objective data. Furthermore, the innovating surgeon must be continuously vigilant and acknowledge competing self-interests such as his/her own financial interests or academic prestige, which may affect the ability to objectively judge the value of a new procedure.

Typically, the innovating surgeon will publish retrospective single institutional outcomes that may engender interest from other surgeons, the early adopters, who may be interested in incorporating the procedure into their own clinical armamentarium. How are these surgeons going to address the ethical issues of patient safety and informed consent? Are their surgical skills equivalent to the pioneering surgeon and will they achieve similar clinical outcomes? How are they going to master the learning curve while simultaneously protecting patients' interests? What are the appropriate markers of having achieved expertise in the new procedure? Do resources exist within the institution or within the health care delivery system to offer the early adopter the opportunity for animal training? Cadaveric training? Simulation training? Should in-OR (operating room) mentoring and preceptorships be a requisite before operating on patients? Are their institutional resources and their team expertise and experience commensurate with the intricacies of the new procedure? As the collective experience with the innovative procedure grows, retrospective analyses of nationwide registries, if they exist, may be a possible method to more rigorously define the efficacy of a new procedure and to assess its role in the therapeutic spectrum. If these results support the innovation, then randomized controlled trials may be undertaken because this currently represents the gold standard of comparative outcome studies. The innovating surgeon then faces yet another ethical dilemma of whether to enroll their patients into a randomized controlled trial, fully believing that therapeutic equipoise between the competing procedures does not exist and in their hands the outcomes associated with the innovation are superior.

# Is Newer Always Better?

There is an overwhelming assumption that newer must be better. This is deeply engrained in our psyche and exploited by marketers frequently framing ad campaigns around the phrase "newer and improved." The public expectations 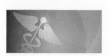 of newer surgical techniques being better are reinforced by the experience in the ubiquitous improvements with each new generation of electronic gadgets, be they our cell phones or computers. Each new version makes the previous models almost obsolete within years or, in some cases, months. The public's experience in the digital world is transferred to health care with similar expectations. Combining this faith in the new with the fact that technology associated with the newer techniques are marvels of engineering design (ie, the daVinci robot) and frequently heavily advertised, although often without a sound basis. Indeed, in a recent *New England Journal of Medicine* editorial, an estimated additional $2.5 billion was added to the national health care tab for robotic procedures without a notable benefit and 50% of hospital Web sites contained unsubstantiated and exotic claims of robotic benefits.[9]

The allure of new high-tech procedures exerts its mesmerizing effects not only on patients but also on providers. The competitive nature of health care and the desire of surgeons to distinguish themselves from their peers produce a hallucinogenic attraction to new technology as a platform to augment the surgeons' prestige in academic circles and establish a reputation of being "on the cutting edge" of the field. It is imperative for the surgeon from an ethical perspective to objectively and honestly evaluate the merits of an innovative approach on its merits and benefits for the patient rather than the surgeon.

# Surgical Innovation and Informed Consent

The informed consent process reflects the providers' commitment to the contemporary ethos of respecting patient autonomy, a fundamental element of bioethics. As such, informed consent was designed to allow the patient to make a rational decision on whether or not the treatment being considered is in his own interest based on accurate assessment of the risks and benefits of the intervention in question, as well as the risks and benefits of alternative, frequently nonsurgical, options. Although intuitively simple, on more in-depth scrutiny, the informed consent process has some ethical challenges. Fundamentally, there must be recognition that, in a fee-for-service health care system, the provider and the patient may have a conflict of interest because the full disclosure of the procedural risks, especially if its benefits are not well defined, may result in a financial loss for the provider inherent in an alternative therapeutic choice. In addition, there is frequent ambiguity and disagreement on the benefits of alternative therapies whose risk-benefit profile is simply not well defined and represents one of the limits of our collective health care knowledge. This stems from the fact that health care, at present, lacks a robust system of capturing nonprocedural-based outcomes across the wide spectrum of providers such that this information is simply not available in a meaningful and precise fashion. In addition, the data that do exist on the risks and benefits of a given procedure seem to be interpreted quite differently by providers with significant interobserver disagreement of the risks and benefits of a surgical procedure. Sacks et al found wide differences in surgeons' perception of operative and nonsurgical alternatives, risks, and benefits, as well as their decisions to offer an operative intervention (49%-85% agreement to offer an operation).[10] Interestingly, the empirically derived surgical risk calculators now available to surgeons (The Society of Thoracic Surgeons Online Risk Calculator and the American College of Surgeons National Surgical Quality Improvement Program Surgical Risk Calculator)[11,12] may aid in surgical decision making by providing objective assessment of perioperative risk based on patient demographics, yet they have been shown not to affect a surgeon's decision to operate.[13] Thus, surgical decision making in the face of ambiguity must inevitably affect the informed consent process. Awareness of these knowledge gaps and cognitive deficits is important to assure a robust and accurate informed consent process and perhaps mitigate the current observation that 25% of Medicare patients will undergo an operation within 3 months of the end of life, arguably futile interventions devoid of any meaningful impact on appreciably extending the patient's life expectancy, to say nothing of the associated incurred cost.[14]

---

## Ethical Conflict Between Surgical Innovation and Clinical Practice Guidelines–Driven Standardization of Care

The ultimate goals of all CPGs are efficient, safe, and fiscally prudent care through adherence to the articulated best practice recommendations and thus in the end, practice pattern standardization. Indeed, CPGs were and continue to be  developed to address controversial relevant clinical scenarios where significant variability in practice exists and leads frequently to disparities in outcomes. For example, in a large nationwide analysis of banked blood utilization in cardiac surgical patients, the transfusion rate ranges from 8% to 93%.[15] Such variability, known to adversely affect efficiency in the manufacturing sector and long since eliminated, stems from the traditional individualist approach to surgery that resulted from an unflinching belief that an individual provider was best suited to provide optimal care. At best, this approach continues to propagate a haphazard approach to clinical care and 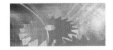 springs from the apprenticeship model of our medical education. We learn from mentors who were trained in the era of the great surgical leaders who espoused an individualistic approach to health care quality driven as much by "cult personality" as by data. Such a mano-a-mano approach to surgical challenges led to distinct schools of thought as what constitutes the best approach to surgical pathology, each with doctrines that have been propagated over multiple generations through our surgical residency training programs. Not infrequently, the adopted approach as the standard of care was driven by the academic prestige and the eloquence of the surgeon rather than objective data. As in other fields, such degrees of variability in health care are not ideal and CPGs have been developed to succinctly articulate the most appropriate approach and to standardize care across the nation. Such efforts have resulted in the development of the joint Society of Thoracic Surgeons and the Society of Cardiovascular Anesthesiologists Perioperative Blood Transfusion and Blood Conservation Guidelines.[16] Whether this effort will bear fruit in decreasing clinician's variability in transfusion practices remains unclear.

Standardization of care, however, by definition, minimizes chances for meaningful innovation. Notably, before the development of the Society of Thoracic Surgeons Database in the 1990s, it was impossible for patients, third-party payers, or regulatory agencies to delineate the average mortality risk in heart surgery across the United States, aside from what was reported in peer-reviewed publications from leading cardiac surgical centers. Nevertheless, 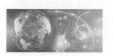 in the health care of previous eras, when standardization was not emphasized, innovative approaches were prolific and significant advances in surgery were made. The disruptive innovations in health care of the last several decades were notable in the development of laparoscopic surgery followed by robotic surgery. It should be pointed out that the first surgeon, an Austrian surgeon named Kurt Semm, to perform a laparoscopic appendectomy in 1980 was heavily criticized by the established surgical experts who failed to realize the impact of this technology on the course of surgical treatment. Innovation by the cardiology community in the late 1970s led to the development of percutaneous platforms for the treatment of coronary artery disease with concurrent tectonic shifts in the surgical treatment of coronary artery disease that still reverberate throughout the cardiovascular community today. Importantly, this approach was incorporated into clinical practice with relatively little regulatory oversight. Indeed, the initial clinical results were hailed as either revolutionary and innovative or dangerous and cavalier (technical success rate of 63%, 36% complication rate)[17] akin to redecorating one's living room with dynamite depending on one's specialty and possible commitment to, and benefit from, the established, principally surgery-based, standard of care. Yet, without these innovative approaches and the associated early risks principally borne by those early recipients of these therapies, the rich benefits enjoyed by today's patients and society of these techniques would not have been possible. Thus, from an ethical perspective of this earlier era, the early patients' risk exposure was accepted by the medical community and was offset by the later generations' beneficiaries across the health care landscape.

The contemporary complexity of health care delivery also contributes to the substantial variability in the delivery of health care, as it is exceedingly difficult to "protocolize" all aspects of clinical practice. Until very recently, there was simply a lack of data-gathering tools to ascertain the extent of that variability and the capacity to correlate it with meaningful patient outcomes. Taking cues from the manufacturing sector, through quality improvement tools such as Lean or Six-Sigma, proved convincingly that variability is a significant obstacle to efficiency and is associated with product defects; health care has recently placed increasing emphasis on standardization of provider practice patterns. This emphasis toward standardization in the pursuit of efficiency and quality is an effort to address the "inconvenient truth" that preventable harm in health care is the third leading cause of patient death,[18] which in large part explains the proliferation of CPGs. The staggering cost of noneffective therapies has been estimated to be a third of the entire health care costs or $1 trillion or $9000 per household.[18] The struggle in health care is akin to the Jeffersonian- versus Hamiltonian-type conflict between independent flexible individual provider innovation and a centrally planned rather rigid set of guidelines often criticized as "cookbook medicine." Given the strong emphasis on individuality in the health care ethos, it is not surprising that significant opposition to the later approach exists among providers.[19] CPGs are viewed as intrusive by multiple clinicians who argue that they reflect and perpetuate established biases of the writing committees and become unbendable dogma and accepted principles when in fact they were not meant to be so, given the complexity of the clinical realities under which they may not be applicable given the large number, if not an infinite spectrum of variables that enter a clinical decision based on the patient's variable presentation.

With the recent availability of robust health care analytics, one has to ask whether variability might be the flip side of innovation if positive patient outcomes can be correlated to a specific iteration of health care practices. Although hypothetically possible, the required sophistication of data analysis to achieve this goal surpasses what is currently available in health care informatics and will likely remain aspirational for the foreseeable future. In the current state of affairs, clinician variability will unfortunately continue to result in higher than necessary error rates, team malalignment, and general chaos as opposed to an esprit d'corps among well-integrated multidisciplinary teams delivering patient-centered care.

A specific example of surgeons ignoring CPG comes from contemporary cardiac surgery. Coronary artery bypass surgery (CABG) is perhaps one of the most intensely studied surgical procedures in the history of medicine. Since its inception in the late 1960s, it has progressed through a number of iterations driven by innovative surgeons. Initially the operation relied on the exclusive use of saphenous vein grafts (SVGs) as conduits 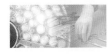 for myocardial revascularization. This initial approach was followed by the adoption of the left internal thoracic artery (LITA) as a solitary arterial graft usually used to bypass the left anterior coronary artery in conjunction with additional SVGs to bypass other diseased coronary targets. The use of LITA in CABG has resulted in improved long-term survival, given the favorable physiologic properties of arterial versus venous grafts resulting in substantially greater LITA patency (90% at 10 years) compared with SVG patency (50% at 7 years). Not surprisingly, this single arterial bypass grafting strategy has been the standard of care since the 1990s, although the transition from all SVG grafting to LITA/SVG has taken over 2 decades to complete. Given the improved outcomes with a single arterial graft, multiple innovators have undertaken to assess whether incremental benefits can be achieved with additional arterial grafts in CABG patients. The principal additional arterial conduits that have been explored are the radial artery (RA) and the right internal thoracic artery. Collectively these newer iterations of the traditional CABG procedure have been designated as multiarterial CABG. Since 2004, a growing body of literature has uniformly confirmed the superiority of the multiarterial CABG in terms of patient survival compared with the traditional single arterial CABG.[20,21] This has resulted in the incorporation of multiarterial CABG into CPGs in the United States and Europe.[22-25] Despite these efforts, the surgical community remains skeptical about efficacy of multiarterial CABG, and only about 10% of all CABG patients are grafted with multiarterial grafts.[26] Arguably our patients are being disenfranchised from an improved long-term survival by surgeons not following CPGs. Our group has been an early adopter of multiarterial grafting in the form of the RA as the additional arterial graft to be used in conjunction with the LITA. Since 1996, our group has progressively increased the utilization of the RA, such that today more than 75% of our patients receive more than one arterial graft. It has been estimated that a similarly robust adoption of multiarterial grafting across the United States would result in 10 000 fewer deaths and an additional 64 000 person life-years over a decade.[27]

Our innovative journey with multiarterial CABG highlights the multiple ethical issues discussed. Our initial interest in using RA was based on a report of excellent long-term RA patency published in 1992.[28] Driven by a commitment to optimizing patient outcomes, we began using RA in a highly selective fashion in relatively younger patients who would have a long enough life expectancy to benefit from the improved durability of the RA compared with the SVG. Being cognizant of the fact that there were 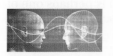 no available data on clinically meaningful outcomes for patients with this technique, our group joined the emerging Society of Thoracic Surgeons National Adult Cardiac Surgery Database (our institution was the fourth in the nation to join this quality effort) to assess our risk-adjusted perioperative outcomes to assure our patients that this technique did not expose them to increased risk of adverse short-term outcomes. We instituted a monthly meticulous review of our perioperative outcomes over the next 10 years, finding that our observed mortality was lower than the predicted mortality, thus consistently achieving superior outcomes. Concurrently, we developed a robust research infrastructure to focus on the impact of RA grafting on long-term survival. In 2004, we published our results, which showed that RA grafting was associated with statistically significant improved survival up to 6 years postoperatively.[21] Thus, within the span of 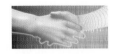 8 years, we were able to convince ourselves that this technique not only did not increase short-term operative risk but also actually extended patients' life expectancy. Based on these results, we transitioned from a selective use of the RA to its routine use with similar improved survival noted among all clinically important patients' subcohorts. We have endeavored to share our enthusiasm for multiarterial grafting with the cardiac surgical community, but in light of the low adoption rate of this technique into the therapeutic armamentarium by cardiac surgeons, we believe that we have a large quality improvement opportunity in contemporary cardiac surgery. Given the impracticality of randomized controlled trials in evaluating competing surgical techniques, we have redoubled our efforts to document the superiority of multiarterial CABG by studying the biggest clinical database developed by the Society of Thoracic Surgeons (STS) comprised of millions of CABG patients. The intent is to assure the cardiac surgery constituency that the results published by our group will be reproducible in a much larger data set and thus assure generalizability to other practice settings. Paradoxically, surgeons when asked to decide on a grafting strategy that they would choose if they needed a CABG, 49% would choose the multiarterial approach.[29] The ethics of clinging to a familiar traditional procedure in the light of consistent emerging data on the benefits of newer versions of the same procedure, without a single report indicating any increased risk, needs closer evaluation.

In summary, surgeons have an ethical obligation to innovate and improve surgical techniques safely, timely, effectively, and transparently. Full disclosure to the patient of the innovative nature of any new procedure is absolutely imperative to facilitate shared decision making based on the best available informed consent. Patients' decisions to opt out of participating in any new procedure must be respected. Surgical innovation is associated with a host of ethical dilemmas that will need to carefully balance a whole host of thorny conflict of interest issues. CPGs represent the most up-to-date, concise, evidence-based treatment recommendations compiled by experts and/or professional societies and thus should be incorporated by clinicians into their practice patterns for the majority of their patients. To be most effective, CPGs need to be deployed with sound clinical judgment. Capricious failure to comply with CPGs represents an ethical "no man's land" and should be avoided.

# References

1. Densen P. Challenges and opportunities facing medical education. *Trans Am Clin Climatol Assoc.* 2011;122:48–58.
2. Weisz G, Cambrosio A, Keating P, et al. The emergence of clinical practice guidelines. *Milbank Q.* 2007;85:691–727.
3. Field MJ, Lohr KN, IoM Committee to Advise the Public Health Service on Clinical Practice Guidelines. *Clinical Practice Guidelines: Directions for a New Program.* Washington, DC: National Academy Press; 1990.
4. Institute of Medicine. *Clinical Practice Guidelines We Can Trust.* Washington, DC: National Academies Press; 2011.
5. Bakaeen FG, Svensson LG, Mitchell JD, Keshavjee S, Patterson A, Weisel RD. The American Association for Thoracic Surgery/Society of Thoracic Surgeons position statement on developing clinical practice documents. *Ann Thorac Surg.* 2017;103:1350–1356.
6. McGlynn EA, Asch SM, Adams J, et al. The quality of health care delivered to adults in the United States. *N Engl J Med.* 2003;348:2635–2645.
7. American College of Surgeons, Code of Professional Conduct. http://www.facs.org.
8. American Board of Internal Medicine. Charter on Medical Professionalism; 2002. http://www.abimfoundation.org/Professionalism/Physician-Charter.aspx.
9. Barbash GI, Glied SA. New technology and health care costs—the case of robot assisted surgery. *N Engl J Med.* 2010;363:701–704.
10. Sacks GD, Dawes AJ, Ettner SL, et al. Surgeon perception of risk and benefit in the decision to operate. *Ann Surg.* 2016;264:896–903.
11. http://riskcalc.sts.org/stswebriskcalc/#/.
12. http://riskcalculator.facs.org/RiskCalculator/PatientInfo.jsp.
13. Sacks GD, Dawes AJ, Ettner SL, et al. Impact of a risk calculator on risk perception and surgical decision making: a randomized trial. *Ann Surg.* 2016;264:889–895.
14. Kwok AC, Semel ME, Lipsitz SR, et al. The intensity and variation of surgical care at the end of life: a retrospective cohort study. *Lancet.* 2011;378:1408–1413.
15. Bennett-Guerrero E, Zhao Y, O'Brien SM, et al. Variation in use of blood transfusion in coronary artery bypass graft surgery. *JAMA.* 2010;304:1568–1575.
16. Ferraris VA, Brown JR, Despotis GJ, et al. 2011 update to the Society of Thoracic Surgeons and the Society of Cardiovascular Anesthesiologists blood conservation clinical practice guidelines. *Ann Thorac Surg.* 2011;91:944–982.
17. Dorros G, Cowely MJ, Simpson J, et al. Percutaneous transluminal coronary angioplasty: report of complications from the National Heart, Lung and Blood Institute PTCA Registry. *Circulation.* 1983;67:723–730.
18. Pronovost PJ. Enhancing physicians' use of clinical guidelines. *JAMA.* 2013;310:2501–2502.
19. Lamos J, Anderson GM, Domnick-Pierre K, Vayda E, Enkin MW, Hannah WJ. Do practice guidelines guide practice? The effect of a consensus statement on practice of physicians. *N Engl J Med.* 1989;321:1306–1311.
20. Lytle BW, Blackstone EH, Sabik JF, Houghtaling P, Loop FD, Cosgrove DM. The effect of bilateral internal thoracic artery grafting on survival during 20 postoperative years. *Ann Thorac Surg.* 2004;78(6):2005–2012.
21. Zacharias A, Habib RH, Schwann T, Riordan C, Durham S, Shah A. Improved survival with radial artery versus vein conduits in coronary bypass surgery with left internal thoracic artery to left anterior descending artery grafting. *Circulation.* 2004;109:1489–1496.

22. Eagle KA, Guyton RA, Davidoff R, et al. ACC/AHA 2004 guideline update for coronary artery bypass graft surgery. *Circulation.* 2004;110:1168–1176.

23. Hillis DL, Smith PK, Anderson JL, et al. 2011 ACCF/AHA guideline for coronary artery bypass surgery: executive summary: a report of the American College of Cardiology Foundation/American Heart Association Task Force on Practice Guidelines. *Circulation.* 2011;124:2610–2642.

24. Windecker S, Kolh P, Alfonso F, et al. 2014 ESC/EACTS guidelines on myocardial revascularization. *Eur Heart J.* 2014;35:2541–2619.

25. Aldea GS, Bakaeen FG, Pal J, et al. The Society of Thoracic Surgeons clinical practice guidelines on arterial conduits for coronary artery bypass grafting. *Ann Thorac Surg.* 2016;101:801–809.

26. Schwann TA, Tatoulis J, Puskas J, et al. World wide trends in multi arterial CABG surgery 2004-2014: a tale of two continents. *Semin Thorac Cardiovasc Surg.* 2017;29(3):273–280. doi: 10.1053/j.semtcvs.2017.05.018.

27. Tranbaugh RF, Lucido DJ, Dimitrova KR, et al. Multiple arterial bypass grafting should be routine. *J Thorac Cardiovasc Surg.* 2015;150:1537–1545.

28. Acar C, Jebara VA, Portoghese M, et al. Revival of the radial artery for coronary artery bypass grafting. *Ann Thorac Surg.* 1992;54:652–660.

29. Catarino PA, Black E, Taggart DP. Why do UK cardiac surgeons not perform their first choice operation for coronary artery bypass graft? *Heart.* 2002;88:643–644.

# 23 The Millennial Surgeon

Lloyd A. Jacobs, MD

PROLOGUE ▶ The great majority of current trainees in the discipline of surgery are of the generation called millennial. It is important to think how this generation may differ from older generations.

The world is currently experiencing a return to subjectivity after 2 or 3 centuries characterized by the ascendancy of objectivity. This reversal began perhaps with Kierkegaard and was continued with Heidegger. The Millennial Generation is currently living the apogee of this trend. They have, therefore, been misunderstood by the generations who have so heavily invested their intellectual and emotional lives in the objectivity of modern science. Contrary to the railing of some, however, Millennials are more than worthy of the legacy of our discipline and its ethics. Millennial surgeons are both skilled and committed.

The great majority of residents and fellows in surgical training programs are of the "Millennial" Generation. Notwithstanding that elders have complained about the youth in their societies since the ancients, it is widely believed that a great gulf exists between the values and ethics of the Millennial Generation and those of generations that preceded it. While I believe that the breadth and depth of this gulf has been exaggerated, those surgeons who are of the Millennial Generation and who participate in a different array of ethical norms must be more fully understood as the great and venerable discipline of surgery is passed to them.

The Pew Research Center has listed a set of definitions of generations. These designations are not of the Center's invention but are more reflective of what has become common usage in our culture. Moreover, the definitions are leaky; there is much spillover related to other socioeconomic and ethnic backgrounds. However, there is enough consistency of ethical stance to warrant some thought. The Pew Research Center[1] lists the generations as follows:

---

## The Generations Defined

### The Millennial Generation
Born: 1981 to 1997
Age of adults in 2015: 18 to 34 years

### Generation X
Born: 1965 to 1980
Age in 2015: 35 to 50 years

### The Baby Boomer Generation
Born: 1946 to 1964
Age in 2015: 51 to 69 years

### The Silent Generation
Born: 1928 to 1945
Age in 2015: 70 to 87 years

### The Greatest Generation
Born: before 1928
Age in 2015: 88 to 100 years

It is immediately evident that most practicing surgeons and surgical faculty members are of the Generation X or Baby Boomer Generation. If there are real cultural and ethical distinctions between the Millennials and those generations, it follows that there are real cultural and ethical distinctions between surgical faculty and attending surgeons and their trainees. Do these distinctions affect the relationships between faculty members and trainees? Do these distinctions affect teaching and learning styles? Do these  distinctions bode well or ill for the future of our discipline? These and other questions will only be answered in time but may deserve some examination because the distinctions not only include differences in cultural foundations but may also be manifested in the daily lives of those involved.

The Millennial Generation has been disparagingly characterized as egotistic, hedonistic, and narcissistic. They are sometimes charged with being uncommitted, selfish, and even lazy. Such characterizations are not only incorrect, but also they are derived from ignorance about the real foundations of the thought paradigms of this group. Moreover, they are gratuitously insulting. If the characteristics ascribed were correct, a dismal future for our discipline would be implied. My own belief is that the youth called the Millennials have much to offer, are clearly possessed of great intellect, and are of an ethical posture, which is slightly different from but is perhaps even more solid than that of "Silents" and "Boomers."

Surgical residents and fellows are, by virtue of their choice of our discipline, conservative in their values. Their ethics and their moral philosophies are often closer to those of earlier generations than to the values and ethics of their Millennial peers. By virtue of the career choice already made, surgical trainees are, to some degree at least, altruistic and beneficent. It is difficult, however, to summarize simply the complex ethics of the Millennial Generation.

Millennials have imbibed deeply the culture of postmodernism. Their ethical foundations are characterized by doubt. They doubt the classical ideas of truth and the certainty of logic and reason; they see humankind as more contingent than substantive. Their worldview is without grounding, without foundation; their world is unstable and indeterminate. At a more mundane-level pedestrian pace, they are more concerned about lifestyle and work-life balance than their forebears. Their minds are perhaps quicker, they tolerate prolixity less, and they place less credence on the grand narratives of Western culture.

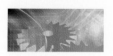

In what is nearly a *coincidentia oppositorum*, earlier generations of surgeons gave of themselves to their discipline in what appeared as almost monomaniacal. Their spouses raised their children. Their outside relationships are thought to have suffered. In some, their devotion was transformed to a harshness, which often manifested itself as an autocratic, hypercritical nature. Whether these weaknesses will develop among the Millennials as they age remains to be seen. Whether Millennials will in the future experience less divorce, substance abuse, suicide, and depression than their forebears remains to be seen.

Much has been written about Millennials and the age of information. The emphasis of learning is slowly changing from the need to hold a great repertoire of facts to an expertise in accessing these facts electronically. Millennials have outstripped their forebears in this regard, and although their expertise is salutatory, it has made some older surgeons suspicious. Furthermore, questions concerning the accuracy of information thus obtained are real. The information available is nearly infinite; the choice of an information source raises serious epistemic questions. It is necessary, furthermore, that the users of electronic information sources develop a hierarchy of degrees of warrant for any proposition given by the testimony of the Internet. The use of electronic devices on rounds or in clinics has seemed discourteous to some faculty mentors and indicative of inattention. Millennials are far more facile than their elders with an electronic medical record, the advent of which has caused great distress to preceding generations.

The most important characteristic of the Millennial is the disbelief of that generation in the grand narratives of our society. They have little belief in the "American Dream." They are skeptical of the notion of continued progress, even of the "upward" progress of surgical sciences. Indeed, they are skeptical of established science as a force of continuous progress for humankind. Their communication comes in small pieces: 280 characters per tweet, television sound bites of news in the range of 60 seconds or less, and so forth. Their world is staccato, abrupt, and disconnected. They change jobs frequently. Their attention span is alleged to be short. There are 3 areas where this shortened cycle time may have an impact on the practice of our discipline.

Teaching surgeons have commented that residents are excellent at specific manual maneuvers but tend to lack on overall sense of the progression of an operation. They respond to individual occurrences but perhaps lose their focus on where an operation is going in its entirety. They may perform and react in "bytes" and miss the context.

The critical care of postoperative surgical patients in the intensive care unit may display a similar trend. Once settled there, we tend to respond piecemeal to isolated, singular occurrences. The oxygen saturation decreases; we increase the positive end-expiratory pressure. The creatinine rises; we respond appropriately. The wound leaks serosanguineous fluid; we react to that occurrence. We tend to fail in the recognition of a "grand narrative" and fail to see the postoperative course in its entirety.

There is no aspect of our discipline where this tendency is more striking than in considering end-of-life issues for the surgical patient. We respond appropriately to the "present illness" and the present complication but may fail to see the patient's life in context. We may fail to contextualize the love, the accomplishments, and the suffering of each patient as unique.

Millennials wish for meaningful work. They wish for meaning in their lives. Millennials are hardworking; it is not true that they have abandoned the "work ethic." However, they cannot tolerate busywork. In addition, Millennials are on a constant search for meaning in their own lives as well as in their occupations. Seventy-five percent of them believe that American culture is inadequately focused on improving the life of all citizens in our society. Surgery has at its foundation a commitment to excellence and beneficence. The very substance of the discipline is in acting for another. 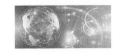 Millennials are passionate about this type of devotion and are willing to sacrifice a great deal for it. The notion of practical ethics for the surgeon provides the meaning that Millennials crave. A surgical life provides the meaning they seek.

The discipline of surgery has survived massive sociologic changes in the past and will do so again. Residents and fellows may wish to think more about the grand narrative of the discipline of surgery through at least 30 centuries. Moreover, as ontogeny recapitulates phylogeny, trainees may wish to think about connectedness, linearity, and context in their careers as working surgeons and in the lives of their patients.

For their part, faculty members and attending surgeons must recognize that Millennials will be our successors whether we wish it to be so or not. They bring to our discipline a focus that is very much needed now at the maturation of the age of modernity and modern surgery. Millennials wish for the life of meaning that a commitment to the discipline of surgery can so richly provide. Millennials are humanists, more deontologists than teleologists in their ethics. A much simplified variant of the "Mayor's dilemma" may illustrate this point. Imagine you are one of the 3 captives of an amoral and ferocious group of captors. They offer you 2 choices; in either choice you will be spared. Kill 1 of your 2 companions with your own hands with weapons of your choice, or witness your captors killing, in your presence, both of your companion prisoners.

A pure teleologist or practitioner of classic decision analysis would choose the first option, the end result of which is 2 persons living. A deontologist who believed the command "Thou shalt not kill" to be absolute, brooking no exception, would choose the latter option, reasoning that he has not killed even though 2 have died.

What is missing in this analysis is the impact on the actor himself/herself. Do we factor in regret, does it count for anything? Or, more pertinent to our health care perspective, do we factor in the likelihood of posttraumatic stress disorder? What of the more personalized sense of guilt or even of sin that option 1 may provoke? Millennials to whom I have posed this dilemma react in a more subjective mode than do members of earlier generations. Millennials are more moved by the impact on the subject here and are more likely to choose option 2 even though it contradicts our prevailing utilitarian ethic. Their holding to an absolute prohibition on killing may seem at first to have only a deontological foundation, but at a deeper level it may be based on the notion that our acts create us and that what we do is our essence, not what we merely believe.

Millennials are different and have much to teach "Silents" and "Boomers." Our passing the discipline of surgery to them can be done with great confidence in their beneficence and commitment.

# Reference

1. Pew Research Center. http://www.pewresearchcenter.org. The Generations Defined; May 8, 2015.

# 24 The Surgeon-Chaplain Relationship

Rev Andrew T. Wakefield, MMP, JD
Thomas W. Wakefield, MD

PROLOGUE ▶ Dr John Flynn was at his wits' end. He had been on in-hospital call the night before but had found it necessary to use alcohol to help him sleep. We left him in the call room at the end of Part 1: Theory, chapter 3. He had awakened feeling fuzzy. The day had been grueling in the extreme. One of his postoperative patients died, and the attending surgeon could not be reached. An intensive care unit nurse had shouted at him while he was trying to intubate an anoxic trauma victim; it was now 7 PM.

The family members of the patient who died were not only saddened, but they were also shocked at the unexpectedness of the death of a loved one. Dr Flynn would have been alone with the now angry family in the absence of the attending surgeon had not a young chaplain joined him in the family waiting room. The chaplain gently and unobtrusively took over the conversation, and Flynn became a listener. The family's anger subsided. The chaplain acknowledged their pain and did not seek to diminish it. Suddenly, Flynn felt himself to be within the energy field of the chaplain and among those being ministered to. Finally, the family appeared to have achieved some level of peace, without Flynn having contributed substantively. The chaplain rose to leave. Flynn closed with the family, promising that the attending surgeon would contact them, and hurried, nearly ran, down the hall to overtake the hospital chaplain. "May I talk to you sometime," was all Dr John Flynn found to say.

Tom and Andrew Wakefield are, like other sets of authors of the chapters in this book, father and son. Both have a deep religious faith, which informs every aspect of their lives and which serves as the basis for their ethics, every day. They have much to offer us.

Rev Andrew T. Wakefield was recently ordained a priest in the Archdiocese of Washington in Washington, DC.

Dr Thomas W. Wakefield is the section head of Vascular Surgery, James C. Stanley Professor of Vascular Surgery, and director of the Samuel and Jean Frankel Cardiovascular Center at the University of Michigan Medical School.

In the time before the Constantinian era, it was considered appropriate for those who provided medical care to offer spiritual advice to patients with incurable diseases.[1,2] In the later Middle Ages, laypersons in various religious traditions who became physicians believed that they were "Collaborators with God."[2,3] The vision of a relationship between medicine and religion was brought to America. Cotton Mather, an 18th-century Puritan, advised physicians to prescribe "admonitions of piety."[2,4] The practice of medicine in the 18th and early 19th century then followed Mather because physicians were urged to adopt professional standards that were based on Christian ideals.[2,5] Benjamin Rush, a prominent physician in Philadelphia, urged his colleagues to show respect for religion in their patient care, and in 1823 a system of medical ethics for New York mentioned that physicians should be aware of "contempt for religious practice and feelings."[2,6] The code of ethics adopted by the American Medical Association later in the 19th century also followed Mather's views.[2,4] Leading American physicians in the first half of the 20th century 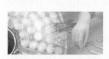 considered religion a large part of medicine, including the famous William Osler. The noted American physician Richard Clarke Cabat, with colleague R.L. Dicks, went on to publish a book in which he provided a model for cooperation between physicians and clergy when caring for patients, focusing on the need to accommodate their religious concerns.[2] Even the Nobel Prize–winning vascular surgeon, Alexis Carrel, wrote a volume on his experience at Lourdes.

However, by the middle of the 20th century, times were changing, and with the ascendency of hard medical science, the feeling was taking hold that there was little room for discussions of the religious commitments of patients and their physicians. It was not acceptable for physicians to mix religion and medical science in discussions with their patients. Although this feeling dominated the second half of the 20th century, a growing body of knowledge suggests patients who have religious commitments 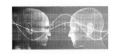 do better medically. "The majority of 350 such studies have found that religious people are physically healthier, lead healthier lifestyles, and require fewer health services."[2,7] Although there is still controversy in this area, a basic issue is not whether spiritual commitments improve the health of patients, but whether the inquiries that surgeons may make into these areas honor their patients as persons. Many patients base their lives on a fundamental belief system, and therefore surgeons need to be aware of and engage at least intellectually in the belief systems of their patients.[2]

The spiritual care of patients is important for their sense of well-being, healing, a shorter hospital stay, less pain, and less nursing time.[8] Spiritual care is arguably best provided when the surgeon creates a partnership with the hospital chaplain, who is trained to engage with patients and their families, to establish trusting rapports, to understand patients' emotional, affective, and spiritual needs, and to respond to patients' verbal and nonverbal communications. Yet despite the unique skills chaplains can bring to a patient's overall care, the relationship between the surgeon and the hospital chaplain can be described as distant and nonexistent at worst, tolerant at best. The majority of patients, however, who receive health care believe in some form of God, and a significant number actively participate in some type of religious tradition.[8] Pastoral care is therefore entirely appropriate for such patients. Patients who do not receive pastoral care from a surgeon-chaplain team may, in turn, seek spiritual guidance from their surgeon alone, who may feel ill-equipped to provide such care. Finally, patients' religious backgrounds often determine how they are or are not receptive to treatment and medical care. Surgeons should be aware of these orientations. Clearly, it is then prudent for the surgeon to join in a close relationship with his/her hospital chaplain colleague to more readily be able to take care of the entire patient and both his/her physical and spiritual needs. The purpose of this discussion is to explore important aspects of effective pastoral care, as well as look at some of the broad areas where a more formal relationship between the entire surgical team, including surgeons, nurses, therapists and so forth and the hospital chaplain service would facilitate and improve the health and well-being of patients.

## Effective Listening

A hospital chaplain or other pastoral care minister may serve an important role in caring for the spiritual, emotional, and affective needs of patients. Patients arrive at the hospital with unique histories, experiences, and relationships 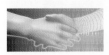 that will have an impact on their physical well-being. In the course of surgical care, chaplains are in a unique position to engage with patients to learn more of their personal story beyond their current surgical and/or medical condition. Health care crises often cause patients to confront existential questions about their lives, and chaplains can assist in offering a consoling and compassionate presence for patients and their families during difficult times.

To offer true pastoral care, surgeons and their chaplain colleagues must be masters of the art of listening. Listening is at the heart of every encounter between a pastoral minister and a patient. This may seem blatantly obvious, but true, genuine, authentic listening is sorely lacking across all sectors of society today, and in health care settings. True, effective listening requires patience, empathy, energy, humility, and openness, qualities that are often downplayed as "soft" or "insignificant" in a world where data, information, and quantitative measures often drive recommendations, decisions, and outcomes, especially in surgical settings. When resources, particularly time, are scarce, effective listening requires slowing down, putting aside distractions, and truly encountering another person exactly where that person is—not where one may assume another is or where one may wish or expect another to be—but exactly in the emotional, spiritual, affective, and physical state that a person presently occupies. In a world where time is billed in increments of minutes and communication occurs instantaneously because of advancements in technology, listening requires a world without limits, without time constraints, without "to-do" lists, and without exorbitant workloads, all of which impede genuine, authentic listening.

The realities of the world and the health care system result in circumstances that challenge the conditions that facilitate listening. Those involved in patient care, including surgeons, therapists, technicians and nurses, as well as chaplains and other pastoral ministers alike, must strive to improve their listening skills. It is only in listening to their patients that they truly encounter their patients and can holistically treat them in body, mind, and spirit. Although the innate importance of listening varies among each type of care provider, all those who work with patients must strive to understand the unique person who seeks their expertise. Listening is foundational and essential for such work.

Listening is at the heart of pastoral ministry. Chaplains and all those called to pastoral care are called to care for the emotional, affective, and spiritual needs of patients. By listening they can truly understand, access, and respond to those needs. When surgeons enter a hospital room, they often have little, if any, idea of the emotional or spiritual state the patient may be in. Hopefully the partnering chaplain has already been aware of the medical condition of the patient; it is, therefore, important that chaplains have a basic knowledge of a patient's medical condition, but the physical condition may often be just one of many layers to the patient. A patient's medical diagnosis, treatment, recovery, and long-term prognosis certainly weigh on him/her, but in the course of a pastoral visit, the chaplain may learn that patients carry many concerns in their hearts and bear many burdens on their shoulders. A hospital stay can be the place where all that weigh on a patient comes to the surface. Surgeons and chaplains must, therefore, be prepared to encounter unexpected patient situations that often extend well beyond the actual medical situation that brought the patient to the hospital.

The chaplain will most often visit the patient without the surgeon. Before stepping into a hospital room, the chaplain must be prepared to put aside his/her own busyness, fatigue, and other distractions and simply be present to the patient he/she is about to meet. Authentic listening happens only when one is fully present to another. A deep breath, quick prayer, or a silent moment of contemplation can help a chaplain step into a hospital room clearheaded, calm, and eager to encounter the patient and truly listen to the patient's story that may unfold. When a chaplain enters a hospital room in this way, he/she is less likely to project his/her own feelings onto a patient or rush through a patient visit in a way that is off-putting to a patient or a patient's family. Rather, a chaplain's calm, warm, and reserved presence can facilitate an atmosphere in which the patient comes to trust the chaplain's intentions and open up emotionally. However, even the most effective chaplains will encounter patients who are resistant to pastoral care, and chaplains must always respect the wishes of patients who do not care to be seen, visited, or prayed with. For such patients, the chaplain can offer pastoral care if the patient were to request it in the future, but the chaplain must never force a pastoral visit onto a patient. Rather, effective pastoral care is always responsive to and respectful of exactly where a patient is in his/her emotional, affective, and spiritual condition. Chaplains must also be respectful of patients' physical conditions and be flexible enough to offer pastoral care at times most conducive to patients' medical schedules.

Consider the example of an elderly patient whom the hospital chaplain meets while conducting pastoral ministry rounds in the hospital. Through taking the time to speak with the patient, the chaplain learns she is a widow and is alone in the hospital, awaiting biopsy results for a possible cancer diagnosis. Certainly the medical uncertainty of her condition causes great suffering and anxiety, but in the course of a pastoral visit, which extends well beyond the mere formalities of introductions and moves into a discussion of 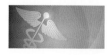 the substantive, deep-seated affections the woman experiences, the chaplain learns that she has been estranged from her daughter for nearly 20 years. This estrangement weighs deeply on the woman's heart and adds increased distress to her stay in the hospital. Such weighty matters make the patient highly emotional, and in the course of the pastoral visit, she is able to express her fears and pain. While talking with the hospital chaplain, she becomes emotionally distraught in thinking about her estranged daughter, which only adds to the concern she carries with her because of the uncertainty of her medical condition. Therefore, it is evident to the chaplain that this woman's suffering exists at many levels, and the chaplain seeks to offer her a sense of hope and compassion for all that she is experiencing. As the chaplain listens to what the patient expresses verbally and observes what she expresses nonverbally about her emotions, the chaplain validates her experience by acknowledging back to her what she says and what she expresses, allowing her to fill in any gaps in his/her understanding of her story, and simply giving her the space and time to share whatever she wishes to share. The chaplain remains engaged with the patient throughout the pastoral visit, but without monopolizing the conversation or probing too deeply, which could inadvertently suggest to the patient that the chaplain is trying to evaluate or diagnose her situation. Rather, the chaplain's job is to offer a compassionate, nonjudgmental, accessible presence for the patient. As it has been revealed in the course of the visit, the chaplain and patient are of different faith traditions, but sensing that prayer may be helpful and comforting to the patient, the chaplain also offers to pray with her toward the end of their visit, and she agrees. The chaplain 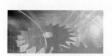 offers a prayer that reflects the magnitude of the suffering the woman has expressed verbally and nonverbally, to which she adds her own words of petition. After praying with the patient, the chaplain assures her of continued prayers and support, and the chaplain offers to check on her again soon. As the chaplain leaves the hospital room to continue rounds, he or she senses the patient seems a little calmer and more relaxed than when first entering her room, as though a burden has been lifted from her shoulders. The chaplain continues on with rounds, visiting other patients in the hospital, but is sure to follow up with the patient in the following days.

In such a pastoral visit as this with an elderly widow, the chaplain offers her a kind and trusting presence. This posture allows her to feel comfortable in sharing what truly weighs on her. The chaplain never leads the woman on in terms of forcing her to speak in any way. Rather, his/her calm and reassuring presence allows the woman to feel completely free to share or hold back whatever she wishes, knowing that the chaplain is there to offer encouragement and support. She senses that the chaplain is not judging her situation or critically evaluating her in any way but is there simply to listen to whatever she wishes to share. The chaplain exudes a sense of calmness and patience, which allows the woman to open up on her own terms. This sense of comfort allows the patient to share the deeper struggles that she has brought with her to the hospital. Only if she senses that the chaplain has truly heard her, will she continue to open up and share. In this visit, she does. In the course of sharing, emotions pour forth from her and she becomes emotionally distraught, as she talks through the deep pain she feels from the difficult situation with her daughter. But her expressions of sadness give way to a sense of calm and increased hope, for in effectively listening to the woman, the chaplain helps her to know that she is not alone in her pain. Rather the chaplain is with her, hearing her, and acknowledging the legitimacy of her affections, and helping her to know that God is with her, walking with her, and helping to bear her burdens. Whatever the outcome of her biopsy will be, the woman is a little bit stronger to face her future than before the chaplain entered the room, and she feels comforted by speaking with him/her. And the surgeon has had the advantage of the assistance of a trusted and trustworthy ally.

## Existential Questions

Hospital stays can bring to light the existential questions all people face during their lives, and medical crises can often expedite these questions in a highly emotional and traumatic way. Regardless of one's faith background, all people confront questions regarding their purpose in life, the relationships that have shaped their experience, the values they hold dear, and questions regarding why they are suffering in the first place. It is often in the midst of suffering that a patient faces these questions and seeks answers, particularly if they have not been faced before. Patients often believe that because of their shortcomings, they are being somehow punished by God for something in their life or that they deserve the pain and suffering they are enduring. Hospital chaplains and other pastoral care workers are in a privileged position to help patients confront the questions that weigh on them and seek further clarity, even resolution.

In representing a particular faith tradition, chaplains can serve an important role for patients of that same tradition. Chaplains may help patients know that God is with them in the midst of their suffering, and they may be a comforting, familiar presence in a hospital environment. Chaplains can help to diffuse the cold, sterile, and institutional atmosphere that patients may perceive in a hospital, particularly if they are alone or seem to have few family members and friends present to support them. As faith representatives, chaplains must be men and women of prayer, spirituality, and contemplation. Patients must sense in a chaplain a close relationship with the divine. When patients can perceive in a chaplain a sense of comfort, trust, and hope in the 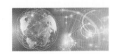 divine, they can more freely wrestle with the progression of their own faith journey and the existential questions their illness brings to light. Although certainly not surgical experts, chaplains are experts in helping patients relate their medical experience to the realm of the existential in which all men and women exist and bring that expertise to their partnership with the surgeon.

Within a shared faith tradition, chaplains can offer sacramental care, prayer, and scriptural guidance. This can provide patients with hope and a deep knowledge that God is with them and their families in the midst of their hospital stay and their subsequent health care. Particularly in faith traditions that place significant importance on sacraments or sacred scripture, chaplains offer very real and tangible reminders of God's grace for patients. For example, in the Catholic tradition, the sacraments are actions of the Holy Spirit at work in the Church, instituted by Jesus Christ himself, and are tangible reminders for the recipients of God's love. Particularly important in a hospital setting is the sacrament of Anointing of the Sick that confers God's healing touch on a patient while forgiving his/her sins. For a Catholic patient to receive this sacrament by a Catholic priest serving as a chaplain can be a tremendous source of renewed hope for that patient and his/her family, whether in illness, undergoing an operation, or preparing for imminent death. The sacrament may be celebrated in conjunction with the Holy Eucharist or Reconciliation, both of which further nourish a patient's soul and repair his/her unity with God. The chaplain may assist the surgeon, therefore, in offering profound consolation during what may be deeply challenging times in the patient's life. The importance of such consolation is immeasurable yet profoundly real in the life of a patient. In representing shared faith traditions with patients, chaplains can remind patients that even from their hospital room, they are vital members of their faith communities, which further brings patients a consoling sense that they are not alone in their physical suffering. Their community of faith is with them and God is with them, walking with them, praying for them, and supporting them in whatever uncertainty they may be experiencing. All human beings are innately relational, and so to be reminded that others are with them in their suffering is not only reassuring for patients but also highly restorative of their own sense of personal dignity. This can have positive consequences for patients' emotional states, making them more hopeful, trusting, and even receptive to their medical care.

If a chaplain represents a different faith tradition from that of the patient, he/she can still help to open channels for the patient to express the thoughts and feelings that weigh on him/her, particularly those that are existential. Take, for example, the pastoral visit of a Catholic chaplain to a Jewish man, who is in the hospital recovering from an operation for leg ischemia. The chaplain stops by the man's room on pastoral rounds to say hello and check on how the patient is doing in his recovery. Because the chaplain is dressed in clerics, the patient knows at first glance that they are from different faith traditions, but he still welcomes the chaplain into the room and engages in conversation.

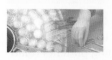 The chaplain, listening attentively to the patient's story and acknowledging the various affects he expresses verbally and nonverbally, offers to pray with the patient at the end of the visit, and he accepts. The chaplain offers an appropriate prayer to God that is meaningful to the patient and respectful of his Jewish faith, and the patient expresses his gratitude for the common prayer. At the conclusion of the pastoral visit, the chaplain assures the patient of his continued prayers, offers to follow up with the patient in the coming days to see how he is doing, and reminds the patient that he/she is always available for a visit if he would like him/her to return.

As evident in this pastoral visit, different faith traditions need not impede effective pastoral care. Certainly there are situations when patients request a chaplain of their own faith background or when a chaplain knows the patient desires specific rites, prayers, or sacraments that he/she is not able to provide. In such situations, the chaplain should strive to facilitate the visitation of another appropriate chaplain. 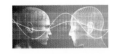 Thus, chaplains must be sensitive to the unique spiritual aspects and limitations of their own faith tradition. Often, however, the chaplain can offer effective pastoral care without regard to the patient's particular religious affiliation, or lack thereof. Pastoral care is about connecting with patients in whatever circumstances they find themselves and helping them to explore the spiritual and existential questions that may arise during hospitalization, questions that are influenced by the cares and concerns patients bring with them into the hospital. Chaplains help patients deal with questions of fear, loneliness, values, meaning, hopelessness, and hope. Although faith can guide and frame these questions in life-giving ways, these questions transcend religious labels. These are questions that all human beings face, and chaplains are particularly equipped to help patients confront them constructively.

Chaplains may also partner with the surgeon in offering pastoral care to patients' family members or friends who may be with them in the hospital. Family members suffer with patients, and chaplains may offer a listening ear and compassionate presence to spouses, children, and others they may encounter. Family members may wish to pray along with a chaplain and a patient, or they may wish to speak privately to the chaplain, perhaps to share their own perspective on the patient's experience or express their own fatigue, exhaustion, or emotional toll. Just as in providing pastoral care for patients themselves, this pastoral care for family members and friends requires the chaplain to be a master of the art of listening.

## Addressing Patient Suffering

Although there are certainly medical conditions, diseases, and illnesses that may seem completely random and unexpected for patients, patients often face recurring medical conditions that can result in continued hospital stays or years-long medical battles. Both types of conditions and particularly the latter cause an emotional toll on patients and their family, which can only further exacerbate the suffering experienced. Long-term conditions, particularly those that may be terminal, can force a patient to confront many existential questions and may take such an emotional toll that the patient may be tempted to give up all trust in the medical care system, particularly if the patient feels as though his/her life has been a broken record of illness, doctors' visits, treatments, and hospital stays. Such conditions may make a patient less inclined toward and perhaps even critical of the prescribed treatment and care, even to the point of refusing to abide by the surgeon's orders. In such a situation the chaplain plays an important role in hearing the patient's concerns and serving as a bridge with the surgical care team of surgeons, nurses, and therapists, all of whom may have responsibilities that preclude them from truly 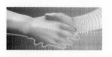 getting to "know" their patient in the complexity of his/her emotional, affective, and spiritual state. The chaplain can serve as a bridge between patients, family, and the surgical care team, assuring patients that others care for them in the midst of their suffering. The chaplain can help articulate the fatigue and emotional toll of patients to those responsible for their surgical care, which may influence the effectiveness of the prescribed treatment.

Often during the course of pastoral care, patients may come to trust a chaplain and confide in him/her their real fears and concerns over their prognosis, and so surgical care providers may wisely consult with the chaplain regarding the patient's condition. Given the time constraints and potentially great differences in position between patients and surgeons or other care providers based on authority, expertise, and education, a patient may feel utterly helpless as surgeons, nurses, therapists, and technicians go about their work. Each patient is unique, with experiences, relationships, joys, and pains of their own, and in the institutional nature of hospitals it is important for all care providers, whether medical or pastoral, to remember the uniqueness of each patient encountered. Some patients may feel that they must simply acquiesce regarding their treatment and passively accept whatever the doctor orders, without voicing their own opinion. Chaplains, by virtue of their position in engaging with patients on affective, emotional, and spiritual levels, may be given glimpses into the true interior state of a patient and so can help guide surgeons and other care providers on how to best reach their patients to ensure they receive the most effective medical care. If a patient seems resistant to treatment or highly skeptical of those whose job it is to care for their surgical condition, a chaplain may know why, and likewise, a chaplain may know the best way to communicate with such a patient. Therefore, effective surgical care envisions chaplains and surgeons in regular dialogue with each other, assessing not only a patient's medical needs but also his/her emotional, affective, and spiritual needs, all of which affect his/her surgical outcome.

## The Surgeon's Role in Addressing Spirituality

Research has shown that spirituality positively affects patient mortality, the ability of patients to cope, and their recovery time from illness. Surgeons involved in patient care can address spirituality in many specific ways. These include practicing compassionate presence; taking the time to listen to their patients' hopes, pains, dreams, and fears; obtaining a spiritual history during the history and physical examination; and being attentive to the full dimension of interaction between patients and their families. The surgeon can also refer

## TABLE 24.1 ▶ THE FICA METHOD OF TAKING A SPIRITUAL HISTORY

| | |
|---|---|
| F | *Faith and belief.* Ask: Are there spiritual beliefs that help you cope with stress or difficult times? What gives your life meaning? |
| I | *Importance and influence.* Ask: Is spirituality important in your life? What influence does it have on how you take care of yourself? Are there any particular decisions regarding your health that might be affected by these beliefs? |
| C | *Community.* Ask: Are you part of a spiritual or religious community? |
| A | *Address/action.* Think about what you, as a health care provider, need to do with the information the patient shared—eg, refer to a chaplain, meditation or yoga classes, or another spiritual resource. It helps to talk with the chaplain in your hospital to familiarize yourself with the available resources. |

Copyright © Christina M. Puchalski, MD, 1996.

the patient to chaplain services for appropriate spiritual care.[9] Thus, it is clear that although the specific role that chaplains play is important in providing effective, holistic care, surgeons also should be concerned with the emotional, affective, and spiritual aspects of patients' lives. A simple way for surgeons to do this is to document the patients' spiritual history as part of their medical history. Using the FICA method, as described by Puchalski (see Table 24.1), is a way to do this.[10] FICA, standing for Faith and Belief, Importance and Influence, Community, and Address/Action, provides a framework for surgeons to inquire into the affective, emotional, and spiritual dimensions of their patients' lives. Physicians may specifically ask what spiritual beliefs help patients cope with difficult times or give meaning to their lives; whether spirituality is important to patients' lives and whether there are any medical decisions that may be affected by these beliefs; and whether patients are part of a religious or spiritual community. Finally, physicians should consider whether their patients should be referred to a chaplain for additional care.[9] All of these questions help ensure that surgeons provide the best possible compassionate care to their patients.

A great majority of patients today wish their surgeon to at least take their spiritual or religious beliefs into account if they become seriously ill, even if they do not openly discuss these beliefs with their surgeon.[11–13] Hemming et al reported the benefits of physicians and chaplains working together. They conducted several focus groups with participants in an interprofessional curriculum between residents in internal medicine and chaplain interns. They found 4 major themes from their work: medical interns learn effective communication skills for addressing spirituality from such a group; chaplain interns were effective in enhancing patient-centered care; chaplain interns provided emotional support to the medical team; and the partnership was effective if there was adequate time for introductions, clear expectations, and opportunities for feedback.[14] In another study, chaplain visits were found to improve the willingness of patients to recommend the hospital based on a positive experience during their hospitalization, seen in both the Hospital

Consumer Assessment of Healthcare Providers and Systems survey and the Press Ganey survey. This was a study of 8978 patients discharged from a tertiary care hospital.[15] In the Press Ganey survey, patients who were seen by chaplains during their hospitalization also stated that their spiritual needs had been met, as well as their emotional needs. In addition, overall patient satisfaction was improved. Although these findings may not result exclusively from chaplain visits, it is clear that chaplains do very well in meeting the spiritual, religious, and emotional needs of patients.[16]

Based on these findings, we recommend that patients should be asked about their religious and spiritual beliefs in several clinical contexts during their hospitalizations, and surgeons should also take these beliefs into account during treatment. The partnership between the surgeon and the chaplain can make all the difference in making this a reality. Some of the situations when this partnership between the surgeon and chaplain may be most needed are at the end of life, at the onset of a long-term surgeon-patient relationship, or when the patient specifically requests pastoral care from a chaplain. Other possible situations in which a dialogue between surgeons and chaplains is helpful include the time before a patient's major operation, after major trauma, or during significant and grave illnesses, all of which may pose particular emotional, affective, and spiritual burdens on

a patient. Importantly, anytime a patient requests pastoral care or begins to discuss issues that his/her surgeon believes a chaplain might be equipped to answer, the surgeon should be responsive and facilitate appropriate care. However, it is extremely important that a surgeon avoid any actions or words that can be misconstrued as suggesting that the patient's care will be compromised in any way by knowing and acknowledging their beliefs. Patients should never feel that their faith is an impediment to their medical care. Additionally, surgeons and chaplains should avoid at all costs any appearance of coercion in the realm of spiritual assessment and direction. Sensitive spiritual care is more appropriately offered by the chaplain with experience in pastoral assessment and care. Finally, we firmly believe that the role of the chaplain in the health care team, although important as documented above, must be patient initiated or patient sanctioned. Pastoral care must never be coerced or forced on a patient. This requires genuine listening to the patient, who must always feel his or her perspective is valued, legitimized, and truly heard by the surgeon, chaplain, and entire health care team. When it comes to issues of spirituality, it is the patient's feelings that are most important, not the chaplain's interpretation of these feelings or the perspective of anyone else.[17] As most referrals for chaplain services come from nurses (27.8%) and patients themselves (22.3%), while few come from surgeons and social workers,[18] it is our hope that by understanding the important role that chaplains play in the health care of patients, surgeons will use their pastoral care services more frequently for the well-being of their patients.[19]

## Conclusion

In conclusion, a close relationship between a surgeon and a patient's larger medical care team including chaplains can improve patient care and offer complete, holistic treatment to the patient in need. Effective care must include the emotional, affective, and spiritual realm, in addition to the specific medical care that patients require, and it requires effective, genuine listening, both by the patient's chaplain and surgeon. We hope that the examples and the aforementioned discussion will describe how a greater and closer relationship between the surgical care team, surgeons, and chaplains can lead to improved patient outcomes and the complete care of the patient in need.

## References

1. Entralgo PL. Professional-patient relationships: historical perspectives. In: Reich WT, ed. *Encyclopedia of Bioethics*. 2nd ed. New York, NY: Simon & Shuster Macmillan; 1995:2076–2084.
2. Cohen CB, Wheeler SE, Scott DA, Anglican Working Group in Bioethics. Walking a fine line: physician inquiries into patients' religious and spiritual beliefs. *Hastings Cent Rep*. 2001;31(5):29–39.
3. Sigerist H. *On the History of Medicine*. Marti-Ibanez F, ed. New York: MD Press; 1960.
4. Mather CA. *Bonifacius: An Essay upon the Good*. Levin D, ed. Harvard University Press; 1966.
5. Pellegrino E. *American Medical Ethics: Some Historical Roots*. Spicker S, Engelhardt HT, ed. Dordrecht: D. Reidel Publishing; 1977.
6. Rush B. *Sixteen Introductory Lectures Upon the Institutes and Practice of Medicine, With a Syllabus of the Latter*. Philadelphia: Bradford and Innskeep; 1811.
7. Koenig HG. Religion, spirituality, and medicine: application to clinical practice. *JAMA*. 2000;284(13):1708. MSJAMA.
8. Thiel MM, Robinson MR. Physicians' collaboration with chaplains: difficulties and benefits. *J Clin Ethics*. 1997;8(1):94–103.
9. Puchalski CM. The role of spirituality in health care. *Proc (Bayl Univ Med Cent)*. 2001;14(4):352–357.
10. Puchalski C, Romer AL. Taking a spiritual history allows clinicians to understand patients more fully. *J Palliat Med*. 2000;3(1):129–137.
11. Anderson JM, Anderson LJ, Felsenthal G. Pastoral needs and support within an inpatient rehabilitation unit. *Arch Phys Med Rehabil*. 1993;74(6):574–578.
12. Daaleman TP, Nease Jr. DE. Patient attitudes regarding physician inquiry into spiritual and religious issues. *J Fam Pract*. 1994;39(6):564–568.
13. Ehman JW, Ott BB, Short TH, Ciampa RC, Hansen-Flaschen J. Do patients want physicians to inquire about their spiritual or religious beliefs if they become gravely ill? *Arch Intern Med*. 1999;159(15):1803–1806.
14. Hemming P, Teague PJ, Crowe T, Levine R. Chaplains on the medical team: a qualitative analysis of an interprofessional curriculum for internal medicine residents and chaplain interns. *J Relig Health*. 2016;55(2):560–571.

15. Marin DB, Sharma V, Sosunov E, Egorova N, Goldstein R, Handzo GF. Relationship between chaplain visits and patient satisfaction. *J Health Care Chaplain.* 2015;21(1):14–24.

16. Flannelly KJ, Oettinger M, Galek K, Braun-Storck A, Kreger R. The correlates of chaplains' effectiveness in meeting the spiritual/religious and emotional needs of patients. *J Pastoral Care Counsel.* 2009;63(1-2):9-1-15.

17. Loewy RS, Loewy EH. Healthcare and the hospital chaplain. *MedGenMed.* 2007;9(1):53.

18. Vanderwerker LC, Flannelly KJ, Galek K, et al. What do chaplains really do? III. Referrals in the New York Chaplaincy Study. *J Health Care Chaplain.* 2008;14(1):57–73.

19. Russell RC. Professional chaplains in comprehensive patient-centered care. *R I Med J (2013).* 2014;97(3):39–42.

# 25 Palliative Care for the Surgeon

Annette K. Collier, MD, FACP

PROLOGUE ▶ Death is an inevitable part of what it is to be human. In many cultures, it is approached as integral to life, and the time of its approach is seen as a rewarding period of understanding and benignity toward those who are to follow. In the Western world, however, death has all too often become a technologic nightmare. The trappings of death often include a respirator, a dialysis machine, and a set of intravenous infusions arranged like a Christmas tree. Dr Annette K. Collier has been a pioneer in countering this trend.

Dr Annette K. Collier is an assistant professor at The University of Toledo College of Medicine.

Balfour Mount, MD, a surgeon, coined the term palliative care in the early 1970s to describe care focused on a patient's goals and quality of life. He encouraged physicians to attend to the whole person and to the patient's experience of illness, not only to the cure of disease. Dr Eric Cassell furthered this challenge[1] when he wrote,

> *"The relief of suffering and the cure of disease must be seen as twin obligations of a medical profession that is truly dedicated to the care of the sick. Physicians' failure to understand the nature of suffering can result in medical intervention that (although technically adequate) not only fails to relieve suffering but becomes a source of suffering itself."*

**199**

The goals of palliative care are to relieve patient suffering and to assure that a patient's care aligns with his/her goals, expectations, and values. The need for palliative care has grown out of the continuously increasing complexity of medicine and the decrease in humanistic aspects of medical care. Dr Ira Byock[2] has stated, "It is harder to be seriously ill—and much harder to die—than ever before." Palliative care has grown out of the realization, and the public demand for choices and better care at the end of life.

What do we know about what is most important to persons facing a serious, life-threatening illness? The top responses outlined in 2000 were (1) pain and symptom control, (2) peace with God, (3) presence of family, (4) mental awareness, and (5) having treatment preferences followed.[3] Yet 1 in 5 deaths in the United States occur in, or immediately following discharge from, an intensive care unit. Most of these deaths have been preceded by life-sustaining measures that prevented interaction with loved ones in the last days of life and were associated with pain and suffering.

Palliative care principles grew out of the hospice movement, but palliative care is not about dying. It is about helping the patient live well with serious illness. The presence of pain, nausea, or anxiety will lessen a patient's quality of life and ability to interact with family and loved ones. Living well, while coping with serious illness, involves expert management of these physical symptoms. Spiritual, emotional, and social suffering must also be addressed to assure that we help a patient live well. Palliative care is practiced with an interdisciplinary team. The team frequently includes a physician, advance practice nurse, registered nurse, chaplain, and social worker. Physicians are obligated to understand the nature of suffering but may not have the skill set to address all the sources of this suffering, such as spiritual, existential, or emotional pain. The diverse expertise of the interdisciplinary team allows caregivers to address all domains of a patient's suffering.

This chapter will review sources of patient suffering and will discuss ways in which physicians themselves may be a source of that suffering. We will consider how self-reflection can prepare a physician to respond to suffering and align with a patient's hopes, fears, and goals. These skills are the core of palliative care.

How do patients suffer? Initially we think of physical pain. Spiritual, emotional, or existential pain is also a source of suffering when patients face serious illness. Illness, regardless of whether it is terminal or a "bump in the road" of otherwise good health, imposes a threat to a patient's personhood. The threat to personhood is a source of suffering. As an example, con-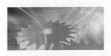sider a young mother who is diagnosed with early-stage breast cancer. She is treated and is given an excellent prognosis for a prolonged disease-free survival. During treatment, she experiences the physical symptoms of pain and nausea. Her role in the family changes during recovery from her operation because she is unable to be fully active in caring for her children. There are financial hurdles for the family because of poor insurance coverage.

Intimacy with her husband changes. She is angry with God and worries about her children's future if the cancer recurs. Thus, despite an illness that has excellent prognosis, the patient has experienced physical, emotional, existential, social, and spiritual pain. She has suffered. Imagine the magnitude of suffering when a patient is facing a terminal diagnosis.

*The Death of Ivan Ilyich*[4] is a poignant literary account of a suffering, dying man. Ivan, a 45-year-old lawyer climbing the professional and social ladders of his time, was afflicted with incapacitating abdominal pain and impending death. Because his symptoms represented not only physical but also existential suffering, Ivan's abdominal pain did not respond to increasing 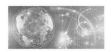 doses of opium or morphine. It was only the touch and physical presence of his servant that offered Ivan any relief from his suffering. Although Ivan suffered great physical and existential pain when facing death, the abandonment by his physician magnified his distress.

> *"What tormented Ivan Ilyich most was the pretense, the lie, which for some reason they (friends, family and his doctors) all kept up, that he was merely ill and not dying."*

Likewise a 6-year-old boy hospitalized for chemotherapy appears sad and withdrawn when working with the art therapist. The little boy's simple, unsolicited sketch depicting a large, smiling physician next to his bed is not a reflection of the "nice doctor" it appears to represent at first glance. Instead, the child describes his doctor as being "bad" because the doctor is smiling while the little boy is hurting. He is experiencing the physical pain of procedures and treatments, the emotional pain of seeing his parents sad and anxious, and the social pain of isolation from school and friends. Again, failure to acknowledge the presence of suffering became a source of suffering itself. The physician is physically present, but the child feels isolation and abandonment because his source of suffering is not addressed.

Physicians are taught to never abandon a patient. Abandonment can be a legal term for terminating the physician-patient relationship in such a way that the patient is denied necessary medical care. Most physicians look beyond the legal definition of abandonment and feel committed to the care of their patients, regardless of how difficult or risky the operation or how complex and prolonged the clinical course may be. This commitment is rooted in a love of their profession, not in the fear of malpractice. While skillfully managing medical and surgical issues at the bedside, physicians may yet be abandoning their patients by not communicating well and by not understanding the impact of the illness on the *person*, not the *patient*, in the bed. This abandonment can be detrimental to the emotional health of the patient and the physician.

A study in the *Archives of Internal Medicine*[5] examined the feelings of abandonment at the end of life from the perspective of patients, caregivers, and clinicians. Most striking was the discrepancy between doctor's and patient's perception of the relationship between them leading up to the patient's death. Many times, what was missing for the patient and caregiver was a sense of closure, an acknowledgment that death was approaching for the patient. This acknowledgment can be an opportunity for both patient and physician to reflect and express gratitude.

Dr Sherwin Nuland[6] points out that the personality traits frequently attributed to surgeons—authority, power, certainty, coolness under fire—do 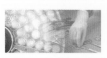 not serve them well, as they seek to look deeper into the patient's experience of illness, especially at the end of life. However, to fulfill the twin obligations of medicine defined at the beginning of this chapter, surgeons should be encouraged and trained in the practice of introspection.

Is it unrealistic or absurd to expect self-reflection in the day of a busy surgeon? Does the surgical personality exclude introspection? Joan Cassell[7] discussed the surgical world of the 1970s and 1980s as "macho" and as displaying traits of arrogance, certitude, and activism. Medical anthropologist Pearl Katz[8] suggested that detachment may be a necessary protection for surgeons experiencing dramatic confrontations with death.

Although this persona is likely to persist in lore and also in practice, the surgeon of today is advised to move beyond this authoritarian, stoic nature. Shared decision making, not paternalism, is the standard that patients expect and deserve. Communication skills must be cultivated to facilitate discussion of options, quality of life, and autonomy. Allowing and encouraging the examination of one's own emotional state will help overcome the detachment, which risks that a dying patient is abandoned at the time of greatest need.

All too often physicians see death as a failure and not as a natural, appropriate, and unavoidable conclusion to the doctor-patient relationship. Doctors are not generally aware of the tremendous value their presence brings at the end of life. They are not aware of how gratifying these conversations can be for the physician who has mastered the skill of communicating empathy and presence. Physicians who routinely transition their dying patients to the care of others have lost an opportunity to examine their own emotional state. This introspection can counter the depersonalization that leads to burnout, a condition reported by 30% to 40% practicing surgeons.[9]

The core principles of palliative care when practiced routinely near the end of life can achieve a "triple win." First and foremost, care is patient centered, and family and caregivers gain the needed support during a difficult time. In addition, our health care system, already strapped with limited resources, would benefit when unwanted medical interventions are avoided. Finally, the fact that the physician and other health care workers can also benefit personally adds an almost magical element to what we have to offer our patients.

*"The capacity to give one's attention to a sufferer is a very rare and difficult thing; it is almost a miracle. It is a miracle."*

*Simone Weil (2000)*

# References

1. Cassel EJ. The nature of suffering and the goals of medicine. *N Engl J Med.* 1982;306:639–645.
2. Byock I. *The Best Care Possible: A Physician's Quest to Transform Care Through the End of Life.* New York: Avery; 2012.
3. Steinhauser KE, Christakis NA, Clipp EC, et al. Factors considered important at the end of life by patients, family, physicians, and other care providers. *JAMA.* 2000;284(19):2476–2482.
4. Tolstoy L, graf. *The Death of Ivan Ilyich.* New York: Health Sciences Pub. Corp.; Print 1828–1910.
5. Back AL, Young JP, McCown E, et al. Abandonment at the end of life from patient, caregiver, nurse, and physician perspectives. *Arch Intern Med.* 2009;169(5):474–479.
6. Nuland SB. A surgeon's reflections on the care of the dying. *Surg Oncol Clin N Am.* January 2001;10(1):1–5.
7. Cassell J. *Expected Miracles—Surgeons at Work.* Philadelphia: Temple University Press; 1991.
8. Katz P. *The Scalpel's Edge: The Culture of Surgeons.* Boston: Allyn and Bacon; 1999.
9. Balch CM, Freischlag JA, Shanafelt TD. Stress and burnout among surgeons: understanding and managing the syndrome and avoiding the adverse consequences. *Arch Surg.* 2009;144(4):371–376.

# 26 Fee-Splitting and Modern Look-alikes

Joseph J. Lach, MD, FACS

PROLOGUE ▶ There have been, regretta-
bly, historical stains on the ethical fabric of our
discipline. Often, these resulted from surgeons
becoming swept up in the flow of overwhelming historical trends. For example, Ferdinand
Sauerbruch was a pioneer in thoracic surgery
but left a historical blot by becoming complicit
with the rise of Adolph Hitler.

Another historical abuse became common in
our discipline during the sweeping rise of capitalism
and the adulation of the businessman.

Fee-splitting is the return of a portion of the surgeon's
fees to the referring physician. Its business purpose is not unlike
a sales commission. Ultimately, the discipline of surgery, in this instance
led by the founders of the American College of Surgeons, was able to stand
against the societal tide of unfettered business practice and end such
transactions.

Similarly, large forces today, related to the insurance industry, the device
industry, and the pharmaceutical industry, again threaten to sweep away the
scruples of the surgical practitioner.

Dr Joseph J. Lach is an assistant professor of surgery at The University of
Toledo College of Medicine.

The surgeon has an obligation to avoid creating or condoning practices that give incentives contrary to the best interests of his/her patients. The unethical division of surgical fees is among such practices. It lives on today, somewhat camouflaged by terms such as "market share" and "incentive." In this section, we examine fee-splitting and explore the ethics and tactics in overt as well as modern, more subtle forms of incentives for surgical referrals. The goal of this section is to remind ourselves that, despite the changing face of surgical practice, the reasons for what we do as surgeons can and should remain clear.

"Fee-splitting," in the sense it is used here, is one of the terms describing the offering or receiving of an inducement to reward a referral. More broadly, it implies the return of some sort of remuneration, money, or something of value, to the person or entity referring the patient. It is a remuneration that was not earned in the caring for the patient by that referring entity but was given to create incentive or coercion for sending the patient to the surgeon. Generally, fee-splitting "exploits the relative ignorance" of the patient. As summarized by Koocher,[1] this practice is unethical for many reasons.

Fee-splitting often leads to unnecessary operations and unjustifiable costs. The surgeon decides, "I'll keep the referring doctor happy as he sends so many patients. Whether or not the patient really needs the operation, I'll do the case and raise my fee to cover the kickback (the 'finder's fee') I pay to the referring doctor." It is the motive for the referral that is suspect, and it is *the motive least in keeping with the patient's best interest* that makes the practice unethical.

Concerns over the custom of fee-splitting in medicine are documented at least as far back as the Middle Ages,[2] and, in his 1803 "Treatise on Medical Ethics," Thomas Percival was still dealing with issues of fee-splitting.[3] In chapter 2, section VI of his seminal work, he praised referring apothecaries and defended the fees paid to them:

> *"And a physician, who knows the education, skill, and persevering attention, as well as the sacrifice of ease, health, and sometimes even of life, which this profession (i.e.,* being an apothecary*) requires, should regard it as a duty not to withdraw, from those who exercise it, any sources of reasonable profit, or the honourable means of advancement in fortune."*

It is virtually certain that, when certain practices such as fee-splitting are legislated against, the practices are usually common.

At the time of its founding in May 1847, the American Medical Association adopted a "Code of Medical Ethics"[4] based almost entirely on the treatises of Thomas Percival. It was the first time in world history that an ethical guide for the practice of medicine had been adopted on a national scale. Two hundred fifty delegates, representing more than 40 medical societies and 28 medical colleges, were in attendance.[5(p115)] However, this Code, adopted only 44 years after Percival's work, contained no specific reference to or condemnation of fee-splitting.

The AMA meeting in May 1903 legislated a number of changes, including the relabeling of the ethics code as "Principles of Medical Ethics." In chapter 2, article VI, section 4 of that publication, and under a heading condemning the giving or receiving of "commissions," was found, at last, a nationally endorsed admonition against fee-splitting[5(pp258–259),6]:

*"It is derogatory to professional character for physicians to pay or offer to pay commissions to any person whatsoever who may recommend to them patients requiring general or special treatment or surgical operations. It is equally derogatory to professional character for physicians to solicit or to receive such commissions."*

Nine years later in June 1912, the next revision of the Principles of Medical Ethics was published. Once again the subject of fee-splitting was addressed.[7] Although the admonition against paying for referrals (commissions) was retained, division of fees was sanctioned if the patient was informed:

*"It is detrimental to the public good and degrading to the profession, and therefore unprofessional, to give or to receive a commission. It is also unprofessional to divide a fee for medical advice or surgical treatment, unless the patient or his next friend is fully informed as to the terms of the transaction. The patient should be made to realize that a proper fee should be paid the family physician for the service he renders in determining the surgical and medical treatment suited to the condition, and in advising concerning those best qualified to render any special service that may be required by the patient."*

Unfortunately, this did not solve the problem. Although the proscription against buying and selling patients had now been stated twice, the practice remained widespread. Likewise, unfortunate was the AMA's inability to enforce any of these guides. By its very nature, it was an entity composed of independent, albeit representative, medical societies from around the country. They imposed no penalty for violation of these principles.

The American College of Surgeons was born in 1913 out of needs unaddressed by the medical organizations of the day. Specifically, the College outlined those needs to be, "defining the qualified surgeon, eliminating financial graft, improving the hospital, and making reforms national in scope... and establishing the legitimacy of any organization that presumed to undertake the first four tasks."[8(p8)]

With the rapid development of safe anesthesia and antisepsis in the early 1900s, there was a rapid increase in the number of people doing surgery. Diseases hidden from view in the chest, abdomen, pelvis, and brain were becoming legitimate targets for treatment and cure.[5(p258)] 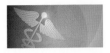 Elective surgery was becoming commonplace if not popular. Further, the surgeon's hour in the operating room grew to be more highly reimbursed than the family physician's hour in the office. Thus, with so many new providers of surgery entering the marketplace and with discrepancies in reimbursement between primary care and specialist creating an ever-widening gulf, there was a growing attraction to fee-splitting.

The American College of Surgeons was in a position to enforce its ethical code. At its first organizational meeting, the College included the proscription against fee-splitting in its Fellowship Pledge[8(p211)]: surgical fees were no longer to be split by the surgeon; referrals were no longer to be purchased.

Despite the opposition by the American College of Surgeons to fee-splitting, for many years there was no significant public opposition to the practice. At the time, only three states had legislated against medical fee-splitting. *Only one court decision, in the Michigan appellate, had judged fee-splitting a breach of the physician's fiduciary duty to the patient (McNair v Parr, Mich., 1913).*[9,10] The opposition to measures to limit fee-splitting was great.

The Chicago Medical Society openly declared the American College of Surgeons to be un-American and inequitable, owing, in no small part, to its stand against fee-splitting.[11(pp130–135,p426)] Resolutions against the College were raised in the AMA national meetings.[12] The American Board of Surgery, founded in 1937 as the certifier of surgeons, fought back and further admonished surgeons themselves by affirming that[8(p212)]:

> *"The Board, believing that the practice of fee splitting is pernicious, leading as it does to a traffic in human life, will reserve the right to inquire particularly into any candidate's practice in regard to this question."*

Early on, the actual techniques for fee-splitting were not very sophisticated,[13(pp36 and 50–57)] but they were effective:

1. The surgeon simply paid the referring physician outright for his/her referral.
2. The referring doctor arranged to be the assistant at operation, and he/she and the surgeon billed the patient as a single entity but did not itemize their fees. Here, the referral was being purchased, and the total bill was usually inflated.
3. The referring doctor was the assistant at surgery, and both he/she and the surgeon submitted itemized bills, but the surgeon gave more of his/her fee to the referring doctor.

The College of Surgeons continued its struggle against these practices for decades, but, by World War II, the practice of fee-splitting was so widespread 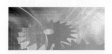 that the College despaired of ever controlling it. To compound the problem, at that time only 50% of country's surgeons were Fellows of the College. It would take till the early 1950s before 23 states, not even half the Union of the time, would have laws dealing with fee-splitting.[8(p212)] It was a small wonder that surgeons who refused to engage in the practice suffered financially.

At the end of the war, the College came into possession of a powerful weapon: one that has come to be known as the "Columbus Plan." In 1945 the Columbus (Ohio) Surgical Society was established by 57 surgeons with its primary purpose being the eradication of fee-splitting. Their tactic was unique. They required an annual audit of their members' accounts, and anyone who tried to deduct the cost of split fees as "business expenses" was reported to the Internal Revenue Service (IRS). Ordinarily, the IRS would not have a cause to intervene, but the Society was able to demonstrate so much opposition to the practice of fee-splitting that the IRS considered those payments to be "against public policy" and therefore not deductible.[8(p213),13(p57)]

Several years later, the IRS Commissioner would rule against 2 opticians who claimed that the tax deductions, which they took for kickbacks to ophthalmologists on glasses sold to their patients, were "business expenses."[14] As in the Columbus Plan, the IRS cited disallowance of expenditures on the grounds that payments (split fees) "violated a fixed public policy" and were medically unethical. The opticians challenged this in the Supreme Court and won, because, at the time they were claiming their deductions, kickbacks had not yet been sufficiently defined as being against public policy.

However, within 5 weeks of that decision, the American College of Surgeons declared its position to both the IRS and to the public, opposing the "secret division of fees between a surgeon and a referring physician as being a violation of medical ethics and inimical to the best interests of the patient, and hence the public."

Furthermore, they proclaimed:

> *"It is the fixed opinion of the Regents that fee-splitting is against public policy. It is against public policy in terms of the Code of Ethics of the American Medical Association, which represents the great majority of American physicians. It is against public policy in terms of the Fellowship Pledge taken by each Fellow of the American College of Surgeons. Obviously, it is against public policy in the 23 states which have laws prohibiting fee-splitting."* The College also took this opportunity to outline its position to its own membership in *"A Statement on Certain Unethical Practices in Surgery."*[15]

To this point, the American College of Surgeons had waged a battle against fee-splitting: on the one hand, by establishing itself as a separate entity with a specific mission to do so, and, on the other hand, by specifically defining what it meant to be a "surgeon." It had incorporated its stand against fee-splitting into the fabric of its membership and had established a mechanism to prosecute by expulsion any violation of this position. It had elicited the support of the American Board of Surgery. It had held forth against very public attacks of organized medicine of the day. It had endorsed the punitive approach adopted by the Ohio surgeons in reporting directly to the IRS anyone who would claim split fees as business deductions.

In 1953, the College played the card it had been hesitant to play: It finally and purposefully brought the struggle against fee-splitting to the arena of American public opinion.[16] In 1953 the opening salvo of that tactical move took place in the geographic center of the United States, the state of Iowa. The problem of fee-splitting in the state of Iowa was so pervasive that the College initiated a "boycott" of the entire state and publicized it.[13(p56)] It voted to defer consideration of all applicants for Fellowship from Iowa until a credentials committee could be formed within the state to examine the dealings of those applicants. For their efforts, they once again drew criticism from their own membership and from many of the medical organizations of the time, but they had the public's attention.[8(p217),11(pp168,255, and 421–427),17]

## Modern-Day Substitutes

The post–World War II growth in health insurance, the attempts to secure health care for the poor, and the introduction of Medicare and Medicaid in July 1965 may appear to have made the issue of overt fee-splitting extinct, but they introduced a new set of substitutes. Today, patients seem to have become the "property" of their insurers. They go where they are told to go. They are seen by the physicians they are told to see. It seems every provider is either "in-plan" or "out-of-plan."

Although subtle in respect to fee-splitting, concerns about the ethical distribution of the surgeon's remuneration were raised again by the young but growing reimbursement plan that was "prepaid health insurance." Originally an extension of accidental loss coverage, prepaid plans grew out of accidental loss coverage offered to employees of the railroads and other industries.[18] However, in the mechanics of day-to-day business and in the absence of computers, multiple billings generated by a single procedure, to include payments to the surgeon and to the assistant, could not be handled by most of the companies in the days before those computers.

Reimbursement for surgery consisted of a single check, sent to the operating surgeon, from which all additional services stemming from the surgery were to be paid. Blue Cross and Blue Shield of Massachusetts could process multiple claims, but they, too, were unwittingly, albeit operationally, complicit in fee-splitting by establishing a flat assistant's fee of 15% of 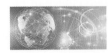 the surgeon's fee. Again, if the assistant was also the referring physician, this created an incentive to send more patients for surgery.[8(p220)]

Those who argued in favor of establishing a flat-percentage assistant's fee took the position that, by assisting in surgery, the referring physician was rendering a service to his/her patient. Actually, though, the "service" was being rendered to the surgeon, both in the consultation with the patient for surgery and in the operating room. Were it not for the innate qualities of each physician, the unspoken rubric might easily have been, "Whether your patient needs an operation or not, the referral for operating on her will be to our mutual benefit."

To understand this, a brief review of the finances of medicine may be helpful. For many years, the principle underpinning the finances of the practice of medicine in the United States has been "fee-for-service": a fee was charged before or after a service was rendered. For generations it has been the obligation of physicians to render their services with expertise and with expedition proportional to the problem and without undue consideration given initially to recovery of their fees. This has contributed to the public's opinion that physicians are honorable and has helped to both idealize and codify the

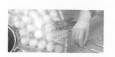 physician-patient relationship. Unfortunately, in some situations, it also left the relationship open to abuse by the patient. In other situations, it gave the physician control of not only the fee but also the extent to which treatment would continue. The norms of the profession and the physician's own conscience would dictate that extent.

Prepaid health insurance was intended to ameliorate some of these issues. Its designers assumed many things which led to unintended consequences. They assumed that self-preservation, rather than excess and dangerous living, would rule those insured; that reason would govern the spending of those dollars; and new drugs or new devices would be given to those most in need. They did not envision hospitals competing for the latest technology and duplicating the same equipment acquired by their competitor across the street; or the absurd costs passed on to the consumer as well as the protectionist policies that have secured the pharmaceutical industry's monopoly and profit margins in this country; or the "malpractice crisis" of the 1970s, 1980s, and 1990s and the wasteful cost of "defensive medicine"; or expectations that there was a cure for everything and, failing that cure, that there would always be someone to blame. They may not have envisioned that they would become the primary fiscal intermediary between the patient and the physician.

Essentially, then, as these health insurance systems evolved, the very nature of the referring entity changed dramatically, and the entity with whom the surgeon "split the fee" became the insurance company. Instead of giving a percentage of his/her surgical fee to the referring doctor, the surgeon agreed to give that percentage to the insurance company in return for being listed on its "provider panel" to have the patient sent to him/her in the first place.[19] Therefore, effectively, the surgeon pays the company for the referral and for a guarantee of being able to keep a portion of his/her fee.

Over time, the inability of health insurance to deal with rising costs led to the introduction of "managed care" and "preferred provider" organizations. In these systems, individual cases are under continuous review if the patients are hospitalized and are subject to a complex pathway for outpatient testing approval. One of the arguments that faced the introduction of Medicare was that it would interfere with the sanctity of the physician-patient relationship. Yet, despite the rules enacted to protect patient privacy, many more layers of bureaucracy and many more people have been added to the cost base of managed care.

If "fee-splitting" amounts to a fee, originally paid to a physician in his/her care of a patient, a portion of which is then paid back (kicked back) to someone who is not treating the patient but who *procures* the patient for the physician, then the advent of the health maintenance organization (HMO), as a spin-off of managed care, may be the single greatest opportunity for abuse.

Here, under the cover of cost-containment, a patient or his/her purchasing organization pays a fee to a third party that or who is not a physician. The third party then distributes a portion of that fee to a physician, who has agreed that the patient's care will be paid out of that fixed amount. Any testing or treatment that is required will come from that fixed amount. Any part of the fee not used in testing or treatment, in a given time frame, is then remitted to the physician as income. The "incentive" here is ostensibly to promote the medical management of health; thus the derivation of the term. The unstated and, hopefully, undesirable result of the arrangement, however, is to discourage the physician from finding anything wrong with the patient.

The Regents of the American College of Surgeons began examining the fee-splitting potential in HMOs in 1985. They recognized the rise of "discount" or "contract" medicine, and they addressed the question of whether discounting of fees, as required by managed care (referred to as "alternative delivery systems"), constituted fee-splitting. Their deliberations led to the amendment of article VII, section I of the Bylaws of the College and to modification of the Fellowship Pledge by referencing governmental proscriptions against medical fraud and abuse dating to 1977:

*"A Surgeon Must Refuse to Split Fees. Fee-splitting as an inducement to refer a patient to another physician is unethical. The premise for referral must be quality of care... Many of the states have laws which forbid any fee-splitting, and there is no state which sanctions it. Additionally,* 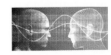 *federal law makes illegal any form of rebate, kickback, or splitting of fees which includes any federal money. Thus, such illegal inducement cannot be considered an item of deductible business expense."*

In making these changes, the College informed its Fellows that the stand against fee-splitting was not intended to influence any Fellow's decision regarding "whether to participate in a particular alternative delivery system which may require discounting of fees."[20] In essence, the College acknowledged the dilemma that managed care systems presented while recognizing that surgeons still needed to work within those systems.

In 1994, the College went a step further by creating a policy outline that both the HMO and the surgeon could follow. In so doing, it acknowledged the stated objectives of the HMOs while simultaneously shedding light on those points at which the surgeon could be confronted by conflicts of interest in his/her financial relationship with the HMO. In its "Statement of Recommendations to Ensure Quality of Surgical Services in Managed Care Environments," the College issued guidelines for "seeking to ensure the maintenance of high-quality surgical care for patients enrolled in managed care systems."[21]

In April 1986, director of the American College of Surgeons, C. Rollins Hanlon, MD, FACS, made a series of observations in his own inimitable style: "Just as students of dishonest business practice have marveled at the endless ingenuity of embezzlers, so have I been amazed at the lengths to which physicians and surgeons have gone in devising innovative ways to split professional fees without appearing to do so." He observed that, at that time, not only were referring doctors being paid for "real or alleged" assisting in the operating room, but they also were receiving a portion of the surgeon's fee for "preop and postop care." He further decried the practice of lithotripsy centers paying for the referral of patients with renal calculi, saying that, even when the referral originated with a urologist, the payment kicked back was out of proportion to the pre–extracorporeal shock wave lithotripsy care the patients were receiving. As these centers were effectively purchasing the patients, the Board of Regents of the College labeled this practice "fee-splitting."[22]

The law cited stemmed from the Medicare and Medicaid Anti-Fraud and Abuse Act of 1977 and the case of the United States v. Greber (760 F.2d 68 (3d Cir.), cert. denied, 474 U.S. 988 (1985) wherein a cardiologist paid kickbacks to his referring physicians while claiming that the payments were also for professional services rendered by the referring doctors. The courts held that a payment to a referring physician is illegal if it is done to encourage future referrals, "even if the payment is compensatory."[23]

Nonetheless, Dr Hanlon also expressed his disappointment that control from outside the profession and most regrettably by statute was needed: "It is unfortunate that the degree of venality evidenced by old and new forms 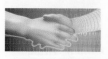 of fee-splitting should have contributed to validating the need for imposing a felony statute on relationships that should be controlled by professional ethics. When we complain about the [impact of the] relentless march of corporate transformation on the practice of medicine and the resultant loss of professional independence, we should not fail to assign some degree of blame to the improper conduct of a minority of physicians."

Another applicable statute is the Physician Self-Referral Law (Stark Law). This prohibits a physician from making a referral for certain "designated health services payable by Medicare or Medicaid" to an entity in which the physician (or an immediate family member) has an ownership or investment interest or with which he/she has a compensation arrangement. An example is the situation in which a doctor refers a Medicare patient for laboratory work or X-rays to a business in which the doctor has an investment interest. A portion of the fee collected for the test is then kicked back to the referring doctor-investor.[24] The American College of Physicians in its Policy Compendium of August 2016[25] points out that fee-splitting can also take the form of financial incentives and even gifts from pharmaceutical or medical device companies; perhaps to induce overutilization of services, in the case of fee-for-service plans, or underutilization, in the case of capitation (HMO) plans. The gifts themselves may take the form of industry support of educational programs, making them especially appealing.

Fee-splitting can take the form of referrals of patients to facilities in which the doctor has invested but does not provide care. Furthermore, the AMA's Opinions on the Physician as Businessperson (Opinion 6.03/11.3.4) specifies that health care facilities (eg, laboratories, clinics, hospitals, and the like) "that compensate physicians for referral of patients are engaged in fee splitting, which is unethical." Payments for the physician's "cognitive services" in these facilities (ie, prescribing for the patient or revising the patient's course of treatment) cannot be made by the facility but only by the patient or the patient's third-party payer.[26,27]

As eloquently stated in the ACP Compendium:

> *"Physicians must practice in a world of increasing complexity and cost pressures. To do so appropriately, they must be conscious of all potential influences and must use ethical judgment and scientifically valid clinical decision-making as their guides. Putting patients first and maintaining professionalism should continue to be the goal of every physician."*[25(p47)]

As set forth at the beginning, it is sincerely hoped that this review serves as a reminder that, despite the changing face of surgical practice, the reasons for what we do as surgeons can and should remain clear. Moreover, surgeons ought to carefully examine all business practices for variations on the fee-splitting theme.

# References

1. Koocher GP, Keith-Spiegel P. *Ethics in Psychology and the Mental Health Professions: Standards and Cases.* New York: Oxford University Press; 2008:166–170.
2. McVaugh MR. *Medicine Before the Plague: Practitioners and Their Patient in the Crown of Aragon, 1285–1345.* Cambridge: Cambridge University Press; 1993:109.
3. Percival T, Russell S. *Medical Ethics: Or, a Code of Institutes and Precepts, Adapted to the Professional Conduct of Physicians and Surgeons.* Manchester, London; 1803.

4. American Medical Association. *Code of Medical Ethics of the American Medical Association: Adopted at the Adjourned Meeting of the National Medical Convention in Philadelphia*. Chicago: American Medical Association Press; May 1847.

5. Rothstein WG. *American Physicians in the Nineteenth Century: From Sects to Science*. Vol. 115. Baltimore: Johns Hopkins University Press; 1985:258–259.

6. American Medical Association. *Principles of Medical Ethics of the American Medical Association*. Chicago: American Medical Association Press; 1903:23–24.

7. American Medical Association. *Principles of Medical Ethics of the American Medical Association, Article VI, Section 3*. Chicago: American Medical Association Press; 1912:269.

8. Nahrwold DL, Kernahan PJ. *A Century of Surgeons and Surgery: The American College of Surgeons, 1913–2012*. Vol. 8. Chicago: The American College of Surgeons; 2012:211–213;217;220.

9. Michigan Reports: Cases Decided in the Supreme Court of Michigan. Vol. 177. ("McNair v. Parr," Michigan, October, 1913, 143N, w. 42); Phelps & Stevens, printers, 1914. Harvard University; 2008:327–336.

10. Michigan Law Review: Vol. XII 1913–1914:227–228. Ann Arbor: University of Michigan Department of Law; 1914, Evans Holbrook, Trustee.

11. Davis L. *Fellowship of Surgeons: A History of the American College of Surgeons*. Chicago: American College of Surgeons; 1960:130–135;168;255:421–427.

12. Baker RB, Caplan AL, Emanuel LL, Latham SR, eds. *The American Medical Ethics Revolution: How the AMA's Code of Ethics Has Transformed Physicians' Relationships to Patients, Professionals, and Society*. Baltimore: Johns Hopkins University Press; 1999:87.

13. Spencer SM. Patients for sale. *Saturday Evening Post*. January 16, 1954;226(29): 36–41;50–57.

14. Supreme Court decision spurs college to oppose tax deduction of split fees. *Bull Am Coll Surg*. July–August 1952;37(2):49–51.

15. A statement on certain unethical practices in surgery. *Bull Am Coll Surg*. July–August 1952;37(2):51–52.

16. *Surgeon Attacks Ethics Violators*. The New York Times, NY Times Special; May 20, 1954:37.

17. *Surgeons' Golden Anniversary, Medical World News*. New York: Maxwell M Geffen Publisher; May 10, 1963.

18. Field MJ, Shapiro HT, eds. *Employment and Health Benefits: A Connection at Risk*. Institute of Medicine Committee on Employment-Based Health Benefits. National Academies Press; 1993 [Chapter 2: Origins and Evolution of Employment-Based Health Benefits].

19. Verrilli DK, Zuckerraan S. Preferred provider organizations and physician fees; Medicare & Medicaid Research Review (Centers for Medicare and Medicaid Services). *Health Care Financ Rev*. Spring 1996;17(3):161–170.

20. Jurkiewicz MJ, Parks P. Fee-splitting: college bylaws clarified. *Bull Am Coll Surg*. November 1985;79(11):19–21.

21. American College of Surgeons. Statement on Recommendations to ensure quality of surgical services in managed care environments. *Bull Am Coll Surg*. December 1994;79(12):30–31.

22. Hanlon CR. Fee-splitting. *Bull Am Coll Surg*. April 1986;71(4):1.

23. United States v. Greber 760 F.2d 68 (3d Cir.), cert. denied, 474 U.S. 988 (1985); Chicago: American College of Healthcare Executives.

24. Avoiding Medicare Fraud & Abuse: A Roadmap for Physicians; Department of Health and Human Services, Centers for Medicare & Medicaid Services; ICN 905645; August 2016.

25. American College of Physicians Policy Compendium. *The American College of Physicians Division of Government Affairs and Public Policy*. Washington, DC; Summer 2016 (updated 8/10/16):47.

26. Chapter 11: Financing and Delivery of Health Care, Opinion 11.3.4—Fee Splitting. In: *AMA Principles of Medical Ethics: II*, p. 11. Chicago: Code of Medical Ethics of the American Medical Association/Council on Ethical and Judicial Affairs; 2017.

27. AMA Code of Ethics Concordance, 2016: Opinion 6.03 (11.3.4)—Fee Splitting: Referrals to Health Care Facilities. *AMA J Ethics*. 2013; Volume 15, Number 2: 136–140.

# 27 Delivering Bad News—Challenges and Opportunities

Roland T. Skeel, MD
Kristi S. Williams, MD

PROLOGUE ▶ There are an infinite number of descriptions of any operation, disease, or prognosis. In choosing from this infinity of tellings, the surgeons' goal should be "therapeutic truth" without sacrificing verisimilitude.

Emily Dickinson, among the greatest of American poets, put it this way: "tell the truth but tell it slant." The slant required is the patient's well-being. "Therapeutic truth" is a form of cognitive psychotherapy.

A recent contribution to this area is the proposal to use more than one of the infinity of tellings: a best-case scenario and a worst-case scenario. Chesney et al[1] report that this approach can be learned with relative ease and that it balances hope with the most fearful of prospects.

There are several father-son teams among the contributors to this book. With Kristi Williams and Roland Skeel, we have a father-daughter team of clinicians with great expertise and equally great experience. They have much to say about the praxis and pace of truth telling; they address in detail the elements of "therapeutic truth."

Dr Roland T. Skeel is a professor of medicine at The University of Toledo College of Medicine.

Dr Kristi S. Williams is a professor of psychiatry at The University of Toledo College of Medicine.

*It is much more important to know what sort of a patient has a disease than what sort of disease the patient has.*

*Sir William Osler*

## Introduction

Physicians and surgeons frequently have not only the opportunity to deliver joyful news to patients, such as in the birth of a healthy baby, but also occasions when they must be the deliverer of bad news, which will bring confusion, anxiety, fear, and sadness to patients and their families. The latter is a stressful time not only for the patient and family but also for the surgeon who has the responsibility to deliver the bad news in a way that is clear and honest, and also empathetic, and does not cause added harm to the patient or the patient's family.

## Ethical Principles

There are few situations in which applying the ethical principles of *beneficence, respect for persons,* and *honesty* is more complex than when the physician undertakes the responsibility to deliver bad news to his/her patient.

Beneficence requires that we try to do what is best for the patient and his/her family, but exactly what that means when giving bad news is not so clear. If we present only the straightforward facts, we would be honest but could leave the patient with anxiety and questions about the meaning of those facts and their consequences. The patient and his/her surrogates need understanding of survival, activities of daily living, family, finances, occupation and quality of life. All these considerations are issues that the surgeon should be prepared to address with the patient and patient's family in as empathetic and compassionate a way as possible, as he/she seeks to avoid doing harm to the patient.

On the other hand, if the bad news is presented in a way that is ambiguous or uses medical jargon, it is unlikely that the patient would gain a clear understanding of what was really going on. Such obfuscation might seem a kinder way to get through the immediate challenge of giving the bad news, but by avoiding telling the patient the news more directly and in terms that are understandable, the surgeon may undermine trust or give false hope to the patient and not fulfill the desired goal of showing respect for autonomy of the patient and his/her right to know with empathetic honesty. Although obfus-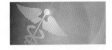cation might be undertaken with a laudable goal of protecting the patient, it may also be viewed as the physician's tendency to protect himself/herself from the pain experienced when having to deliver bad news in a more candid way. The surgeon may obfuscate to make the conversation personally less painful and less time-consuming.

## The Bad News Spectrum

Not all "bad news" is the same. Informing a patient that a fingernail must be removed, an appendectomy must be performed, or he/she must have 6 weeks of intravenous antibiotics can be classified on the lower end of the bad news spectrum; while these events may not be pleasant for the patient, they are not likely to have long-term implications. In contrast, there are many types of bad news that can be devastating to the patient and his/her family and that require skill and compassion to deliver empathetically yet truthfully. These categories, in no particular order, include the following:

- The death of a child, spouse, parent, or other loved one
- A new diagnosis of cancer or recurrence of a cancer
- The necessity for amputation
- The diagnosis of a degenerative neurologic condition
- The diagnosis of human immunodeficiency virus infection

Each of these situations is unique, yet there is a commonality as how to best approach the patient and family; how best to help them to understand 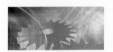 the surgical condition and the potential options if options are present; and how to help them to cope emotionally and intellectually with the bad news they have just received. Learning how to break bad news is an important lesson for any physician[2] and particularly for surgeons who are often faced with this challenge.

## How, When, and Where to Deliver "the Bad News"

It is nearly always best to deliver bad news in person. Although this is not always possible, the surgeon or other physicians should make sufficient time in their schedule to be present for the patient and family. Although it is entirely appropriate—and a good learning experience—for house staff to deliver or participate in the delivery of bad news, it should not be delegated to others because the attending or responsible surgeon is "too busy" or uncomfortable giving the bad news.

Usually, it is preferable to deliver the bad news as soon as it is clearly known. This was well illustrated by Joel Vernick and Myron Karon in their seminal article, "Who's Afraid of Death on a Leukemia Ward?"[3] They found that even children with leukemia dealt better with the death of one of their friends on the leukemia ward at the National Institutes of Health when they were told the truth compassionately by the first staff member to see them after the death, rather than having the truth withheld by phrases such as "she was transferred to the 12th floor last night."

There is no single best place to deliver painful and distressing information. Best is a quiet place or a private room where the patient and family can believe that the news is not being shared with others who do not have the need to know. Cell phones should be muted to let the patient and family know that during this time, their needs are paramount and that they have your undivided attention. Let others in the area, nurses, and other staff not involved in the discussion know that the meeting is taking place, so that you will not be disturbed unnecessarily.

## Who Should Be Present?

Often patients and families will know ahead of time that there is important "news" that is about to be given and will already have gathered together those whom they wish to be present to hear what is said. If this has not already occurred, it is often best to inform the patient ahead of time that their situation will be explained and ask whether they wish to have others present to hear. Not infrequently, one may have patients or family say that they want the physician to wait until other family members are present before the physician talks with the patient; this should be respected, even though it might mean that the discussion must be deferred to a less convenient time for the surgeon. Some patients may also wish to have a spiritual counselor or their favorite nurse present when the bad news is anticipated. The medical team does best to defer to the patient's wishes. It is about them, not about us!

## Preparing the Patient and Family

Depending on the situation, it is often possible and beneficial to prepare the patient for bad news that may follow. This might consist of telling the patient before obtaining a specimen for biopsy of the lung, for example, that the reason is to determine whether a cancer or an infection problem is responsible for the mass on the chest X-ray or computed tomography scan. This helps to prevent the diagnosis from coming to them totally unexpectedly. Similarly, if a patient has presented with a neurologic syndrome for which the neurologist suspects multiple sclerosis, letting the patient know the range of potential 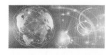 findings on the computed tomography scan or the magnetic resonance imaging scan—while in itself anxiety provoking—can be helpful in preparing the patient.

Preparing the patient and the family in this way also carries its own potential to exacerbate anxiety, and the surgeon should recognize that many people have a more difficult time with the unknown than they do with a known, definite diagnosis. The surgeon should take sufficient time when having this preparatory discussion to:

- let the patient know that it is important to carefully examine all relevant evidence before coming to a conclusion about the nature of their illness;
- assure them that all testing will be done as expeditiously as possible, but that the risks of jumping to conclusions are greater than taking the time to get it right;
- let the patient know what can be done if the worst is found;
- tell them that they will be informed as soon as the surgeon is sure; and
- reassure the patient and family that they can reach the surgeon at any time if questions arise before the meeting intended to discuss the findings in detail.

## How to Deliver the Bad News

When the time has come and the patient, family, or other representatives have gathered, the first step is to greet all of those present and introduce yourself to those who may not know you. Sit down and face the patient and family. Try to have an open posture, and do not cross your arms (too authoritative and may be threatening) or put your foot across your opposite knee (too casual—not serious and can be perceived as physical barrier between you and others) when having this serious conversation. This will let them know that for this time, you are there for them and not there just to give them a diagnosis and get out of the door. Be aware of your own body language.

If they have been prepared ahead of time for a potential "bad news" discussion, this is the time to transition that preparation by saying something like, "As you might remember, we said we're going to do the biopsy to determine whether the nodule we saw in the lung was infection, cancer, or some benign problem. Unfortunately… or, I'm sorry to have to tell you… we found on the biopsy that cancer cells were in that nodule." At that point, rather than launching into a full explanation of what that means, it is critical to be attentive to the nonverbal body language as well as verbal response of the patient and 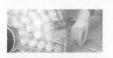 family before speaking further. This might be termed the "iterative approach to giving bad news." What you say further may be determined by the specifics of the diagnosis, prognosis, and treatment, but how it is said must be modulated by how the patient and family respond. Kirk et al[4] delineated process attributes that patients receiving palliative care for cancer want to be told. The attributes they suggest are to (1) play it straight, (2) make it clear, (3) show you care, (4) give the patient and family enough time, (5) pace the information, and (6) reassure that you will not abandon the patient/family as illness progresses.

These attributes apply well to delivering bad news. Baile et al[5] have given the acronym SPIKES to their protocol for giving bad news.

SPIKES Protocol

*S*—Set up the interview: Mental and physical preparation
*P*—Perception: Assess what patient knows
*I*—Invitation: Ask how much patient wants to know
*K*—Knowledge: Give the medical facts
*E*—Emotional: Respond to patient's emotions
*S*—Strategy and Summary: Discuss follow-up steps

Each of these principles provides helpful insights regarding approach and technique for helping patients and their families as you take on the responsibility of delivering bad news.

One sensitive and critical issue is whether or not and in what circumstances it is desirable to have more physical contact with a patient beyond a handshake. In nearly all circumstances, it is important to take the cues from the patient. Thus, if the patient reaches out to the physician to take his/her hand or give a hug, and if the physician feels comfortable, it is often 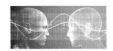 helpful to provide the patient that tangible reassurance of caring. Remember, however, this is for the patient's well-being, not the physician's. Other factors that should be taken into account include how well the patient and family are known to the physician, and the age and sex of the physician and patient. The physician can be empathetic without physical touch, and many patients, particularly from other cultures, may be distressed by the physician to showing physical manifestations of affection.

Depending on how well the patient and family were prepared ahead of time, their personal and family history, their psychologic makeup, and the severity of the bad news, the conversation may head in many different directions, and the physician must be prepared to adjust to the exigent milieu and not simply rush through a planned delivery of the diagnosis, management, and likely outcome.

Studies have shown that once a person hears a "bad news" diagnosis, he/she often does not hear or remember anything else in the conversation. Having family members or friends present can help this. It may also help if they are allowed to record what the physician says. Reiteration of the relevant key points is also helpful. As once was said, "I tell them what I'm going to tell them; I tell them; then I tell them what I told them." It is important not to try to give too much information at one sitting. Nonetheless, there are key pieces of information that the patient and family will want to know and are helpful to convey:

1. What is the specific diagnosis or problem? Give it a name that they can write down, remember, and "research" for themselves.

2. What are the physician's expectations about the potential course of the disease? Remember we usually do not have a crystal ball, so avoid getting too definitive about prognosis.
3. What are the options and recommendations for treatment of the underlying problem, the alleviation of symptoms, and improvement of quality of life? Reassure them that you will work with them each step of the way.
4. Give them reason for hope and optimism, which they need to counterbalance their intuitive pessimism on hearing the bad news. It can help to assure them that you will always tell them the truth, but your approach is one of realistic optimism. Let them know you and your staff will be there for them, and they will not be left to deal with their situation alone.
5. What are the next steps to be taken?
6. Write down the name and phone contact information of a specific person whom they can call if questions arise and to set up another meeting if appropriate. Patients and family members need time to process the information given and to gather their thoughts and develop questions.

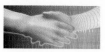

## Learning How to Do It Well

Giving bad news is a challenge for surgeons, particularly early in their career. It is not something that comes naturally to anyone but can get better with time and with practice. One helpful technique is to listen and observe carefully to mentors who appear to do it well, to learn how they perform in these difficult situations. It is also worthwhile to make note of times when the process does not go well and to analyze what problems might have been avoided. Some younger surgeons have found that it is worthwhile to practice giving bad news to a "standardized patient"[6] while having the session videotaped.[7] This affords an opportunity for the "patient" to give feedback to the physician about how the process felt to them and what went well or not. It also allows a review of the video with a mentor or among colleagues whose observations can suggest information about the physician's delivery and his/her response to the patient's reactions.

## Dealing With Expected and Unexpected Consequences

Responses by patients and families have a wide range; many are predictable, such as sadness and tears, numbness or courageous defiance, denial or wanting a second opinion. Having a box of tissues available to wipe away the tears as well as a nurse or other assistants to help provide comfort is always a good idea. At times, there may also be unexpected responses that may be a challenge for the surgeon to handle effectively. These may include uncontrolled wailing, storming out of the office, or irrational anger at the surgeon. One of the first of these that I (Dr Roland T. Skeel) saw was the response of a mother who was informed by a resident that her 10-year-old son had died of acute leukemia and sepsis. Her unexpected reaction was to land a right hook on the jaw of the resident as her expression of pain and anger at the son's death. There were other situations where unrelenting wailing continued for hours. Some patients will walk out as soon as they have heard the initial bad news. Others will deny the possibility of what they have heard and insist on a second opinion.

When confronted with any of these unexpected responses, the surgeon must remember that each patient and family member brings his/her own history, culture, personality, and social structure to the hearing of bad news, and the physician's responsibility is not to judge the reaction but to try to understand and help the patient and family however he/she can. In so doing, we support the obligations of beneficence and respect for the autonomy of the individual persons as well as the principle of justice within the social structures we have established for attending to both the physical and psychologic care of our patients.

# References

1. Chesney TR. Training surgical residents to use a framework to promote shared decision making for patients with poor baseline prognosis experiencing surgical emergencies. *J Am Coll Surg.* 2016;223(4 suppl 1):549.
2. Buckman R, Kason Y. *How to Break Bad News: A Guide for Health Care Professionals.* Baltimore: Johns Hopkins University Press; 1992.
3. Vernick J, Karon M. Who's afraid of death on a leukemia ward? *Am J Dis Child.* 1965;109:393–397.
4. Kirk P, Kirk I, Kristjanson LJ. What do patients receiving palliative care for cancer and their families want to be told? A Canadian and Australian qualitative study. *BMJ.* 2004;328(7452):1343.
5. Baile WF, Buckman R, Lenzi R, Glober G, Beale EA, Kudelka AP. SPIKES—a six-step protocol for delivering bad news: application to the patient with cancer. *Oncologist.* 2000;5(4):302–311.
6. Rosenbaum ME, Kreiter C. Teaching delivery of bad news using experiential sessions with standardized patients. *Teach Learn Med.* 2002;14(3):144–149.
7. Supiot S, Bonnaud-Antignac A. Using simulated interviews to teach junior medical students to disclose the diagnosis of cancer. *J Cancer Educ.* 2008;23(2):102–107.

# 28 Fundamental Principles of Leadership Training in Surgery and the Moral Imperative

Shiela Beroukhim, MD
Hollis W. Merrick, III, MD
Francis Charles Brunicardi, MD

PROLOGUE ▶ The prevention of job-induced emotional exhaustion, all too common among surgeons, is an obligation of every surgeon and specifically a goal of leaders in our discipline. Surgeons, particularly young surgeons, are often admonished to assume responsibility for their own resilience; however, this approach may possess little value. Far more efficacious are acts and utterances of persons in leadership roles: section heads, chairs, or others. Institutional changes in technology or work expectations are important, but an emphasis on interdependence, congruence of goals, and resolution of ethical ambiguity is even more important. All of these are fostered by an inspirational style of leadership as opposed to an authoritarian style. In the end the demonstration of ethical behaviors and utterances are essential strategies for the prevention of job-induced emotional exhaustion.

Shiela Beroukhim is a medical student at the David Geffen School of Medicine at the University of California, Los Angeles.

Dr Hollis W. Merrick is a professor emeritus in the Department of Surgery at The University of Toledo College of Medicine.

Dr Francis Charles Brunicardi is a professor and chairman of the Department of Surgery at The University of Toledo College of Medicine. He assumed this role after a long career of contributions to our discipline.

He is the senior editor of Schwartz's *Textbook of Surgery* and has a special interest in surgical leadership.

## Abstract

Everyday new medicinal drugs are developed, advanced surgical techniques are established, and insurance policies are further modified. Physicians and surgeons have a duty to lead their health care teams in adapting to the rapidly changing field of medicine while continuing to deliver excellent care to patients. This is the great leadership challenge facing physicians and surgeons today. We searched the literature using PubMed and Google Scholar for articles on leadership training in the field of surgery and the effects of leadership on the quality of health care delivered in hospitals and clinics. Our review of the literature shows that training residents to attain leadership skills ultimately leads to substantially improved outcomes across multiple aspects of health care. However, many surgical residency programs need to more strongly emphasize leadership training to help surgeons prepare for their role as leaders. In an effort to mold the abstract concept of leadership into a more tangible and teachable topic, we define the 5 most important attributes of leadership and the moral imperative as demonstrated by one of the greatest leaders in history, Dr Martin Luther King, Jr, and show how each individual attribute leads to improved quality of health care. We also provide examples of current residency programs, which have successfully implemented leadership training as well as objective methods of measuring leadership qualities. Ultimately, training surgeons to become skilled leaders and mastering the ethical and moral skills required in modern medical care are important components of residency programs' commitment to delivering only the highest quality of care for patients.

## Introduction

A surgical team consists of the attending surgeons, surgical residents, nurses, anesthesiologists, surgical technicians, medical students, and patients and their families. It is self-evident that in this highly dynamic and functional setting, effective patient care demands active guidance and leadership from the surgeon. It is imperative that we offer substantive training in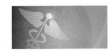

leadership, more than what can be garnered by observation, yet most surgical residency programs have not implemented specific training in leadership, and young surgeons across the country think that their residency curricula lack sufficient leadership training.[1,2] In a university survey, the majority of senior surgical residents judged themselves to be lacking in leadership and managerial skills.[3] In this chapter, we address this need in leadership training in surgical residency training programs by defining leadership's most important attributes, outlining the benefits of leadership training in surgical residency curriculum, and offering suggestions on how to measure leadership to ensure that its training produces visible and tangible results.

The goal of leadership training is to improve quality of care and patient safety. Of critical importance, multiple quality and safety reporting systems, holding hospitals and physicians accountable to these higher standards of care, are now in effect all over the nation, the proliferation of which are intensifying the demands being placed on physicians to excel in performance. Although most surgeons are aware of the technical skills by which they are evaluated, many are not familiar with the nontechnical skills or with the organizations that focus primarily on evaluating nontechnical skills. For a holistic view of the extent to which surgeons are evaluated by these systems, a comprehensive list of the different systems evaluating surgeons nationwide is listed in Table 28.1. This is the first time ever that a comprehensive list of the various organizations and methods by which physicians and hospitals are evaluated, and by which reimbursement rates are determined, is provided in a single paper. It will help surgeons understand the context of the current environment in which they work. As the table shows, many of these organizations' assessments of physicians directly take into consideration both technical surgical and nontechnical skills. In fact, nontechnical skills, such as communication, have been repeatedly proven to directly impact measures of technical surgical skills, such as patient outcomes. Surgeons must use this information to optimize their performance via best practices, high performance, and efficiency, all delivered and best summarized under the rubric of modern leadership skills. By training res-
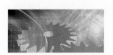
idents based on a model of leadership in the field of medicine, residency programs will be preparing future surgeons to tackle the leadership challenge of providing excellent care in the modern world of rapidly increasing medical scientific information and increasing demands to include patients in a shared decision-making process.

## Key Aspects of Leadership

A surgeon is expected to master the medical knowledge, skills, and manual dexterity required for his/her field of specialty. In addition, a surgeon's navigation of both surgical and nonsurgical medical treatments by nature casts him/her into a leadership role in the field of medicine, in general, and in each

TABLE 28.1 ▶ MULTIPLE ORGANIZATIONS HAVE BEEN CREATED TO EVALUATE BOTH THE TECHNICAL AND NONTECHNICAL SKILLS OF SURGEONS. THIS IS THE FIRST TIME A COMPREHENSIVE LIST AND DESCRIPTION OF THESE ORGANIZATIONS HAS BEEN PROVIDED IN A SINGLE PAPER

| Organization Name | Description | Main Skills, Conditions, or Qualities Evaluated | Evaluation of Technical Skills? | Evaluation of Nontechnical Skills? |
|---|---|---|---|---|
| Hospital Consumer Assessment of Healthcare Providers and Systems (HCAHPS) | A public reporting initiative that measures patient perspectives on and satisfaction with hospital care based on qualities of health care that patients view as important. | Communication with nurses, communication with doctors, responsiveness of hospital staff, pain management, communication about medicines, discharge information, care transition | No | Yes |
| Clinical and Group Consumer Assessment of Healthcare Providers and Systems (CGCAHPS) | A public reporting initiative that measures patient perspectives on and satisfaction with care provided in an office setting based on qualities of health care that patients view as important. | Access to care, provider communication, test results, office staff, overall provider rating | No | Yes |
| Datix, Incident Reporting | A database of incidents that improves reliability of physicians by improving rates of reporting, promoting ownership of mistakes, and improving patient safety. | System issues, patient safety and quality issues, provider behavior, leadership style | Yes | Yes |
| Patient Advocacy Reporting System (PARS) | A system that compiles patient complaints into a complaint index for each physician for comparison with other medical group members and to help identify high malpractice–risk physicians who may benefit from peer intervention. | Unprofessional behavior deemed as disrespectful and rude | No | Yes |

*Continued*

**TABLE 28.1 ▶ MULTIPLE ORGANIZATIONS HAVE BEEN CREATED TO EVALUATE BOTH THE TECHNICAL AND NONTECHNICAL SKILLS OF SURGEONS. THIS IS THE FIRST TIME A COMPREHENSIVE LIST AND DESCRIPTION OF THESE ORGANIZATIONS HAS BEEN PROVIDED IN A SINGLE PAPER—cont'd**

| Organization Name | Description | Main Skills, Conditions, or Qualities Evaluated | Evaluation of Technical Skills? | Evaluation of Nontechnical Skills? |
|---|---|---|---|---|
| Coworker Observation Reporting System | A system in which physicians document the unprofessional conduct of a coworker to provide nonjudgmental and timely feedback and to encourage self-reflection and change. | Unprofessional behavior deemed as disrespectful and unsafe | Yes | Yes |
| American Board of Surgery (ABS) Maintenance of Certification (MOC) Program | A program that documents a surgeon's ongoing commitment to professionalism, lifelong learning, and practice improvement through self-report. | Restrictions on medical license, restrictions on hospital privileges, continuing medical education, self-assessment of continuing medical education, cognitive expertise, ongoing participation in quality assessment program relevant to the surgeon's practice | Yes | Yes |
| Hospital Compare | A database that is part of the Centers for Medicare & Medicaid Services (CMS) Hospital Quality Initiative and provides information on hospital performance and quality of care based on consumer perspectives so that patients can assess and compare hospitals. | Hospital Compare is based on data from HCAHPS and evaluates hospitals by the same guidelines as HCAHPS | No | Yes |
| Federation of State Medical Boards (FSMB) | An organization representing all state medial and osteopathic boards in the United States that license physicians and sponsors the United States Medical Licensing Examination. | Medical knowledge, patient complaints, violations of the law | Yes | Yes |

**TABLE 28.1** ▶ MULTIPLE ORGANIZATIONS HAVE BEEN CREATED TO EVALUATE BOTH THE TECHNICAL AND NONTECHNICAL SKILLS OF SURGEONS. THIS IS THE FIRST TIME A COMPREHENSIVE LIST AND DESCRIPTION OF THESE ORGANIZATIONS HAS BEEN PROVIDED IN A SINGLE PAPER—cont'd

| Organization Name | Description | Main Skills, Conditions, or Qualities Evaluated | Evaluation of Technical Skills? | Evaluation of Nontechnical Skills? |
|---|---|---|---|---|
| Internet clinical scores | A database of direct patient opinions of physicians, provided through various sources, including Healthgrades.com, RateMDs.com, and Yelp. | Professionalism, communication, timeliness | No | Yes |
| Hospital-Acquired Condition Reduction Program | A government program that provides incentives for hospitals to reduce the number of undesirable patient conditions resulting from their stay in the hospital and that could have been avoided by adjusting hospital reimbursement rates accordingly. | Foreign objects retained after surgery, air embolism, blood incompatibility, pressure ulcers, falls, poor glycemic control, catheter-associated infections, surgical site infections, deep vein thrombosis, pulmonary embolism, pneumothorax | Yes | No |
| American College of Surgeons National Surgical Quality Improvement Program (ACS NSQIP) | A program that collects information on and provides a risk-adjusted ranking of preventable surgical complication rates to encourage providers to improve care. | Surgical complications rates, surgical site infections, urinary tract infections, readmission rates, surgical outcomes | Yes | No |
| Centers for Medicare and Medicaid Services Surgical Care Improvement Project (CMS SCIP) | A collaborative health care organization that collects data on surgical complication rates based on established guidelines. | Rates of infection, cardiac, venous thromboembolism, vascular, and respiratory complications of surgery | Yes | No |

TABLE 28.2 ▶ LEADERSHIP ENTAILS FIVE MAIN QUALITIES AND THESE ARE DIRECTLY APPLIED TO THE FIELD OF MEDICINE

| Leadership Skill | Description and Application in the Field of Medicine |
| --- | --- |
| Vision | The act of establishing tangible goals of care for patients on both a daily basis and for long-term purposes. |
| Effective communication | Establishing an open, respectful, and nonjudgmental forum for communication between different members of the health care team and with the patient. |
| Willingness to lead | Taking on full responsibility for the care of patients and remaining ethical, professional, and committed despite the especially challenging rigors of joining the field of surgery. |
| Willingness to learn | A commitment to lifelong learning of the latest scientific, medical, and surgical updates to deliver optimized patient care. |
| Conflict resolution | The art of resolving conflicts in a peaceful and ethical manner in team settings. |

patient case he/she manages, in particular. This begets the question, what qualities make for a great leader? From a previous study of one of the greatest leaders in history, Dr Martin Luther King Jr, also coauthored by one of this chapter's writers, we have selected 5 qualities that make for a most effective and successful leader.[4] These qualities, as demonstrated by Dr King himself, include the following: a shared vision, effective communication, willingness to lead, willingness to learn, and ability to resolve conflicts. Table 28.2 compiles these skills of leadership and provides a brief description of each. As detailed below, surgeons should strive to maintain all of these qualities as they address challenges in the medical field and conflicts during surgery.

## Vision

During the Civil Rights Movement of the 1950s-1960s, Dr Martin Luther King Jr shared his dream that his country would "rise up and live out the true meaning of its creed: 'We hold these truths to be self-evident that all men are created equal.'"[5] His vision united people of different genders, races, and beliefs behind his leadership in the race for freedom for all of humanity. Similarly, the most fundamental principle of leadership in the field of surgery is establishing a common vision to unite and direct the health care team. An immediate example of how a vision helps to guide the medical team comes in the form of morning rounds, during which surgeons and surgical trainees establish daily inpatient goals; establishing goals in even this simple fashion helps direct the team toward a common purpose for the entire day.

Studies across several major medical centers support the importance of a unifying vision to lead the surgical medical team. One study done in a medical center showed that team briefings with great detail in regard to equipment, surgery stages, and patient background information immediately before the operation are associated with a 25% reduction in the incidence of nonroutine, potentially harmful events during the operation.[6] In a separate cohort study, when the care team in an intensive care unit setting, including surgeons, shared specific daily goals with the health care team through a goals form discussed verbally, this increased resident and nurse understanding of the goals of care and significantly reduced patient length of intensive care unit stay.[7] Yet another study evaluating team behavior during nearly 300 general surgery cases found that surgical teams that exhibited more teamwork behaviors consistent with a common goal were at lower risk of experiencing death or complications.[8] These findings are perhaps not surprising; after all, surgery is a dynamic event with all members executing complex tasks simultaneously. Lack of coordination can lead to adverse events within the hospital, which these studies show can be overcome with detailed daily and preoperative briefings. These studies demonstrate how a standardized, well-developed vision for the surgical team is absolutely vital for patient safety and is a key principle of surgical and moral leadership.

Residency programs can equip surgical residents with the habits necessary, such as establishing a team vision, to lead effectively in a surgical setting by giving them the opportunity to conduct preoperative team briefings. In support of such training, one health organization conducted a study in which surgeons in 108 of their facilities were involved in a formal team-training program, which included the resident surgeon holding pre- and postoperative briefings with the surgical team. In 74 of the facilities that had undergone the training program at the time, an 18% reduction in annual mortality rate was noted.[9] As this study shows, programs can train their residents toward establishing an effective vision that provides an outline of the team strategy; the vision defines which tasks are important and which tasks are not, allowing team members to perform their separate duties effectively and ultimately as a unit and with purpose.[10]

It is important to also recognize that teaching the art of establishing a vision can further strengthen residency programs by helping to fulfill several of the core competencies established by the Accreditation Council for Graduate Medical Education (ACGME). These core competencies are listed in Table 28.3. First, by establishing daily goals of care for patients, surgeons increase the effectiveness of patient care by uniting the health care team behind the same goals for each patient. Second, the unity provided 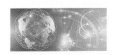 by establishing a common vision will lend itself to greater professionalism among team members as well as with the patients. Third, the specific act of establishing a vision requires open communication among the health care team and encourages communication with the patient to ensure that the health care team's vision for the care of a patient is in line with the patient's vision of care as well. We will continue to address throughout this chapter how each aspect of leadership addresses multiple aspects of the ACGME core competencies.

TABLE 28.3 ▶THE ACCREDITATION COUNCIL FOR GRADUATE MEDICAL EDUCATION IDENTIFIES SIX CORE COMPETENCIES BY WHICH GRADUATE MEDICAL EDUCATION PROGRAMS ARE EXPECTED TO EVALUATE TRAINING RESIDENTS

| Core Competency | Description |
| --- | --- |
| Patient Care | Care must be compassionate and effective for treating health problems. |
| Medical Knowledge | Knowledge must be up to date on both established and new medical and social knowledge regarding patient care. |
| Practice-Based Learning and Improvement | Investigate and improve the practice of care and incorporate new scientific evidence into patient care. |
| Interpersonal and Communication Skills | Communicate effectively with patients and health care staff. |
| Professionalism | Commit to professional responsibilities, adhere to ethical principles, and act with sensitivity toward diverse patient populations. |
| Systems-Based Practice | Be aware of system resources and use these resources appropriately to optimize patient care. |

# Effective Communication

Referring back to our example of great leadership, Martin Luther King Jr also championed yet another aspect of leadership, the ability to communicate effectively. King united his followers under his vision of equality for all through several forms of communication, including passionate speeches in church gatherings and protests, books providing guidelines for social movements, and letters written personally to supporters and opponents alike. Without clearly expressing his goals and plans through these various media, King would not have been as successful in motivating his followers to unite under his extraordinary vision. Similarly, surgeons, as leaders in the medical care of patients, also have a duty to communicate effectively with both the rest of the health care team and their patients. Otherwise, their goals and plans for the care of their patients may not live up to their potential.

# Effective Communication With the Health Care Staff

In recent years, new focus has been directed toward communication techniques between surgeons and other members of the health care team and the correlation between communication and medical errors in recent years. A book on medical errors and safety in the health system points out that medical errors cause 100 000 deaths annually and are the eighth leading cause of death in the United States.[11] Ensuing studies have shown that communication errors between health care staff are one of the most common causes of medical error.[12,13] Furthermore, the Joint Commission recognized miscommunication as the leading cause of adverse events such as delays in patient care, the waste of surgeon and staff time, and medical errors affecting patients.[14]

Several studies have demonstrated that implementing opportunities for effective communication between health care professionals will result in improved patient care and, additionally, less medical litigation.[15,16] In a study discussed earlier, for instance, the modest act of explicitly stating daily goals in a standardized fashion significantly reduced patient length of intensive care unit stay and increased resident and nurse understanding of goals of care.[7] Additionally, certain protocols have been established to ensure open communication in the operating room such as the "time out," during which all team members introduce themselves and critical information needed to complete the operation is expressed verbally before beginning the operation. Another study found that following a checklist consisting of preoperative verification of the person, procedure, and site; marking the operative site; and a time out results in significantly decreased patient complications and mortality.[17]

One particularly concerning aspect of miscommunication among health care staff is that many of the errors born out of miscommunication are not due to simply poor communication but are the result of hierarchical roles in the field of surgery and a fear of backlash for speaking up.[13,18] This finding is not entirely surprising given the highly hierarchical and command-and-follow nature of surgery. It also highlights the particularly significant obligation of current and incoming surgeon leaders to begin fostering a friendlier environment both inside and outside of the operating room so that communication is not hindered but encouraged. To overcome current barriers, surgeons and trainees need to move toward communicating in an open manner and remain receptive to the concerns of all team members.

The above findings should motivate residency programs to begin integrating standardized and team-based communication practice as a vital leadership skill. Such a program can be modeled after a recent pre- and postinterventional collaborative study.[19] The interventions were initiated in response to previous findings that failures in communication between attending surgeons and residents are associated with increased morbidity.[20] In the collaborative study, policies and educational initiatives intended to increase an open and encouraging environment for resident-attending surgeon communication included periodic reminders and a pocket information card for residents.[19] The study found that the interventions resulted in increased resident-attending surgeon communication and ultimately resulted in significant alterations in patient management.[19] 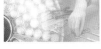 We hope these findings inspire more residency programs to begin incorporating communication skills into the core curriculum as a means to reduce harmful communication breakdowns between surgeons and residents and ultimately as an effective way to improve patient care.

## Effective Communication With Patients

On an analogous note, just as communication between different members of the health care staff is critical, equally important is effective communication between the surgeon and the patient. We live in an age in which patients have more access than ever before to medical knowledge from the World Wide Web, and patients have an increasing desire that their physicians and surgeons fully inform them of their illnesses and treatment goals.[21,22] Patients' increased knowledge puts them in a position of power and in effect makes them partners in the care of their own health. Although surveys report that physicians and surgeons are predominantly content with and even praise their ability to communicate with patients, patients in the same patient-physician relationship are actually discontented with the level of communication; there is thus a wide disparity between how well physicians and surgeons think they are able to communicate with their patients and how satisfied patients are with their level of communication.[23] These findings are significant in at least three aspects: patient health outcomes, malpractice litigations, and financial reimbursement.

First, when physicians demonstrate empathy, actively work on knowing their patients on a holistic level, and engage in shared patient-doctor decision making, patients are more likely to trust their physicians, believe that their surgeons have their best interests in mind, disclose personal information in regard to their health, and have confidence that treatment plans will be effective.[24,25] This scenario results in a win-win situation, enhancing patient health outcomes while also in the long run saving time for the physician and reducing physician burnout and turnover.[16,24]

Second, surgeons can significantly reduce malpractice litigations brought against them by demonstrating empathy toward their patients and maintaining an open and honest relationship with them.[26,27] In fact, there is a direct association between poor doctor-patient communication and litigation, although willingness to disclose has not been established to correlate with risk of litigation.[28,29] One study looking at why patients do not always sue in adverse outcomes found that patients' decision to litigate was most often associated 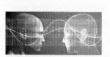 with a "a perceived lack of caring and/or collaboration in the delivery of health care," as well as poor delivery of information.[30] Good bedside manners have, in reverse, been found to decrease patients' desire to carry out litigation against the physician or the hospital, even in the event of adverse medical outcomes.[31]

Third, hospitals and clinics are reimbursed from the government largely based on their performance on surveys administered by the Clinician and Group Consumer Assessment of Healthcare Providers and Systems (CGCAHPS) and Hospital Consumer Assessment of Healthcare Providers and Systems (HCAHPS). With up to 2% of revenue at risk, physicians and hospitals will want to improve their CAHPS scores. These surveys are tailored to find what patients value most in physicians, and they have found that patient satisfaction—and whether a patient would recommend a physician to another—correlates most highly with doctor communication, overriding as well patients' judgment of their physician's surgical skills.[32] Although residency programs and hospitals should absolutely continue evaluating surgical skill based on factors such as mortality and complication rates, they must be mindful that there are factors other than surgical outcomes that are driving patients' perception of their care.[33] These factors are incorporated into the CAHPS surveys to ultimately determine hospital and reimbursement rates based on patient's satisfaction with and perception of care. With millions of dollars in revenue at stake, surgeons now have both moral and financial obligations to focus on communication, openness, and honesty with their patients, while working to also refine their surgical skills and techniques.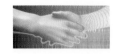

In light of the above findings, the ACGME mandates residency programs and train physicians in patient communication skills.[34] However, nontechnical skills are still largely overshadowed by technical surgical skills in residency programs, leading some to falsely believe that nontechnical skills such as good bedside manners cannot be taught.[1] This belief has been disproven as communication courses in other fields of medicine have been entirely successful in teaching nontechnical skills. For instance, a 1-month rotation for primary care residents at 2 separate universities consisted of seminars discussing and demonstrating patient-centered interview models followed by practice role-playing of the model and then use of the model with real patients.[35] These sessions focused on emotion handling, patient education, and management of psychosocial problems common in primary care settings. A randomized, controlled study of the program found that trained residents were superior to untrained residents in their confidence in psychologic sensitivity, data gathering, and somatization management of real patients. Moreover, patient participants over all 4 years of the study reported increased satisfaction and well-being in their health status. This study, in addition to many others across the country, demonstrate that communication skills can be taught and surgical programs must begin to prioritize nontechnical skills in their obligation to ultimately improve patient health outcomes.[36–38]

Once again, this specific aspect of leadership, in addition to improving health care outcomes, also addresses the core competencies of the ACGME. Most obviously, it directly mirrors the core competency of communication. Additionally, by emphasizing the importance of communication with patients and their family members, training programs will also help residents develop the skill of demonstrating compassionate patient care, whereas learning to communicate with the rest of the health care team also promotes professionalism. Establishing a forum of open communication and respect between different members of the health care team is also key in establishing an open space where surgeons can learn from past mistakes in a practice-based learning manner.

## Willingness to Lead

A willingness to lead speaks to the active commitment necessary for effective leadership. Leaders need to dedicate themselves to honing and practicing 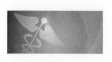 leadership skills, which may seem cumbersome to the surgeon with multiple demands on his/her time. Nonetheless, it is an essential attribute found in great contemporary leaders. Consider, for example, Dr King. King led the Civil Rights Movement at a time where his vision of equality would lead to harassment, imprisonment, and threats to himself and those dear to him.[4] Yet King's commitment to and faith in equality was unshakeable.

In the field of medicine, it is difficult to overstate how critical this unwavering and steadfast commitment to lead is for surgeons as well. Surgeons are put under tremendous stress, most especially during surgical operations. Some tangible examples of stressors include bleeding, time pressure, complexity of the surgery at hand, and problems with equipment.[39] Beyond the operating room, surgeons have the additional stressors of having to make the decision on which procedures to approve and which to deny, holding family meetings where sometimes they must share bad news and not infrequent roadblocks with insurance policies. It is the surgeon's responsibility to bear the torch of hope as he/she leads the rest of his/her medical team to provide the best medical care possible.

Most paradigms of leadership training in the field of surgery are purely through observation and emulation, which does not hone a surgeon's willingness to lead. However, there are some current residency programs in other fields of medicine that not only offer a formal curriculum in leadership training but also strongly encourage trainees to take on a leadership role even during their time as a resident. These paradigms of leadership can serve as a model for similar curricula in surgical residency programs. Consider, for instance, an Internal Medicine residency program in Louisiana. Nearly a decade ago, the program was turned over to the residents, making it the only resident-run program in the United States.[40] Acceptance alone to this program ensures a commitment and a willingness to lead.

Although it certainly is not an easy task and may even not be entirely feasible for surgical residency programs to mirror this Internal Medicine program, small steps can nonetheless be taken in the same direction. For instance, trainees can be encouraged to take on a stronger and more commanding role in terms of scheduling patients' operations and determining the specific techniques to perform them. Most often, operations are scheduled by the attending surgeon; additionally, the resident working under that attending surgeon is expected to perform the operation in the method the attending surgeon has become accustomed to and likely mastered over the course of his/her career. Instead, to prepare trainees to undertake the responsibility of taking all aspects of patient care into their hands, however, attending surgeons must become more flexible in allocating such decision-making powers to trainees, although of course under their careful guidance.

This aspect of leadership, the willingness to lead, is particularly key in addressing the first ACGME core competency. By taking full responsibility for their patients, residents are encouraged to truly bear the weight of caring for their patients and not just as surgical bodies that they will operate on but also as patients whose care they must oversee both preoperatively and postoperatively. It also more solidly allows residents to approach the art of surgery and medicine in a practice-based manner. A willingness to lead also entails a commitment to professional responsibilities that extend beyond applying surgical skills in the operating room. Finally, by carrying greater responsibility for the care of their patients, residents will be encouraged to follow a systems-based practice, whereupon they will learn and be more aware of the various resources they can reach out to and rely on for optimizing patient care.

## Willingness to Learn

In the field of medical surgery, a willingness to lead denotes an additional responsibility: lifelong learning. Everyday advances are made across multiple platforms in medicine, and surgeons have a duty to keep up with the latest findings relevant to their specialty. Consider, for instance, that advances in molecular biology and cell signaling are resulting in the evolution of personalized medicine and surgery.[9] Genetic factors have already been implicated in the recovery of patients after cardiac surgery, in the surgical approach to familial endocrinopathy syndromes, and in the surgical management of familial renal cancer, among many other diseases and treatments.[41-44] Surgeons, with their patients' best interest in mind, must make all efforts to keep up with these findings because they will certainly have repercussions for patients' treatment goals and plans. In addition to developments in scientific knowledge, technologic advances in minimally invasive and robotic surgery are also transforming the field of surgery. Laparoscopy and endovascular techniques are now the standard of care for many diseases, leading to shorter hospital stays, faster recovery times, and fewer postoperative complications for the patient, and surgeons have an obligation to continue to be updated on these advances.[45-47]

To this end, the American Board of Surgery requires all surgeons to complete meaningful continuing medical education to maintain surgical certification.[48] As the American Board of Surgery recognizes, it is by means of a commitment to a lifetime of medical and surgical learning that surgeons can truly adhere to the words of the Hippocratic Oath, "I will apply, for the benefit of the sick, all measures which are required."[49]

As discussed above, a willingness to learn does denote dedicating time to becoming well informed about the latest tangible advances in medicine. However, it also denotes an additional dedication to taking the time to learn about one's patients as individuals. Sometimes, this entails also taking the time to learn about the goals and desires of the patient's family members.

This patient- and family-centered approach runs counter to the often-taught method of learning broadly about various cultural groups grouped together mostly due to racial or religious similarities.[50,51] This former style of patient care leads to stereotyping and judgment of patients based solely on their ethnic origin, ways of dressing, and religious customs, all of which are features that go little beyond what is superficially visible to the eye.[50] A more open and inviting approach to patient care is taking the time to learn about each patient as an individual. Although individuals are influenced by their cultural, racial, and religious origins and backgrounds, each person is unique and will want to navigate his/her illness differently based on his/her unique experiences, beliefs, and even age, all of which the surgical physician must attempt to gain insight into.[52] Notably, Accountable Care Organizations have also adopted this strategy of patient care, requiring physicians to actively engage patients in their health and ultimately aiming for higher patient satisfaction through a patient-centered approach to medicine.[53]

Multiple sources can be found on stepwise instructions for a patient-centered approach to health care; these can be summarized as listening to the patient's views and concerns, using open communication to both explain your perception of the situation and simultaneously acknowledge the patient's view of the situation, recommending treatment, and then negotiating with the patient.[54]

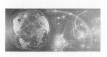 Of particular note, we fully acknowledge that the surgeon's schedule is already a demanding one; however, this patient-centered approach to patient care is not meant to be a long and laborious process but instead a simple means of showing compassion, sensitivity, and partnership toward the patient. We also discussed earlier that surveys report that patients value verbal communication more than technical skills when developing trust in surgeons. This patient-centered approach will thus not only allow patients to feel that they are being heard and respected but can also lead to higher patient satisfaction ratings for their surgeons, improved health outcomes, and increased revenue reimbursements to hospitals and clinics from the government.[24,55]

Importantly, a willingness to learn most directly tackles the ACGME core competency of keeping up to date on medical knowledge in addition to addressing practice-based learning. A commitment to learning about the patient's goals and desires, moreover, addresses not only compassionate patient care but also professional patient care because it encourages sensitivity toward diverse patient populations.

## To Resolve Conflict/Teamwork

In a recent survey at a major medical center, surgical residents reported overall not feeling confident across multiple aspects of leadership, and the skill in which the most residents reported not feeling competent in was conflict resolution.[56] This finding is significant because the very nature of surgery—with a surgical team comprising surgeons, nurses, surgical trainees, anesthesiologists, and surgical technicians—calls for intimate teamwork and peaceful conflict resolution across multiple aspects of a patient's care. As leaders in their medical teams, surgeons must take responsibility to display excellent skills in resolving conflicts that may arise in such intimate work environments. Although an authoritative attitude may be reasonable in certain settings, such as in emergency critical cases during which surgeons are expected to make decisions rapidly, this approach is not as effective in most cases of conflict. The command-and-follow culture of surgery is dangerous because it can paint surgeons as nonapproachable, further cultivating a work environment in which communication is discouraged. As discussed earlier, failures in communication, particularly in the setting of conflict, are consistently reported as one of the top contributors to surgical errors.[12]

A recent multistate survey of operating room staff across 60 hospitals offers further insight into why an authoritative style of leadership is dangerous in the field of surgery. The study's most compelling finding was that most surgeons were satisfied with their teamwork skills and rated the quality of their own collaboration at 85%, whereas operating room nurses rated the same surgeons at a significantly lower rate—48% to be specific.[57] Further discussions with the surgeons and nurses revealed that surgeons rated a team as more cooperative when nurses followed instructions and anticipated the surgeons' needs, whereas nurses rated the surgeons low in cooperation because they felt their input was not respected in the operating room.[58] The feedback from the nurses highlights the risks of the command-and-follow nature of surgery: When nurses feel their inputs are not appreciated, they are less likely to speak up when they spot an error. Moreover, such job dissatisfaction leads to higher turnover rates among nurses.[58]

The results of the multistate study are further enlightening because they tease out an important aspect of leadership, in general, and teamwork, in particular: Conflict resolution should always begin with self-reflection. This concept is yet another one that Martin Luther King Jr exemplified. Rooted in Christian love and inspired by the Gandhian method of nonviolence, King's entire leadership and movement were built on the foundations of peaceful conflict resolution and negotiation.[4] Likewise, in the lifelong effort to improve patient care, surgeons have an obligation to abandon the current hierarchical leadership style and instead lead on a stage open to negotiation and dialogue between operating room staff.

In light of these findings, the AGCME recognizes the importance of conflict resolution skills in resident training and recommends surgical trainees to train in various conflict resolution techniques to become surgical leaders in the future.[34] Although many techniques exist toward establishing conflict resolution, they generally focus on maintaining objectivity, elevating the 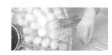 conflict above personal differences, and refocusing on the common vision.[59] Specifically, when a conflict emerges between two parties, both sides must be given the opportunity to express their position, and then surgeons must take the responsibility to carefully examine the relevant facts to negotiate a solution that is both independent of any personal interests and curated toward the end goal of improving patient care. Overall, conflict resolution techniques require a measure of flexibility, and demand that surgeons should view conflicts as though they are opportunities to learn. Fortunately, surgeons are not strangers to the commitment to a lifetime of learning, as evidenced by their decision to enter the field of medicine.

We want to emphasize here an additional quality necessary for effective conflict resolution: professionalism, which, as it pertains to the medical field, is defined as the demonstration of the principles of ethical behavior (ie, informed consent, patient confidentiality) and integrity that promotes the highest level of medical care. The sheer gravity of professional and ethical behavior in conflict resolution, in particular, and in the medical field, in general, can simply not be overstressed, and the ACGME has already recognized professionalism as a core competency required for surgeons to abide by.[34] We, the authors, initially debated whether to create an entirely separate section for ethical behavior because it is so important to have an attribute; we ultimately decided to include it in the section of conflict resolution as questions of ethics often challenge us when conflicts arise.

Furthermore, surgeons are often presented with ethical dilemmas in which a black-and-white approach to morality does not necessarily apply. For instance, innovative surgical therapies and techniques, advanced palliative surgery, and transplant procedures require careful ethical scrutiny and often encroach on morally ambiguous territory.[60,61] Unfortunately, however, there is currently no set curriculum within residency programs in the United States, which is accepted nationwide regarding training residents in medical ethics and most programs do not adequately emphasize ethics in the curriculum.[62] Nonetheless, most residency program directors do agree that a specific focus on ethics education would benefit residents.[63]

In one particular surgical training program, residents take a case-based approach to discuss ethical dilemmas monthly in a fascinating multidisciplinary forum composed of nurses, medical students, residents, fellows, and attending surgeons from multiple disciplines as well as the ethics committee and chaplains.[64] This interactive approach encourages attendees to exercise their minds in matters of ethics, preparing them with confidence for when they come to face these challenges in their practice. A separate study designed specifically for surgical intensive care unit residents used a similarly case-

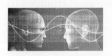

based approach centered on real historical cases.[65] The study found that after the surgery-based ethics program, ethical dilemmas were addressed earlier and more frequently in the medical records than before the program. In addition, the length of stay for patients with at most 30 days of stay in the intensive care unit was cut in half, showing concrete and positive health outcomes of an ethics-centered approach to the medical surgical care of patients. Given these results, surgical residency programs must begin moving toward implementing a regular ethics course into the curricula. As demonstrated by the studies above, a case-based approach is an effective method of teaching ethics; such an approach can further be supplemented with OSCEs (objective structured clinical examinations) for both further practice of dealing with ethical dilemmas and a method of measuring the improvement in residents' ability to handle such issues in a safe and standardized environment.[66]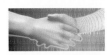

Referring back to the ACGME core competencies, the art of conflict resolution is key to emphasizing a professional and ethical approach to health care, in both resolving conflicts and making important decisions involving the entire health care team. It also provides a model by which physicians and residents can more comfortably investigate surgical errors and complications to carry out effective practice-based learning.

## How to Measure Leadership Outcomes in Health Care

There is an unmistakable and growing body of evidence, discussed above at length, that leadership training improves the quality of care in health care systems. It is for these reasons the ACGME has also recognized leadership qualities such as surgical judgment, technical skills, and nontechnical skills, among other factors, as core competencies in medical training.[1,34] Unlike the scientific measurement of surgical judgment and technical skills, however, objective measurement of the nontechnical skills listed above is a much more difficult endeavor. It is, however, very much possible. We provide here the most comprehensive list yet provided of the various methods already applied by some residency programs in Table 28.4.

One means by which leadership can be qualified and quantified, as listed in Table 28.4, is through questionnaires such as the Multifactor Leadership Questionnaire (MLQ), the NEO Five-Factor Inventory, and the Surgeon's Leadership Inventory (SLI). The MLQ, commonly used in other industries, is based on the theory that leadership can follow either a transactional or a transformational mode; whereas leadership based on transaction focuses on completing tasks and rewarding the completed tasks, leadership based on transformation focuses more on the motivation behind completing the tasks and emphasizes a positive and encouraging working environment for the team.[67] In a study applying the questionnaire to 5 surgeons in a single hospital, surgeons who scored higher on the transformational section—showed that they focused more on promoting an encouraging and open environment for all the attending surgeons, residents, nurses, and other staff in the operating room—correlated with teams in which there was greater communication.[68] These findings are significant in light of research showing that lack of communication is often a leading factor in surgical errors and can help guide feedback for the teams in which there was less communication overall.

TABLE 28.4 ▶ RESIDENCY PROGRAMS CAN OBJECTIVELY MEASURE TRAINEE IMPROVEMENT IN LEADERSHIP QUALITIES THROUGH VARIOUS METHODS. WE PROVIDE THE MOST COMPREHENSIVE LIST TO DATE OF THE WIDE SPECTRUM OF METHODS ALREADY EMPLOYED BY SOME RESIDENCY PROGRAMS

| Method of Leadership Measurement | Description |
| --- | --- |
| Multifactor Leadership Questionnaire (MLQ) | The MLQ is a questionnaire based on the differences between transformation and transactional approaches of leadership. It identifies leadership qualities through rater's beliefs about effective leadership. |
| NEO Five-Factor Personality Inventory (NEO) | NEO explores different facets of 5 different personality traits—neuroticism, extraversion, openness to experience, agreeableness, and conscientiousness—through a questionnaire. |
| Surgeon's Leadership Inventory (SLI) | The SLI is a questionnaire based on literature on leadership in surgery and surgeon's leadership behaviors observed in the operating room. It includes 8 elements of surgeon's leadership in the operating room, which include maintaining standards, managing resources, making decisions, directing, training, supporting others, communicating, and coping with pressure. |
| Patient Feedback | Patient complaints are inversely related to leadership effectiveness and can thus be used as opportunities to improve and as a measure of leadership. |
| Objective Structured Clinical Examination (OSCE) | The OSCE can be administered in a controlled environment with attending feedback on various aspects of leadership tackled in the practice cases. Videotaped sessions provides further opportunities for improvement as residents will be able to later observe their own behaviors and reflect on ways to improve their approach to the case presented. |
| Consumer Assessment of Healthcare Providers and Systems (CAHPS) | CAHPS surveys are based on aspects of health care that matter most to patients, such as physician communication. The results are made public and can be used to shed light on areas of leadership physicians can improve on to work toward a patient-centered approach to care. |

In a larger study of a group of 65 surgical residents in a university medical center, administration of the MLQ showed a significant association between transformational leadership and overall perceived team effectiveness and resident satisfaction.[69] The questionnaire additionally found that the residents surveyed placed less value than the national average on individualized consideration, in which leaders seek to help teammates fulfill individual desired needs; this finding helped identify an area of leadership training on which the program can focus to help further cultivate a more supportive team atmosphere among the training residents. The NEO Five-Factor Personality Inventory (NEO), a widely used personality assessment tool, was also administered to the same group of residents.[70] The inventory, which assesses personality on 5 broad strokes, including neuroticism, extroversion, openness, agreeableness, and conscientiousness, found that the surgeons scored above the national average on most of the factors tested but below average on agreeableness, which is a measure of altruism and tolerance, among other related factors. This finding correlated well with and thus confirmed the results of the MLQ administered to the same group of residents and thus further helped identify areas of leadership for which the residency program could develop interventions.

The SLI can similarly be used to help guide residency programs.[71] It is in fact more specific to the field of surgery and grades surgeons on 8 different elements of leadership, including making decisions, managing resources, directing, training, supporting others, and communicating. As with the MLQ and NEO questionnaires, the SLI can be used to assess the growth of leadership ability in surgery residents. Table 28.5 provides a list and description of the different elements assessed by the SLI.[71]

In addition to measuring leadership through computerized models, an effective and perhaps complementary method of measuring leadership is to include patient feedback and complaints. In a study done in the United Kingdom, data from 86 hospitals showed that increased leadership effectiveness is associated with lower patient complaints.[72] Patient complaints, a usually neglected area, can thus be used to assess leadership quality in the health care system. To further complement this method, residency programs can administer OSCEs to their trainees and use standardized objectives as measures of their improvement in the leadership qualities discussed while simultaneously providing opportunities for residents to further practice and hone their leadership skills in a safe and controlled environment with feedback from colleagues and attending surgeons. Finally, hospitals and clinics can use CAHPS survey results, made public to hold health care systems accountable and to incentivize them to enhance the quality of care they deliver, to assess whether patient satisfaction rates improve when training in nontechnical skills is emphasized in their programs.

## Conclusion

Previously, surgeons were evaluated based solely on their ability to operate and their medical knowledge. Although surgical skill is absolutely vital in the operating room, the modern health care environment is changing rapidly and surgeons are faced with the great leadership challenge of learning to 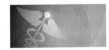 adapt—and continuing to take charge—in this complex, ever growing health care team.

Leadership is an act of both directing and motivating different parts and persons of a team toward an established goal. As defined in this chapter, this form of transformational leadership consists of 5 core elements: established

TABLE 28.5 ▶THE SURGEON'S LEADERSHIP INVENTORY CAN BE USED
TO ASSESS LEADERSHIP SKILLS IN PHYSICIANS, AND IT IS SPECIFICALLY
TAILORED TOWARD ASSESSING THE NONTECHNICAL SKILLS OF PHYSICIANS
IN THE SURGICAL FIELD

| Element | Description |
| --- | --- |
| Maintaining standards | Practicing safe and quality patient care by following established protocols and asking for help when needed. |
| Making decisions | Making informed judgments and communicating decisions with relevant personnel. |
| Managing resources | Appropriately assigning resources and tasks to team members. |
| Directing | Clearly communicating expectations and instructions and demonstrating confidence in leadership ability. |
| Training | Educating and training team members when the opportunity arises. |
| Supporting others | Offering assistance where appropriate and encouraging open communication. |
| Communicating | Sharing information in a timely manner and encouraging input from others. |
| Coping with pressure | Showing flexibility when required to meet goals. |

vision, effective communication, willingness to lead, willingness to learn, and conflict resolution. Although surgeons across the United States generally recognize the importance of these attributes, a leading cause of surgical errors continues to be a lack of sufficient leadership and communication. These findings emphasize the need for training focused on leadership skills in surgical residency curricula. A number of residency programs in the United States that already address leadership training can serve as paradigms after which other surgical training programs can model a similar program. The surgery department at a major medical center, for instance, recently introduced a focused program for enhancing teamwork through alignment of goals, improved communication, and increased integrity ultimately to improve quality of patient care and maximize efficiency through time management.[73] Results from surveys taken before and after the program showed that after the completion of the program, surgical residents reported significantly increased satisfaction with members of their team across multiple factors, including having an encouraging team overall and understanding the goals of the team. These findings are encouraging and should further motivate residency programs to implement formal leadership training courses.

An additional forum—outside of a formal leadership training class—in which surgeons can further gain leadership training is in the operating room. During an operation, a surgeon must maintain the role of a leader to calmly and effectively deal with any situation that could arise. The necessity for surgical residents to get the opportunity to control the procedure is vital to their leadership training. However, attending surgeons on average direct operations 79% of the time, and operating room staff continue to direct inquiries toward the attending surgeon even when residents are designated the role of the operating surgeon.[74] Although it is difficult to relinquish duties to a less experienced resident during a surgery, it must be done in order for the resident to receive proper leadership training.

Overall, it is important for surgical residency programs across the United States to emphasize leadership training in the curriculum so that surgeons can attain the tools to ultimately successfully lead health care teams in the hospital and in their own practice. A surgical team will produce best patient outcomes when the surgeon commits to an established vision, an effective communication, a willingness to lead, a willingness to learn, and a peaceful conflict resolution. These skills—stemming from honesty, open-mindedness, flexibility, compassion, and the ability to be a role model for a health care team—will help provide a culture of increased team chemistry, improved quality of care, and enhanced patient safety. Ultimately, they will help physicians face the great leadership challenge of today with success.

# References

1. Combes JR, Arespacochaga E. Physician competencies for a 21st century health care system. *J Grad Med Educ*. 2012;4(3):401–405. doi:10.4300/JGME-04-03-33.
2. Cantor JC, Baker LC, Hughes RG. Preparedness for practice. Young physicians' views of their professional education. *JAMA*. September 1, 1993;270(9):1035–1040. PubMed PMID: 8350444.
3. Hanna WC, Mulder DS, Fried GM, Elhilali M, Khwaja KA. Training future surgeons for management roles: the resident-surgeon-manager conference. *Arch Surg*. October 2012;147(10):940–944. PubMed PMID: 23117834. doi:10.1001/archsurg.2012.992.
4. Brunicardi FC, Cotton RT, Cole GW, Martinez G. The leadership principles of Dr. Martin Luther King, Jr. and their relevance to surgery. *J Natl Med Assoc*. January 2007;99(1):7–14. PubMed PMID: 17304963; PubMed Central PMCID: PMC2569605.
5. King Jr ML. *I Have a Dream*. Speech at Lincoln Memorial. Washington, DC. August 28, 1963. American Rhetoric. Web. March 25, 2013.
6. Einav Y, Gopher D, Kara I, et al. Preoperative briefing in the operating room: shared cognition, teamwork, and patient safety. *Chest*. February 2010;137(2):443–449. PubMed PMID: 20133291. doi:10.1378/chest.08-1732.
7. Pronovost P, Berenholtz S, Dorman T, Lipsett PA, Simmonds T, Haraden C. Improving communication in the ICU using daily goals. *J Crit Care*. June 2003;18(2):71–75. PubMed PMID: 12800116.
8. Mazzocco K, Petitti DB, Fong KT, et al. Surgical team behaviors and patient outcomes. *Am J Surg*. May 2009;197(5):678–685. PubMed PMID: 18789425. doi:10.1016/j.amjsurg.2008.03.002.
9. Neily J, Mills PD, Young-Xu Y, et al. Association between implementation of a medical team training program and surgical mortality. *JAMA*. October 20, 2010;304(15):1693–1700. PubMed PMID: 20959579. doi:10.1001/jama.2010.1506.
10. Souba WW. The 3 essential responsibilities: a leadership story. *Arch Surg*. June 2010;145(6):540–543. PubMed PMID: 20566973. doi:10.1001/archsurg.2010.82.

11. Institute of Medicine (US) Committee on Quality of Health Care in America, Kohn LT, Corrigan JM, Donaldson MS, eds. *To Err is Human: Building a Safer Health System.* Washington, DC: National Academies Press (US); 2000. PubMed PMID: 25077248.

12. Gawande AA, Zinner MJ, Studdert DM, Brennan TA. Analysis of errors reported by surgeons at three teaching hospitals. *Surgery.* June 2003;133(6):614–621. PubMed PMID: 12796727.

13. Sutcliffe KM, Lewton E, Rosenthal MM. Communication failures: an insidious contributor to medical mishaps. *Acad Med.* February 2004;79(2):186–194. PubMed PMID: 14744724.

14. Williams RG, Silverman R, Schwind C, et al. Surgeon information transfer and communication: factors affecting quality and efficiency of inpatient care. *Ann Surg.* February 2007;245(2):159–169. PubMed PMID: 17245166; PubMed Central PMCID: PMC1877003.

15. Ambady N, Laplante D, Nguyen T, Rosenthal R, Chaumeton N, Levinson W. Surgeons' tone of voice: a clue to malpractice history. *Surgery.* July 2002;132(1):5–9. PubMed PMID: 12110787.

16. Stewart MA. Effective physician-patient communication and health outcomes: a review. *CMAJ.* May 1, 1995;152(9):1423–1433. PubMed PMID: 7728691; PubMed Central PMCID: PMC1337906.

17. Treadwell JR, Lucas S. Preoperative checklists and anesthesia checklists. In: *Making Health Care Safer II: An Updated Critical Analysis of the Evidence for Patient Safety Practices.* Rockville, MD: Agency for Healthcare Research and Quality (US); (Evidence Reports/Technology Assessments, No. 211.). March 2013 [chapter 13]. Available from: https://www.ncbi.nlm.nih.gov/books/NBK133353/.

18. Leonard M, Graham S, Bonacum D. The human factor: the critical importance of effective teamwork and communication in providing safe care. *Qual Saf Health Care.* October 2004;(13 suppl 1):i85–i90. PubMed PMID: 15465961; PubMed Central PMCID: PMC1765783.

19. Arriaga AF, Elbardissi AW, Regenbogen SE, et al. A policy-based intervention for the reduction of communication breakdowns in inpatient surgical care: results from a Harvard surgical safety collaborative. *Ann Surg.* May 2011;253(5):849–854. PubMed PMID: 21173696. doi:10.1097/SLA.0b013e3181f4dfc8.

20. Davenport DL, Henderson WG, Mosca CL, Khuri SF, Mentzer Jr RM. Risk-adjusted morbidity in teaching hospitals correlates with reported levels of communication and collaboration on surgical teams but not with scale measures of teamwork climate, safety climate, or working conditions. *J Am Coll Surg.* December 2007;205(6):778–784. PubMed PMID: 18035261.

21. Diaz JA, Griffith RA, Ng JJ, Reinert SE, Friedmann PD, Moulton AW. Patients' use of the Internet for medical information. *J Gen Intern Med.* March 2002;17(3):180–185. PubMed PMID: 11929503; PubMed Central PMCID: PMC1495021.

22. Powell JA, Darvell M, Gray JA. The doctor, the patient and the world-wide web: how the internet is changing healthcare. *J R Soc Med.* February 2003;96(2):74–76. Review. PubMed PMID: 12562977; PubMed Central PMCID: PMC539397.

23. Ha JF, Longnecker N. Doctor-patient communication: a review. *Ochsner J.* Spring 2010;10(1):38–43. PubMed PMID: 21603354; PubMed Central PMCID: PMC3096184.

24. Dorr Goold S, Lipkin Jr M. The doctor-patient relationship: challenges, opportunities, and strategies. *J Gen Intern Med.* January 1999;(14 suppl 1):S26–S33. Review. PubMed PMID: 9933492; PubMed Central PMCID: PMC1496871.

25. Kerse N, Buetow S, Mainous AG III, Young G, Coster G, Arroll B. Physician-patient relationship and medication compliance: a primary care investigation. *Ann Fam Med.* September–October 2004;2(5):455–461. PubMed PMID: 15506581; PubMed Central PMCID: PMC1466710.

26. Swaminath G. Doctor-patient communication: patient perception. *Indian J Psychiatry.* July 2007;49(3):150–153. PubMed PMID: 20661374; PubMed Central PMCID: PMC2902081. doi:10.4103/0019-5545.37309.

27. Smith DD, Kellar J, Walters EL, Reibling ET, Phan T, Green SM. Does emergency physician empathy reduce thoughts of litigation? A randomised trial. *Emerg Med J.* August 2016;33(8):548–552. PubMed PMID: 27002161. doi:10.1136/emermed-2015-205312.

28. Robbennolt JK. Apologies and medical error. *Clin Orthop Relat Res.* February 2009;467(2):376–382. PubMed PMID: 18972177; PubMed Central PMCID: PMC2628492. doi:10.1007/s11999-008-0580-1.

29. Levinson W, Roter DL, Mullooly JP, Dull VT, Frankel RM. Physician-patient communication. The relationship with malpractice claims among primary care physicians and surgeons. *JAMA.* February 19, 1997;277(7):553–559. PubMed PMID: 9032162.

30. Beckman HB, Markakis KM, Suchman AL, Frankel RM. The doctor-patient relationship and malpractice. Lessons from plaintiff depositions. *Arch Intern Med.* June 27, 1994;154(12):1365–1370. PubMed PMID: 8002688.

31. Moore PJ, Adler NE, Robertson PA. Medical malpractice: the effect of doctor-patient relations on medical patient perceptions and malpractice intentions. *West J Med.* October 2000;173(4):244–250. PubMed PMID: 11017984; PubMed Central PMCID: PMC1071103.

32. Dyer N, Sorra JS, Smith SA, Cleary PD, Hays RD. Psychometric properties of the Consumer Assessment of Healthcare Providers and Systems (CAHPS®) Clinician and Group Adult Visit Survey. *Med Care.* November 2012;(50 suppl):S28-S34. PubMed PMID: 23064274; PubMed Central PMCID: PMC3480671. doi:10.1097/MLR.0b013e31826cbc0d.

33. Kennedy GD, Tevis SE, Kent KC. Is there a relationship between patient satisfaction and favorable outcomes? *Ann Surg.* October 2014;260(4):592–598, discussion 598–600. PubMed PMID: 25203875; PubMed Central PMCID: PMC4159721. doi:10.1097/SLA.0000000000000932.

34. Accreditation Council for Graduate Medical Education. *Common Program Requirements: General Competencies* [Internet]. Chicago, IL: ACGME; 2007:2.

35. Smith RC, Lyles JS, Mettler J, et al. The effectiveness of intensive training for residents in interviewing. A randomized, controlled study. *Ann Intern Med.* January 15, 1998;128(2):118–126. PubMed PMID: 9441572.

36. Fallowfield L, Jenkins V, Farewell V, Solis-Trapala I. Enduring impact of communication skills training: results of a 12-month follow-up. *Br J Cancer.* October 20, 2003;89(8):1445–1449. PubMed PMID: 14562015; PubMed Central PMCID: PMC2394345.

37. Lewin SA, Skea ZC, Entwistle V, Zwarenstein M, Dick J. Interventions for providers to promote a patient-centred approach in clinical consultations. *Cochrane Database Syst Rev.* 2001;(4):CD003267. Review Update in: *Cochrane Database Syst Rev.* 2012;12:CD003267. PubMed PMID: 11687181.

38. Smith RC, Marshall AA, Cohen-Cole SA. The efficacy of intensive biopsychosocial teaching programs for residents: a review of the literature and guidelines for teaching. *J Gen Intern Med.* July 1994;9(7):390–396. Review. PubMed PMID: 7931749.

39. Arora S, Sevdalis N, Nestel D, Woloshynowych M, Darzi A, Kneebone R. The impact of stress on surgical performance: a systematic review of the literature. *Surgery*. March 2010;147(3):318–330, 330.e1–6. Review. PubMed PMID: 20004924. doi:10.1016/j.surg.2009.10.007.

40. Jeff Wiese. *Tulane Internal Medicine Residency Program*. Tulane Internal Medicine Residency Program. Tulane Internal Medicine Team, n.d. Web. February 1, 2017. http://www.tulanemedicine.com/.

41. Fox AA, Shernan SK, Body SC. Predictive genomics of adverse events after cardiac surgery. *Semin Cardiothorac Vasc Anesth*. December 2004;8(4):297–315. Review. PubMed PMID: 15583791.

42. Perry TE, Muehlschlegel JD, Body SC. Genomics: risk and outcomes in cardiac surgery. *Anesthesiol Clin*. September 2008;26(3):399–417. PubMed PMID: 18765214; PubMed Central PMCID: PMC2744392. doi:10.1016/j.anclin.2008.04.002.

43. Shapiro SE, Cote GC, Lee JE, Gagel RF, Evans DB. The role of genetics in the surgical management of familial endocrinopathy syndromes. *J Am Coll Surg*. November 2003;197(5):818–831. Review. PubMed PMID: 14585420.

44. Barrisford GW, Singer EA, Rosner IL, Linehan WM, Bratslavsky G. Familial renal cancer: molecular genetics and surgical management. *Int J Surg Oncol*. 2011;2011:658767. PubMed PMID: 22312516; PubMed Central PMCID: PMC3263689. doi:10.1155/2011/658767.

45. Buia A, Stockhausen F, Hanisch E. Laparoscopic surgery: a qualified systematic review. *World J Methodol*. December 26, 2015;5(4):238–254. PubMed PMID: 26713285; PubMed Central PMCID: PMC4686422. doi:10.5662/wjm.v5.i4.238.

46. van Bree SH, Vlug MS, Bemelman WA, et al. Faster recovery of gastrointestinal transit after laparoscopy and fast-track care in patients undergoing colonic surgery. *Gastroenterology*. September 2011;141(3):872–880.e1–4. Erratum in: *Gastroenterology*. March 2012;142(3):676. Multiple author names corrected. PubMed PMID: 21699777. doi:10.1053/j.gastro.2011.05.034.

47. Mentula P, Sammalkorpi H, Leppäniemi A. Laparoscopic surgery or conservative treatment for appendiceal abscess in Adults? A randomized controlled trial. *Ann Surg*. August 2015;262(2):237–242. PubMed PMID: 25775072. doi:10.1097/SLA.0000000000001200.

48. *American Board of Surgery CME Requirements for Recertification*. June 24, 2014; Available from: http://wwwabsurgery.org/default.jsp?exam-moccme.

49. Miles SH. *The Hippocratic Oath and the Ethics of Medicine*. Oxford: Oxford University Press; 2004. Print.

50. Kagawa-Singer M, Kassim-Lakha S. A strategy to reduce cross-cultural miscommunication and increase the likelihood of improving health outcomes. *Acad Med*. June 2003;78(6):577–587. PubMed PMID: 12805036.

51. Betancourt JR. Cultural competence—marginal or mainstream movement? *N Engl J Med*. 2004;351:953–954.

52. Epner DE, Baile WF. Patient-centered care: the key to cultural competence. *Ann Oncol*. April 2012;(23 suppl 3):33–42. PubMed PMID: 22628414. doi:10.1093/annonc/mds086.

53. Burke T. Accountable care organizations. *Public Health Rep*. November–December 2011;126(6):875–878. PubMed PMID: 22043105; PubMed Central PMCID: PMC3185325.

54. Berlin EA, Fowkes Jr WC. A teaching framework for cross-cultural health care. Application in family practice. *West J Med*. December 1983;139(6):934–938. PubMed PMID: 6666112; PubMed Central PMCID: PMC1011028.

55. Hamelin ND, Nikolis A, Armano J, Harris PG, Brutus JP. Evaluation of factors influencing confidence and trust in the patient-physician relationship: a survey of patient in a hand clinic. *Chir Main*. April 2012;31(2):83–90. PubMed PMID: 22365321. doi:10.1016/j.main.2012.01.005.

56. Itani KM, Liscum K, Brunicardi FC. Physician leadership is a new mandate in surgical training. *Am J Surg*. March 2004;187(3):328–331.

57. Makary MA, Sexton JB, Freischlag JA, et al. Operating room teamwork among physicians and nurses: teamwork in the eye of the beholder. *J Am Coll Surg*. May 2006;202(5):746–752. PubMed PMID: 16648014.

58. Lu H, While AE, Barriball KL. Job satisfaction among nurses: a literature review. *Int J Nurs Stud*. February 2005;42(2):211–227. Review. PubMed PMID: 15680619.

59. Lee L, Berger DH, Awad SS, Brandt ML, Martinez G, Brunicardi FC. Conflict resolution: practical principles for surgeons. *World J Surg*. November 2008;32(11):2331–2335. Review. PubMed PMID: 18787896. doi:10.1007/s00268-008-9702-x.

60. Kavarana MN, Sade RM. Ethical issues in cardiac surgery. *Future Cardiol*. May 2012;8(3):451–465. PubMed PMID: 22642634; PubMed Central PMCID: PMC3374583. doi:10.2217/fca.11.91.

61. Reitsma AM, Moreno JD. Ethics of innovative surgery: US surgeons' definitions, knowledge, and attitudes. *J Am Coll Surg*. January 2005;200(1):103–110. PubMed PMID: 15631926.

62. Downing MT, Way DP, Caniano DA. Results of a national survey on ethics education in general surgery residency programs. *Am J Surg*. September 1997;174(3):364–368. PubMed PMID: 9324157.

63. Helft PR, Eckles RE, Torbeck L. Ethics education in surgical residency programs: a review of the literature. *J Surg Educ*. January–February 2009;66(1):35–42. Review. PubMed PMID: 19215896. doi:10.1016/j.jsurg.2008.10.001.

64. Klingensmith ME. Teaching ethics in surgical training programs using a case-based format. *J Surg Educ*. March–April 2008;65(2):126–128. PubMed PMID: 18439534. doi:10.1016/j.jsurg.2007.12.001.

65. Holloran SD, Starkey GW, Burke PA, Steele Jr G, Forse RA. An educational intervention in the surgical intensive care unit to improve ethical decisions. *Surgery*. August 1995;118(2):294–298, discussion 298–299. PubMed PMID: 7638746.

66. Chipman JG, Beilman GJ, Schmitz CC, Seatter SC. Development and pilot testing of an OSCE for difficult conversations in surgical intensive care. *J Surg Educ*. March–April 2007;64(2):79–87. PubMed PMID: 17462207.

67. Rowold J. *Multifactor Leadership Questionnaire: Psychometric Properties of the German Translation*. Menlo Park: Mind Garden, Inc.; 2005.

68. Hu YY, Parker SH, Lipsitz SR, et al. Behavior in the operating room. *J Am Coll Surg*. January 2016;222(1):41–51. PubMed PMID: 26481409; PubMed Central PMCID: PMC4769879. doi:10.1016/j.jamcollsurg.2015.09.013.

69. Horwitz IB, Horwitz SK, Daram P, Brandt ML, Brunicardi FC, Awad SS. Transformational, transactional, and passive-avoidant leadership characteristics of a surgical resident cohort: analysis using the multifactor leadership questionnaire and implications for improving surgical education curriculums. *J Surg Res*. July 2008;148(1):49–59.

70. Horwitz IB, Horwity SK, Brunicardi FC, Awad SS. Improving comprehensive surgical resident training through use of the NEO Five-Factor Personality Inventory: results from a cohort-based trial. *Am J Surg*. June 2011;201(6):828–834.

71. Henrickson PS, Flin R, McKinley A, Yule S. The Surgeons' Leadership Inventory (SLI): a taxonomy and rating system for surgeons' intraoperative leadership skills. *Am J Surg*. June 2013;205(6):745–751.

72. Shipton H, Armstrong C, West M, Dawson J. The impact of leadership and quality climate on hospital performance. *Int J Qual Health Care.* December 2008;20(6): 439–445.

73. Awad SS, Hayley B, Fagan SP, Berger DH, Brunicardi FC. The impact of a novel resident leadership training curriculum. *Am J Surg.* November 2004;188(5):481–484.

74. Parker SH, Flin R, McKinley A, Yule S. Factors influencing surgeons' intraoperative leadership: video analysis of unanticipated events in the operating room. *World J Surg.* January 2014;38(1):4–10. PubMed PMID: 24114366. doi:10.1007/s00268-013-2241-0.

# Ethical Considerations for Surgeons: Financial Conflicts of Interest

William S. Messer, Jr, PhD

PROLOGUE ▶ The higher education institutions of the United States have seen, in recent years, a great increase in emphasis on the transfer of technology out of the university and into the for-profit public sector. This trend has resulted, in part at least, from a growing recognition that the economic health of the country is and has been dependent on the small, innovative business enterprise. This movement has been particularly strong in the health arena; health care and its derivative device and pharmaceutical enterprises are among the most promising industries in the current economy. The negative inadvertent consequences of this trend have been the creation of an entirely new set of complex relationships with the for-profit world and the potential for surgeons to become massively wealthy from an invention.

A new set of experts has arisen within institutions who are focused on technology transfer negotiations and law. Venture capitalists have become interested in health care and surgery more specifically, and a national organization of technology transfer experts has become organized.

The new enterprises and relationships have brought into being a long list of new potential conflicts of interest.

Dr William S. Messer is a professor in the departments of pharmacology and medicinal and biological chemistry in the College of Pharmacy and Pharmaceutical Sciences at The University of Toledo.

## Abstract

Financial conflicts of interest, whether perceived or real, present significant challenges to physicians and have broad implications on patient care, professional relationships, and, in academic medical center settings, training of medical students and residents. The Affordable Care Act has required the establishment of a transparency program designed to clarify the financial relationships between physicians, teaching hospitals, and the pharmaceutical and biomedical device industries. Many scientific societies require physician scientists to declare their financial conflicts of interest in presentations or publications. These recent changes to reporting requirements related to con- 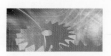 flicts of interest highlight the importance of transparency to the medical field. Patients, and society at large, have a right to know if their physicians have received support from pharmaceutical or biomedical manufacturers. The scientific community also should recognize the source of funding for published research to properly evaluate and interpret reported scientific data.

Concerns regarding financial conflicts of interest center around the type of support received by physicians and the influence payments by the industry might generate. In addition, as physician scientists become engaged in translational research leading to intellectual property and entrepreneurial efforts, licensing revenue from patents and financial stakes in start-up companies raise additional challenges for physicians, especially those with academic ties. Although financial conflicts of interest raise questions regarding the role of physician scientists in the generation of new knowledge and the development of new treatments for disease, it is very often appropriate for physicians to engage in such activities. Identification (disclosure) and management of financial conflicts of interest are key considerations to maintain compliance with existing laws and institutional policies and to assure public trust.

## Introduction

Financial conflicts of interest arise when individuals making decisions can be influenced by financial considerations that may or may not be apparent to those impacted by the decisions. For example, a physician may consider using one of two types of implants for a surgery. The surgeon may decide based on sound scientific principles to choose one of the available implants rather than the other, but what if the surgeon holds a financial interest (eg, stock option) in the company that manufactures the chosen implant? Even if there is a strong rationale for choosing one implant over the other, the ability to receive a financial gain represents a conflict of interest that could influence the decision. In the worst case, a physician could let financial considerations outweigh other factors, such as patient safety or cost. Therefore, financial conflicts of interests need to be addressed appropriately through disclosure and management processes; these will be outlined in detail later in the chapter.

Distinctions have been made between potential and real conflicts of interest and between real and perceived conflicts of interest. McCoy and Emanuel argue that there are no "potential" conflicts of interest.[1] For physicians, any financial influence that could have an impact on patient care, professional judgment, or medical student training should be treated as a real conflict of interest. The modifier "potential" implies ambiguity, as if some might consider a financial relationship, such as a consulting fee from a pharmaceutical company, as a real conflict of interest, while others might not. This is not the case; any financial relationship creates a conflict of interest that must be addressed. The nature of the conflict of interest will determine the potential impact of the financial conflict of interest and guide the steps to address the conflict.

Are perceptions of conflict of interest as important as actual conflicts of interest? If a conflict of interest exists (an actual conflict of interest) and it is perceived as a conflict of interest, then steps can be taken to manage the conflict. The perception does not alter the impact of the conflict of interest. However, if a conflict of interest does not exist, yet is perceived by others to exist, such perceptions can undermine confidence in a physician's judgment.[1]

Several studies have addressed the impact of interactions with the pharmaceutical industry on attitudes and behavior of physicians, as reviewed by Wazana.[2] Meetings with representatives from the pharmaceutical industry were associated with requests to include drugs from the pharmaceutical company in the formulary, despite little evidence of the relative merit of such drugs over existing drugs. Interactions with pharmaceutical representatives also influenced prescribing practices with impact on the cost of medications, a preference for new drugs, and a decreased preference for generic drugs. Accepting samples and receiving industry-paid meals also were associated with preferences for, and rapid prescriptions of, new drugs and addition of drugs to formularies, respectively. Funding for travel, continuing medical education sponsorship, and receipt of honoraria or research funding also were found to be associated with increased prescribing rates and/or requests for including drugs in formularies. Taken together, the data indicate that interactions with the pharmaceutical industry can have an impact on the attitudes and behaviors of physicians.

## Personal Conflicts of Interest

Conflicts of interest arise from a wide variety of circumstances (see Table 29.1). Physicians may be asked to serve as consultants for companies in the biomedical or pharmaceutical fields. In academic medical centers, physicians may receive research funding from a pharmaceutical company or a biomedical device manufacturer to participate in clinical trials. Surgeons may develop new techniques or new technologies leading to patents and companies that seek to commercialize such innovations. Regardless of the nature of the relationship, any payment from companies to physicians creates the potential for a personal financial conflict of interest.

Such financial conflicts of interest create competition between a physician's obligations to patients and the physician's economic interests.[3] This is a matter of personal integrity. Can the patient trust the physician to practice medicine and engage in research with the highest level of ethical standards?

Financial conflicts should be addressed as soon as they are recognized. Although such conflicts can present problems for individuals, they are not inherently wrong; moreover, they can be difficult to avoid. As outlined previously, financial conflicts of interest may arise from research and development activities and efforts to test new hypotheses regarding the best methods to treat patients. Yet studies indicate that industry-sponsored research is more likely to result in conclusions more favorable to the sponsor than research funded through other mechanisms.[4] Conflicts of interest should not prevent physicians from participating in the advancement of medical practice but must be disclosed and managed properly to prevent financial factors from influencing medical research or patient care and eroding patient and public trust.

As outlined in the Introduction, perceptions of conflicts of interest may not be accurate.[1] For example, a physician may receive a consulting fee for

**TABLE 29.1 ▶TYPES OF PERSONAL FINANCIAL CONFLICTS OF INTEREST**

| Type | Description |
| --- | --- |
| Consulting payments | Physicians approached by a company to help evaluate technology or to determine the best marketing strategy for a new device or pharmaceutical. |
| Speaking fees | Physicians asked to speak at a conference in exchange for an "honorarium" that is paid by a company. |
| Research funding | Physicians conduct a pilot clinical trial with a new drug or new device. The research study may be funded through mechanisms that include payments to physicians for initiating the study. |
| Patents and licensing | Physicians develop innovative approaches for treatment resulting in patent applications and licensing of technology to start-up companies or the pharmaceutical and medical device industries. These relationships may result in physicians receiving some type of financial gain. |

advising a pharmaceutical company regarding its marketing campaign for a new drug. Some might perceive the relationship as a financial conflict of interest, but this would be false. Yes, the physician receives a financial gain, but if the payment does not impact the physician's practice or professional judgment, then there is no real conflict of interest. If, however, the physician receives a consulting fee for advising the pharmaceutical company on its marketing strategy and writing a position paper extolling the benefits of the new drug for a journal, the financial gain presents a real conflict of interest. The payment has the potential to influence the physician's professional judgment, and the financial conflict of interest should be disclosed to the publisher of the paper and to its readers.

In academic settings, physician scientists often are reimbursed for their involvement in research studies, especially clinical trials. Such payments could undermine the research to be conducted and bias results toward outcomes favorable to the sponsor.[5] Steps to reduce bias are critical for minimizing the impact of financial conflicts of interest on research outcomes. Disclosures of conflicts of interest represent important first steps, yet other approaches are needed. In particular, it is important to identify ways to remove systematic bias from studies, for example, by assigning patients to groups randomly and blinding patients and caregivers to treatments. Such steps often require additional efforts on behalf of research scientists, yet they can be very helpful in reducing bias and limiting the impact of financial conflicts of interest.

## Institutional Conflicts of Interest

Beyond personal conflicts of interest, institutions may have relationships with companies that provide financial benefits (see Table 29.2). For example, a company might sponsor a seminar series or grand rounds for a department. Biomedical companies may offer scholarships or support residency programs through donations to academic medical centers, colleges, or departments.

TABLE 29.2  ▶ TYPES OF INSTITUTIONAL FINANCIAL CONFLICTS OF INTEREST

| Type | Description |
| --- | --- |
| Sponsorship | Company sponsorship of continuing medical education, departmental seminars, or college events. |
| Scholarships | Company support for graduate or medical student stipends or residency programs. |
| Research funding | Pharmaceutical and biomedical company support for clinical trials of new medicines or devices. Companies also can fund basic and applied research in faculty research laboratories. |
| Licensing | Company licenses patents for technology developed by institutions. |

These relationships may be established with specific guidelines covered in a memorandum of understanding that outlines how the funds are to be used and any restrictions that may be placed on the relationships.

Institutional financial conflict of interest considerations go beyond the personal involvement of individual physicians and can become more complicated because of the pervasive nature of institutional/industry relationships. In some instances, physicians or other scientists at a university might develop technology (eg, a potential drug therapy or vaccine) that is licensed to a spin-off company that is owned in part or in full by the inventor. In such circumstances, a physician might receive payments from the company for consulting or activity on a research grant while the university receives licensing or royalty payments. If the company supports research activities at the university, additional financial conflicts of interest might arise as the university could receive financial benefit from the successful development of new technologies.

As a result, institutions have established policies and procedures to identify and manage conflicts of interest. At academic institutions, committees are established to help manage financial conflicts of interest. As outlined below, identifying financial conflicts of interest is an important first step. A committee of academic peers can play a vital role in helping to identify appropriate measures to limit the impact of financial conflicts of interest on research outcomes, patient care, and student education.

## Legislation Covering Conflicts of Interest

In 2010, the Physician Payments Sunshine Act, a part of the Affordable Care Act, required medical product manufacturers and group purchasing organizations to report financial payments to physicians and teaching hospitals. In 2013, the Centers for Medicare and Medicaid Services began collecting data and making the information available on a public Web site. In the first 5 months of the program (August through December of 2013), $3.4 billion financial interactions (including general financial interactions, research-related financial interactions, and ownership or investment interests) were reported by 1347 companies to 470 000 physicians and 1019 teaching hospitals. In 2014, $6.5 billion financial interactions were reported from 1444 companies to 607 000 physicians and 1121 teaching hospitals.[6]

A review of the reported data from 2013 and 2014 indicates that the vast majority of payments cover food and beverage (83.5% and 87.0% of payments respectively), although the value of payments covering food and beverage is 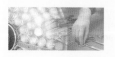 lower than other types of payments—9.4% and 8.8% from 2013 and 2014, respectively.[6] Although a relatively minor proportion of the payments (<0.2%), royalty or license payments represented over 30% of the value of payments in both 2013 and 2014. Consulting payments represented 16.1% of the value of payments in 2013 and 14.4% of the value in 2014. Services other than consulting covered 20.4% of the value in 2013 and 24.7% in 2014. Thus, licensing and royalty payments and services (consulting or otherwise) represented over 65% of the value of payments to physicians in 2013 and 2014.

Between 2013 and 2015, of the 5 physicians receiving the highest payments, each received more than $28 million because of inventions or from being owners or officials of companies purchased by other pharmaceutical companies.[7] The impact of such large payments likely should be considered in a different light than the smaller payments associated with covering food and beverages.

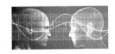

These data highlight the types of financial arrangements with companies that could impact physician activities. Royalties and licensing payments should receive more attention because of the relatively high value of such payments to those few engaged in such activities. Special steps to limit the consequences of such financial arrangements can help manage the impact of financial conflicts of interest as outlined below.

## Best Practices

Several medical societies have weighed in with guidelines addressing financial conflicts of interest for their members. The Institute of Medicine examined conflicts of interest in medical practice, research, and education and published a detailed report providing comprehensive approaches for identifying and managing conflicts of interest.[8]

In 2010, the Society for Vascular Surgery approved a set of guidelines to address the management of conflicts of interest.[9] Although the guidelines primarily cover financial conflicts of interest for the Society, they provide a useful outline for both individual and institutional approaches to deal with conflicts of interest. In particular, general principles include the tenets of developing programs independent of company influence, transparency in disclosing financial relationships, separating grant and medical education control from company control, and limitations on displays of corporate logos. The North American Spine Society also has developed programs to eliminate financial conflicts of interest where possible and to manage such conflicts when they cannot be avoided.[10]

## Identifying and Responding to Financial Conflicts of Interest

The Institute of Medicine recommended a 6-step process to identify and manage conflicts of interest as outlined in Table 29.3.[8] These steps require mechanisms for collecting information about conflicts of interest, establishing policies for dealing with potential financial conflicts of interest, and

**TABLE 29.3** ▶ IDENTIFYING AND RESPONDING TO POTENTIAL FINANCIAL CONFLICTS OF INTEREST[8]

| Step | Description |
|---|---|
| 1. Disclosure | Obtain information about financial conflicts of interest. |
| 2. Evaluation | Evaluate the disclosure to determine if a financial conflict of interest exists and collect additional information as needed. |
| 3. Elimination or exclusion | Determine if involvement in activity is inconsistent with existing policies or if substantial risks should limit participation. |
| 4. Management | As appropriate, develop a plan to manage the conflict of interest. |
| 5. Monitor | Monitor adherence to the management plan or exclusion from activities. |
| 6. Compliance | Determine nature of noncompliance and appropriate response (and follow-through). |

identifying individuals or committees responsible for oversight of conflicts of interest. The latter individual or committee must have institutional support for managing and monitoring conflicts of interest and for addressing problems stemming from noncompliance with institutional policies.

At an institutional level, identifying and addressing conflicts of interest requires support from organizational leaders, particularly with increased pressures related to the levels of support for research and the increased costs of medical education.[11] Adoption of policies outlining the institutional philosophy and approaches for identifying and managing conflicts represents an important first step for leadership. Equally important is a clear commitment to addressing conflicts of interest issues as they arise. For example, leaders need to ensure that clinical trials are conducted free from bias when the technology being evaluated derives from physician scientists at the institution. Open, public discussions of conflict of interest issues can help establish an institutional culture that recognizes the impact of conflicts of interest, encourages disclosures of potential conflicts of interest, and provides appropriate resources for managing identified conflicts.

## Disclosures of Conflicts of Interest

As outlined previously, transparency in disclosing financial relationships is an important principle for properly handling financial conflicts of interest. One of the first steps in dealing with a financial conflict of interest is to disclose the conflict. Academic medical centers have policies that require disclosure of financial conflicts of interest. The disclosure of a conflict of interest leads to an inquiry into the nature of the conflict and a determination of whether a conflict is perceived or real. Specific events, such as submission of a grant proposal or human subjects protocol, also can trigger an inquiry.

It should be emphasized that a disclosure of a financial conflict of interest is not an admission of guilt. It is simply a statement that there is a relationship that may pose a real or perceived financial conflict of interest. The disclosure should reveal the nature of the interaction with outside parties, the level of financial arrangements, and whether services were performed (or will be performed) for remuneration. For payments to physicians, the amount received from a specific company would be disclosed. If a physician holds a financial interest in an outside company, the nature of the relationship (eg, owner or investor) and the size of the investment (percentage ownership and estimated value of the company) should be provided.

## Exclusions of Conflicts of Interest

Although disclosures of conflicts of interest may serve as the first step in addressing and managing financial conflicts of interest, excluding financial conflicts of interest reflects an alternative approach for both individuals and institutions. For example, some academic medical centers have eliminated the practice of receiving gifts (whether monetary or in the form of merchandise such as pens and stationery) from pharmaceutical companies to avoid that type of financial conflict of interest. That approach avoids the questions of whether or to what extent receipt of such gifts influences physician behavior.[12] These exclusions may be limited to the receipt of gifts but still allow other types of interactions, including research grants or participation in clinical trials.[11]

## Managing Conflicts of Interest

Once financial conflicts of interest have been disclosed, steps should be taken to manage those conflicts. Critical issues to address include how the conflicts of interest are made transparent to relevant parties (ie, patients, the scientific community); supervisory roles of physicians in training students, residents, and other scientists (eg, postdoctoral fellows); and clear guidelines for publications and patient care. In academic settings, a committee is often established to review and manage potential conflicts of interest to ensure that these issues are addressed fully.

Of particular importance is the management of financial conflicts of interest that could impact patient outcomes. Lo and Grady suggest that physicians receiving very large payments should be excluded from committees that make decisions regarding clinical practice guidelines, purchase of operating room supplies, and hospital formularies to limit overt influence on decisions impacting large numbers of patients.[7] In a similar fashion, physicians receiving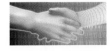

payments because of royalties, licenses, and/or stock options should not be directly engaged in clinical trials (as principal investigators collecting data or evaluating patient outcomes) evaluating their technologies. Such physicians could be engaged as consultants to provide necessary expertise while limiting direct involvement in the conduct of the trial.

Another critical issue, particularly in academic medical centers, is to manage the impact of conflicts of interest on the training of students and residents. Engagement in research and scholarship is an important part of medical, graduate, and undergraduate education. Students and residents involved in research often face pressure from faculty scientists to deliver research results in a timely manner. In addition, students and residents may feel pressured to obtain results that are favorable to the sponsor, even when not explicitly directed to do so by their faculty mentor. Alleviating such pressures requires some flexibility and creativity on the part of faculty mentors and foresight, planning, and direction at an institutional level.

From a faculty researcher's perspective, a key step is to set the right level of expectations for the research project from the outset. A clear statement regarding the scope of the research and the approach to be taken goes a long way toward establishing the importance of research integrity as the research project is initiated. In addition, faculty mentors can look for ways to make  data collection more objective rather than subjective. Using instruments that automatically record data rather than subjective questionnaires helps reduce potential bias. When it is not possible to avoid subjective measures, extra steps to blind investigators to treatments can be helpful. For example, having one investigator collecting the data and another investigator scoring patient behavior in a blinded fashion provides a useful way to limit investigator bias and promote research integrity.

At an institutional level, as financial conflicts of interest are identified, faculty mentors can be encouraged to work with faculty colleagues who help monitor the interactions between the faculty mentors and their students and residents. This may be done as part of the financial conflict of interest management plan. The faculty colleague could be a member of a committee assigned to manage conflicts of interests and his/her role might include evaluation of ongoing practices in data collection, review of protocols and manuscripts for evidence of research bias, and provision of guidance and assistance for students and residents who may feel caught between the interests of scientific research and those of the sponsor or the investigator.

## Summary

Maintaining an environment of research integrity is vital to the proper conduct of research and the appropriate training of students and residents. The disclosure and management of conflicts of interest are critical components of rigorous research programs that reduce investigator bias and build an environment that develops and maintains patient trust. Institutions play an important role in establishing the proper environment for addressing issues related to financial conflicts of interest. Institutional leaders (presidents or chief executive officers, vice presidents of research, and deans of medical colleges) should take proactive roles in highlighting the importance of research integrity, developing appropriate policies regarding financial conflicts of interest, setting up committees to address such conflicts, and establishing procedures to guide researchers through the processes associated with disclosure and management of conflicts of interest.

# References

1. McCoy MS, Emanuel EJ. Why there are no "potential" conflicts of interest. *JAMA*. 2017;317(17):1721–1722.
2. Wazana A. Physicians and the pharmaceutical industry: is a gift ever just a gift? *JAMA*. 2000;283(3):373–380.
3. Jones JW, McCullough LB, Richman BW. Consultation or corruption? The ethics of signing on to the medical-industrial complex. *J Vasc Surg*. 2006;43(1):192–195.
4. Lundh A, Sismondo S, Lexchin J, Busuioc OA, Bero L. Industry sponsorship and research outcome. *Cochrane Database Syst Rev*. 2012;12:MR000033.
5. Bero L. Addressing bias and conflict of interest among biomedical researchers. *JAMA*. 2017;317(17):1723–1724.
6. Agrawal S, Brown D. The physician payments sunshine act—two years of the open payments program. *N Engl J Med*. 2016;374(10):906–909.
7. Lo B, Grady D. Payments to physicians: does the amount of money make a difference? *JAMA*. 2017;317(17):1719–1720.
8. Lo B, Field MJ. *Conflict of Interest in Medical Research, Education and Practice*. Washington, DC: National Academies Press; 2009.
9. Elliott BM. Conflict of interest and the Society for Vascular Surgery. *J Vasc Surg*. 2011;54:3s–11s.
10. Schofferman JA, Eskay-Auerbach ML, Sawyer LS, Herring SA, Arnold PM, Muehlbauer EJ. Conflict of interest and professional medical associations: the North American Spine Society experience. *Spine J*. 2013;13(8):974–979.
11. Pizzo PA, Lawley TJ, Rubenstein AH. Role of leaders in fostering meaningful collaborations between academic medical centers and industry while also managing individual and institutional conflicts of interest. *JAMA*. 2017;317(17):1729–1730.
12. Fineberg HV. Conflict of interest: why does it matter? *JAMA*. 2017;317(17):1717–1718.

# 30 The Unspoken Surgical Curriculum

Lloyd A. Jacobs, MD

PROLOGUE ▶ A significant portion, perhaps a majority, of the ethical precepts of our discipline reside in a subterranean repository of presupposition, intuitions, and sensitivities. Although these foundations of our ethics are largely inaccessible, they color every decision of ours. Moreover, it is important to remember that every act or utterance of the surgeon in the presence of his/her patient has ethical import; it is good or not good. For example, the choice between a Whipple procedure and a palliative gastroenterostomy is as much an ethical choice as is the decision concerning the degree of clarity one should give.

The subterranean repository of ethical foundations is created and modulated most powerfully by metaphor and metonymy as opposed to declaration. A smile or a grimace communicates more directly to this repository than do the data. Much of what the surgeon is learning during training and throughout a long career is of this nature and is so communicated.

Surgeons have an obligation to know themselves in every aspect for two reasons. First, they must equip themselves to make the best moral decisions, of which they are capable, for their patients. Second, they have an obligation to care for their own health and well-being. However, much of what a surgeon learns and knows is not immediately accessible or retrievable, and if retrievable is unsayable, because there are no words or the culture forbids its enunciation. In this regard, surgeons are like every other human person: They carry within themselves a large subterranean cache of mental models and thought forms. More simply, this cache is the repository of descriptions of how one believes the world of reality is constituted. The surgeon has an obligation to periodically inventory this repository to the extent that is 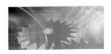 possible, with a view to determining the windage this unspoken knowledge may produce on his/her decisions.

However, how can that inventory be undertaken? How can one come to know the contents of his/her own memory banks? Deep introspection or complex analysis is time-consuming and of doubtful value. One discovers one's own motives or propensities exactly as one discovers these qualities in another person. You are to become an observer of your own conduct, your own utterances, and your own demeanor, posture, and physiognomy. From these data, one learns the inner qualities of one's self and such qualities in others. Ultimately, the surgeon has a duty to strive to see himself/herself as others see him/her.

There are a number of arenas in which these notions find application. One of the most interesting and relevant is the ability to see, an ability on which the surgeon relies heavily. The thrust of this train of thoughts is the assertion that there is no uninterpreted visual experience and that incoherent patterns of light and darkness are constructed in one's occipital cortex into a visual representation of reality, according to one's own understanding of the nature of reality. We see what we expect to see. If one's only tool is a hammer, the whole world looks like a nail.

More seriously, perception in the operating room depends on already existing thought forms and visual models already within the observer's mind. To the medical student or intern the opened body cavity presents only a scene of amorphous red, a prospect of blood and gore. To the trained surgeon the visual patterns are put together very differently. Structure emerges; order and pathology are visually apparent.

This visual phenomenon is well recognized in the world of visual art, where the visual experience is believed to be based on reciprocity between the artist and the viewer. The painting is incomplete without the beholder. This phenomenon is recognized in disciplines other than surgery:

*"The microscopist sees coelenterate mesoglea, his new student sees only a gooey, formless stuff."*[1]

An important part of what one learns in the long training to become a surgeon is of this nature and is unnoticed during acquisition, inaccessible on demand, and unsayable even when recognized. The teaching in this realm of knowledge has been termed "the unspoken curriculum." Some of the topics taught within this unspoken curriculum are a bias to action that almost uniformly is part of a surgeon's presuppositions. Regret, and the surgeon's reaction to it, is taught as a part of this curriculum. Respect for life, particularly when it is difficult in the face of mean spiritedness or poor hygiene, 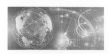 is taught or not taught here. Self-knowledge concerning one's emotions is taught largely as a part of this unspoken curriculum. The tools of this pedagogy are metaphor, stories, and fiction, but the most powerful teacher of all is emulation. Thus the attending surgeon or advanced resident has an obligation to be aware of what he/she exemplifies to his/her learners.

Let us merely list some of the lessons taught in the unspoken curriculum. Equanimity merging into passionlessness is taught. Almost any display of emotion is derogated. Stamina in the face of fatigue and sleeplessness is greatly valued. The idea of a limitation of the hours in a workweek is contrary to our value system and is to be circumvented whenever possible if detection is unlikely. Defensiveness is bad. Lying is good or bad only in relation to the risk of detection. Regret is weakness.

The unspoken curriculum has presented an almost impossible ambiguity about teamwork. Our actions and our preachments are widely divergent. Modern medicine and surgery has specifically evolved into widely ranging areas of knowledge and practice. Multidisciplinary teams are clearly necessary. Within our own discipline, there are many branches of endeavor; one resident cannot be physically present in the operating room, the intensive care unit, and the emergency department at the same time. Interdependence is essential. Still the resident presenter at a conference is expected to "own" the situation and to be aware of every detail of the patient's health. Furthermore, he/she is completely alone at the podium, with the whole department, even the rotating students, arrayed opposite him. The ambiguity produced by these practices powerfully populates the subterranean cache of the presenter, to the detriment of his/her own health and commitment to the chosen field's lifework.

Dr Martin Gray was in slow traffic as he approached St. Mark's Hospital. He seethed in silence even though he was alone in the car. He jogged in the parking lot and was in the family waiting room outside the operating room only perhaps 20 minutes later than he had promised.

The patient was already in the preoperative holding area. The anesthesiologist had made it clear that he was waiting. The family was hesitant. "What exactly is the operation?" "How then will her food pass through?" "Will she need blood?" "What if we leave it alone?"

Dr Gray was startled at his own tone and even more surprised when he heard words come from his mouth to say: "but we can't do nothing!" He pulled himself up short. He remembered hearing the phrase "bias to action." He thought of the operating room staff and the anesthesiologist waiting for him. He was startled, but he continued. "She will die. It would be unconscionable!"

The Hippocratic tradition asserts that the physician and the surgeon should have "a love of mankind." In almost every tradition since that time, in almost every treatise or medical ethics, the surgeon is enjoined to beneficence, with a clear injunction to love. What is difficult here is that the unspoken curriculum does not always teach love of one's neighbor, and the subterranean cache of thought forms may come to contain condescension or even contempt. Some patients are insufficiently washed to preclude an odor. Many are loquacious beyond measure. The mental model produced by these experiences may not be lovable.

Our spoken culture speaks of patient-centeredness; the unspoken curriculum teaches, often by example from older surgeons, a dismissive or deprecating stance toward patients. This may be perceived, particularly by the young trainee, as uncaring and as a lack of respect for life. Moreover, the ambiguity experienced by the surgeon may be the source of depressive feelings, the meaninglessness of life, or worse.

Regret if resolved is probably healthy. Unresolved regret is a common inhabitant of the subterranean world we have described. Actions are most often judged to be good or right in this era by their outcomes or at least by their intended outcomes. If, therefore, a specific act promotes or is intended to promote human flourishing, it is deemed to be good; if it promotes more evil than good, it is on balance: it is not good, not right. Regret as a consequence of our actions has historically been marginalized and has received far less attention than it has deserved. This may, of course, be due in part at least to disagreement about regret. Some view it as dysfunctional and wrong. Others believe it to be salutatory: essential to building on the thought structures of the past and for future acts and experiences and essential for one's integrity. Clearly, regret is an outcome and outcomes are familiar to surgeons; the judgment of decision makers on the basis of the outcome is familiar if not welcome. Regret may be such judgment externalized; if Freud was correct in his structure of mind, regret may be the voice of the superego. Alternatively, regret may be a mere epiphenomenon: The noise that attends the retrofitting of memory to be consistent with our own and our peer's expectations. Given this ambiguity let me assert clearly: regret is essential to the surgeon. It builds the mental structures under which subsequent experience is to be filed. It is a form of metaphor, "imagine if I had done differently," and metaphor is a powerful producer of presuppositions and paradigms, which then determine what we see and what we hear. Preexisting thought forms are essential to perception at all, and regret is a construction that facilitates seeing and hearing initially and facilitates the formulation of perception subsequently. Regret has, therefore, a powerful epistemological function. Along with other emotions and knowledge sources it preformulates what one comes to believe; it justifies or does not justify the knowledge gained by experience. Regret is a part, and a significant part, of the mental function that warrants or 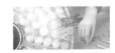 does not warrant the mental models that constitute the surgeon's experience. It is an essential part of a great surgeon. Learn to listen to your inner voice of regret. Try to make a conscious decision whether extinction is appropriate or if you should adjust your acts.

However, regret has inherent dangers. First, the keepers of the discipline of surgery treat it ambiguously. We are told "forget it," "get over it." Most of all we repudiate regret by our actions; we return immediately to the operating room for the next case and celebrate a "don't look back" attitude. However, simultaneously, the keepers of the culture of surgery use regret and use its metaphors as powerful behavioral checks and prods to guide trainees and each other onto the "right" road.

The repudiation of regret, at least at the professed level, as Janet Landman[2] has asserted, is part of a larger tendency in surgery specifically and modern science more generally, to derogate and marginalize the role of emotion in the life of the surgeon and in modern society. Emotion is not recognized for its great hermeneutical power.

Regret has an even more nefarious impact. It may become irresolvable, recurrent, and insistent. Reasonable, healthy regret does not persist. There are many ways to assist in its resolution and extinction; the most important is the collegial analysis and support in the well-run mortality and morbidity conference with which all surgeons are familiar.[3] Personal mental exercises may also be helpful. The extinction of painful emotion over time is a part of the healing function of a healthy mind. Failure of the extinction of an emotion may be a product of stress, or lack of respite, and the absence of time for resolution. These are, of course, vulnerabilities of the surgeon.

What is this discussion of regret doing in a book on Ethics for the Surgeon, beyond the notion that regret is one outcome of an act that invites all of us to judge the rightness of that act? Just this: regret is seen as contrary to the ethos found within most surgical institutions. Regret is seen as self-indulgent and therefore characteristic of an egoistic ethical posture. However, unresolved regret is a common stressor for surgeons, and extreme instances may lead to depression or substance abuse. Its recognition and resolution is an ethical obligation.

# References

1. Laycock SW. *Mind as Mirror and the Mirroring of Mind: Buddhist Reflections on Western Phenomenology.* Albany: State University of New York Press; 1994.
2. Landman J. *Regret.* New York: Oxford University Press; 1993.
3. Jacobs LA. *The Surgeon and the Spirit.* Cincinnati: Compass DataWorks; 2016.

# 31 Resident Supervision

Amir A. Ghaferi, MD, MS
Athanasios Bramos, MD

PROLOGUE ▶ The intergenerational transmission of the knowledge base of the discipline of surgery presents particular difficulties
because of its emphasis on handiwork. The longest paragraph in the Hippocratic Oath, as it is
usually rendered, has to do with what is called
an "art." It must be noted, however, that in a subsequent paragraph, the Oath appears to exclude
surgeons from its admonitions, and perhaps its
emphasis on teaching. Still, the training of surgeons
constitutes the single largest ethical challenge for our
discipline.

Through the centuries since then, surgery has been passed
from generation to generation by the apprentice model. That model was
formalized in our own time by the idea of a learner being "resident" in a hospital for a period of time. Current changes in the public's perception of health
care, the way it is paid for, and the complexity of its technologies have rendered the apprenticeship model vulnerable to significant criticism. Worse, no
good and complete alternative to that model is available at present. Our society and our discipline will face difficult moral decisions in this arena, which
increased regulation may not be able to resolve.

Dr Amir A. Ghaferi is an associate professor of surgery and business, chief
of general surgery at the Ann Arbor Veterans Administration Health System,

director of bariatric surgery, and director of the Michigan Bariatric Surgery Collaborative at the University of Michigan.

Dr Athanasios Bramos is a resident in the Department of Surgery at The University of Toledo College of Medicine.

In 1901, the American Surgical Association met in Baltimore, Maryland. As a part of that meeting, Dr William Stewart Halsted demonstrated the performance of a radical mastectomy. The resident involved was James F. Mitchell. Five decades later, Mitchell at another meeting of the Association related the incident and quoted Halsted as having said: "Mitchell, you operate, I'll stand by." Mitchell continued, "So I did the operation." Apparently, Halsted stayed throughout the operation as Mitchell describes his speaking to the visitors. Furthermore, Mitchell made it clear that Halsted was "...dressed, had on his gloves and everything..."[1]

This vignette involving the surgeon who is widely credited for initiating the surgical residency also illustrates one of its principles: the advanced surgical resident is to be given great operative responsibility. 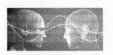 Later, in 1955, Halsted's most illustrious successor, Alfred Blalock of the Blalock-Taussig blue baby operation, in an address to the Clinical Congress of The American College of Surgeons spoke as follows:

> *"...it is unnecessary to say to you that the essence of a good residency training program is the graded and increasing responsibility in the care of patients by trainees."*[2]

It has been harmful to our discipline and to individual surgeons that surgeons have nearly always, in every era, found it necessary and expedient and perhaps appropriate to fail to disclose to patients the exact role trainees will play during their operative and postoperative care. Great ethical tension has resulted from this situation for more than a century.

This ethical dilemma does not, for the most part, belong to the individual surgeon; it belongs to our discipline as a whole. The recognition of the imperative nature of our mode of learning was spoken of by Aristotle:

> *"Anything that we have to learn to do we learn by the actual doing of it: people become builders by building..."*

The experiential training provided by actual operative responsibility is increasingly difficult to achieve because of societal changes, as well as changes in the art of surgery itself. It was at the same meeting of the American Surgical Association that Dr Hugh H. Young, subsequently a foremost urologist, raised a question about the diminishing "opportunities for training..." in surgery. This decrease in "training opportunities" results in part from salutatory social trends, including the advent of medical insurance provided by both private and governmental sources, and the advocacy for and the achievement of greater distributive justice across all segments of American society.

Surgery itself has experienced evolution, which has made experiential training more difficult. Laparoscopic, robotic, and catheter-based procedures render more difficult the supervision of handiwork so essential to the trainee's development. At the same time, many surgeons of good will and good conscience are convinced that "the greatest good for the greatest numbers" of human beings is served by allowing advanced residents to operate with a high degree of independence. However, patients, although they may recognize the correctness of this notion in principle, are often unwilling to be themselves participants.

At the same time, surgical training has been transformed over the last decade. The long hours of every other night call are far away, and all the residents must average a maximum of 80 hours per week. There is more emphasis toward creation of a culture of safety that also addresses the trainee's well-being. However, both fellowship program directors and residents agree that the current graduating surgeons are far less confident than their predecessors of the "good old days." Residents feel inadequately prepared for independent practice and operative autonomy.[3,4] There is much more supervision than there was in the past. In the 21st century, the residents almost never operate completely independently, without an attending surgeon present. As surgeons, we want to do the best for our patients, we want to refine and improve our technical skills, and this takes practice and long hours. The public demands experience and, at the same time, governing bodies impede the resident's education with duty-hour restrictions resulting in some curtailment of experience.

Some surgical educators have held out hope that adoption of technical learning in simulated environments might ameliorate this situation. Although simulation cannot fully substitute for the actual experience of operating, it provides residents some of the necessary technical skills needed to execute complex operations. As such, simulation can contribute much to the development of dexterity and is an excellent learning environment for junior trainees. The operating room experience can then provide an environment to hone those skills in patients and understand the intricacies of integrating various learned techniques into a fluid operation.

Residents have, for decades, rated rotations at an affiliated Veterans Administration (VA) hospital as highly desirable. This has remained true for decades, even with significant changes in regulations about resident supervision. In the past, the reason for this perennial rating was simple. Residents were less closely supervised at VA hospitals compared with university and 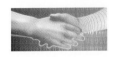 other private institutions. Attending surgeons would sometimes allow residents to conduct operations without being physically present or while they were readily available in the building. Of note, this practice was also pervasive in many academic medical centers and other residency training programs, such as the Johns Hopkins program mentioned earlier. However, there were many policy changes in the VA and the private sector that resulted in the need for closer and more physically present supervision.

Medicare was introduced in the United States in 1965. In 1994, the Medicare inspector general initiated an audit at multiple prestigious institutions titled: Physicians at Teaching Hospitals.[5] These audits were predicated on the concept that hospitals were reimbursed for services performed for patients by residents under Part A of Medicare and that attending physicians were reimbursed for the same services under Part B of Medicare. Fundamentally then, the Physicians at Teaching Hospitals audits sought evidence of double billing for a single procedure. In practice, the auditors demanded evidence of actual supervisory performance by the attending surgeon.

Multiple academic medical centers settled claims by the government for millions of dollars. Suddenly a new era had begun, in which "graded and increasing responsibility" was not merely an imperative that caused an ethical dilemma but also a legal issue with millions of dollars at stake. This era has continued from that time until this, with no clear solution in sight.

The greatest damage to our discipline wrought by this situation has resulted from the widespread misunderstanding of medical and surgical training it has fostered. Dr Anna Reisman, an internist at the Yale School of Medicine, should have understood how academic medical centers operate, given her academic role. Still she was vexed when she learned that it had been a trainee who had tried and failed 3 times to successfully perform her needed amniocentesis. She wrote: "We felt bamboozled."[6] Of course, the level of supervision remains the question.

In the address referred to above, Alfred Blalock went on to say that in a good residency, in the final period of training, the trainee is the patient's physician or surgeon. Although this is not legally possible in the strictest sense in any clinic or hospital in the United States currently, much of our discipline continues to strive toward that ideal. As teaching surgeons we understand the limitations of providing trainees autonomy, but we also believe that building a strong foundational trust and respect from patients is something our trainees should strive for in every case.

Today's patients have little tolerance for the "importance of training" argument that experiential training provides the greatest good for the  greatest numbers. They are concerned that they will be treated as a "guinea pig" or not receive the highest level of care. However, there is no evidence to support this notion. Rather, there are significant data to suggest that patients cared for in environments with trainees and other advanced practice providers—such as nurse practitioners or physicians assistants—receive superior, safer care.[7] It is incumbent on the attending surgeon to convey this to his/her patients and to promote the rightful and important education of future surgeons.

However, this ethical dilemma does not, for the most part, belong to the individual surgeon; it belongs to our discipline as a whole. We must collectively solve or at least ameliorate it. Fortunately, such amelioration is well under way with the development of a new model of the surgical team.

Overall, resident participation appears to slightly increase morbidity but slightly reduce mortality. Resident involvement may increase hospital costs. Currently, equipoise exists on the question of whether the involvement of trainees in operations is salutatory or harmful. Retrospective studies that focused on specific operations found that with higher level residents, 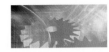 the level of the supervision provided by the attending surgeon and the willingness to intervene during the operation decreased. Resident participation was also correlated with longer operative duration and higher complication rates such as surgical site infections.[8] In addition, the increasing technical role played by the resident in combination with the reduced level of supervision may lead to higher rate of technical complications.[9] Other studies using the National Surgical Quality Improvement Program database throughout the years across surgical subspecialties concluded that resident participation increases complication rates slightly and that there is a direct correlation with the postgraduate year of training. However, having residents at the frontline of postoperative care may confer a mortality benefit at least for these patients undergoing more complex operations.[10–12] Tertiary centers with sicker and more complex patients are more likely to have residents, and therefore these population differences may account for the observed outcomes.

Other disciplines also have demonstrated their best results when performance is by an intergenerational team. A new model of supervision within the team will require new skills from the teaching surgeon. The ability to allow the resident great independence all the while being actively engaged will not be easy to acquire. The teaching surgeon must develop enhanced skills at coaching and mentoring while giving full credence to the resident as an autonomous person. Standardization in medicine has been shown to result in improved outcomes. For example, during the placement of a central line, the adoption of a universal protocol decreased central line–related infections. Similarly, the introduction of a simple preoperative checklist reduced operative morbidity and mortality. The introduction of guidelines to direct care from multiple medical societies is another attempt to standardize the provision of care and decrease errors in patient management. Therefore, it is reasonable for a surgeon to try to standardize his/her surgical team. The use, for example, of a physician extender that is not liable to the quality variability of a rotating resident is a reasonable strategy to maximize effectiveness. Multiple studies have shown better outcomes of surgeons and institutions with a high volume of complex surgical procedures such as pancreatoduodenectomies and esophagectomies.[13] Experience is irreplaceable.

The general public must be educated in the acceptance, indeed, the desirability, of such teams, not by utilitarian arguments, but by evidence that such teams produce the best possible results. The intergenerational teams, characteristic of our discipline, have brought surgical care to heights never imagined a few decades ago. However, our representation of such teams to our patients and their families, as well as to payers and governments, has not kept pace. Resident supervision must be guided by an ethical posture for our discipline, perhaps more than for the individual surgeon.

# References

1. Ravitch MM. *A Century of Surgery: The History of the American Surgical Association, 1880–1980.* Philadelphia: J.B. Lippincott Company; 1981:253.
2. Ravitch MM, ed. *The Papers of Alfred Blalock.* Baltimore: The Johns Hopkins Press; 1966:1786.
3. Mattar SG, Alseidi AA, Jones DB, et al. General surgery residency inadequately prepares trainees for fellowship: results of a survey of fellowship program directors. *Ann Surg.* 2013;258:440–449.
4. Bucholz EM, Sue GR, Yeo H, et al. Our trainees' confidence: results from a national survey of 4136 US general surgery residents. *Arch Surg.* 2011;146:907–914.
5. Report from the United States General Accounting Office to the Chairman, Subcommittee on Health, Committee on Ways and Means, House of Representatives. MEDICARE—Concerns With Physicians at Teaching Hospitals (PATH) Audits; July 1998.
6. Reisman A. How many have you done? *JAMA.* 2016;316(5):491.
7. Ghaferi, Osborne NH, Birkmeyer JD, et al. Hospital characteristics associated with failure to rescue from complications after pancreatectomy. *J Am Coll Surg.* 2010;211(3):325–330.
8. Kiran RP, Ahmed Ail U, Coffey JC, et al. Impact of resident participation in surgical operations on postoperative outcomes: National Surgical Quality Improvement Program. *Ann Surg.* September 2012;256(3):469–475.
9. Scarborough JE, Pappas TN, Cox MW, et al. Surgical trainee participation during infrainguinal bypass grafting procedures is associated with increased early postoperative graft failure. *J Vasc Surg.* March 2012;55(3):715–720.
10. Castleberry AW, Clary BM, Migaly J, et al. Resident education in the era of patient safety: a nationwide analysis of outcomes and complications in resident-assisted oncologic surgery. *Ann Surg Oncol.* November 2013;20(12):3715–3724.
11. Saliba AN, Taher AT, Tamim H, et al. Impact of Resident Involvement in Surgery (IRIS-NSQIP): looking at the bigger picture based on the American College of Surgeons NSQIP database. *J Am Coll Surg.* January 2016;222(1):30–40.
12. Raval MV, Wang X, Cohen ME, et al. The influence of resident involvement on surgical outcomes. *J Am Coll Surg.* May 2011;212(5):889–898.
13. Birkmeyer JD, Siewers AE, Finlayson EV, et al. Hospital volume and surgical mortality in the United States. *N Engl J Med.* April 11, 2002;346(15):1128–1137.

# 32 Team Building and the Role of the Team in Surgery

Jai Prasad, MD

PROLOGUE ▶ One of the great conundrums of the discipline of surgery is how alone the surgeon is when operating and how enmeshed he/she is in society generally. Law, custom, standards, and regulations circumscribe the surgeon's every act or utterance, but the surgeon is alone in disappointment and regret. The societal strictures are almost all cast negatively: avoid lawsuits, do not do this, do not do that. If we are to lessen the impact of acedia and reduce the burden of burnout in our discipline, we must foster a higher level of supportive kinship. The team development that Dr Prasad discusses must support the surgeon as well as the more obvious recipients of our beneficence.

Dr Jai Prasad is a resident in the Department of Surgery at The University of Toledo College of Medicine.

We are in an era of high-throughput medicine. There is an emphasis on efficiency and productivity in the care of patients within both the hospital and the outpatient settings. This stretches physicians thin, leading over time to high rates of burnout, depression and dissatisfaction.

As a resident in surgery, first in the United Kingdom and then in the United States over the past 12 years, I have witnessed this change of the health care landscape and have felt its effects. From the lowest on the totem pole of surgical training, an intern straight out of medical school, to chief resident in surgery, I have worked with a dizzying array of physicians, residents, nurse practitioners, physician assistants, nurses, and a host of other supporting clinical and administrative staff.

The concept of teamwork was always brought forward early and emphat-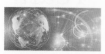ically throughout the course of this journey. Applications for residency expect examples of teamwork, and interviewers would search through one's accomplishments looking for such instances.

Teamwork and its association with reduced adverse events is well documented. This has become especially important with the focus on high-throughput medicine, that is, emphasis on outpatient surgical procedures, decreasing length of stay, reducing hospital readmissions, and increasing productivity of outpatient clinics in an era of increasing comorbidities, safe working hour initiatives, aging population, and increasing costs.

With this context, I am going to attempt to put forth my experiences in building a team and fostering effective teamwork within a surgical residency program.

## The Challenges

### Hierarchy

The surgical residency system, regardless of where it is practiced or what it is called, is embedded in hierarchy. This hierarchy is a wrench in the works for a high-throughput clinical expectation and in its true form impedes an efficient process. On the other hand, this hierarchy has been historically very effective in training perioperative management to junior surgical trainees and training senior surgical trainees in the operating room. The hierarchy functions also in some ways as a sieve such that the information reaching upstream is sequentially filtered to the most relevant. The sieve does sometimes also function to eliminate useful information. The challenge, therefore, for an effective team consisting of surgical learners is to transcend and embrace this hierarchy at the same time.

### Flux

I was once told, "Residents are like a box of chocolates; you never know what you're going to get." Residency, by design, requires a multitude of clinical experiences, which requires that residents change across subspecialties and service lines frequently as early as 3 or 4 weeks. This creates unique challenges in incorporating effective teams within an academic surgical environment. For me, this has been the most challenging aspect of surgical training. Residents are expected to function at the same capacity on the last day of week 4 on service A and the first day of week 1 on service B. Maintaining morale, efficiency, safety, and effectiveness of the teaching and clinical environment across this flux is critical to building effective teams.

## Training and Safety

Good and effective teams have to foster the training of surgery residents and provide safe care to patients. I have found it challenging to incorporate both of these goals within an effective team. Building efficiency within an effective team has the potential to lead to a lack of safe redundancy, leaving fewer holes to align in a "Swiss cheese model" of adverse events. The same efficiency and effectiveness may limit surgical residents' participation and may adversely affect their training. For instance, the focus on high throughput in the outpatient setting limits the time that a resident may spend evaluating, presenting, and learning from the clinical encounter. The irony lies in the fact that the team's effectiveness adversely affects its own core values and objectives.

## Building Effective Teams in Surgery

A chief resident's role is one of quandary. As the senior most resident, usually a few months to a year away from being classed as a fully trained surgeon, he/she performs the role of a chief operating officer, reporting directly to the attending or faculty surgeon of record for the patient. The chief surgery resident is expected to diagnose and formulate comprehensive treatment plans for patients, teach and supervise residents and other learners, and coordinate with various other specialties involved in the care of patients. In this capacity, in the final 2 years of my residency, I had the chance to develop and build multiple teams across various academic surgical services learning in the process the ways and means to overcome challenges and build effective and efficient teams.

## Formulating the Vision

I begin by defining the team and its role as early as possible. This ideally occurs before or the day the team starts working together. The core team usually consists of the chief resident, 1 or more junior residents, and midlevel providers (such as nurse practitioners and physician assistants). Other team members may include social workers, other clinical and nonclinical support staff, nursing staff, and medical students.

The vision reflects an amalgamation of the values and objectives of the team members and reflects a shared blueprint toward the functioning of the team. The vision may include but not be limited to the team striving toward safe and effective patient care, teaching and training its members, serving the well-being of its members, and respecting diversity. It is imperative that all the team members buy into this shared vision and believe in it for the team to function effectively. Reinforcing this vision regularly allows the team to remain focused and helps develop camaraderie. This relationship between team members then fosters interdependence, creating seamless workflows and a blurring of boundaries between defined roles and allowing the team to function more efficiently with a greater degree of satisfaction.

Intriguingly a team that fosters its team members and allows them the space and the opportunity to develop becomes more efficient with better results. Consider the difference in an experienced senior resident and an 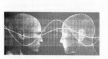 intern, fresh from medical school, going through the same degree of this flux. It is likely that this flux is going to have a different effect on the intern, who would be far more likely to get overwhelmed and overworked and suffer with decreases in efficiency in a traditional hierarchy within the high-throughput character of current medicine. A shared vision that recognizes the need to foster and develop the intern's capability is likely to lead to safer and more effective patient care with seamless workflows and blurred boundaries between the roles of the individual team members.

## Mutual Trust and Communication

Trust is developed by a combination of honesty and reliability. Open communication between team members is important and should be the norm. This is especially important in high-stakes situations such as the operating room and in time-critical environments such as the emergency department and intensive care units where surgeons frequently find themselves looking after patients.

Trust and communication are interdependent. Open, frequent communication cannot exist without mutual trust and respect. An example of this interplay can be found in the morning rounds and formulating plans of care for the patients on a service list, also known colloquially as "run the list." Rather than a top-down approach with the chief resident making the plans, we encourage the junior residents and interns to initiate the formulation of a management plan, followed by sequential inputs of any supporting team members. This empowers junior residents and other team members, giving them ownership, respect, and autonomy supervised by the leading chief resident.

## Accountability

With trust, open communication, and shared vision comes accountability toward that vision. A team has to have a mechanism built-in that allows for team members to know when their action or inaction has let the vision down. This is fostered by a mutual trust and respect and is best engaged by self-correction. This in itself would be the perfect team where an adverse event or near-miss prompts immediate self-reflection with the team members supporting each other and learning from the circumstance.

A patient is discharged with a leukocytosis incorrectly attributed to a urinary tract infection when the actual problem was an anastomotic leak realized on a readmission within 24 hours. The intern on the team mentions that the rising leukocytosis was noted; however, the pressure to discharge with an expiring precertification to a skilled nursing facility prompted the trend to be missed. The chief resident making the call on the discharge immediately brings this to the attention of the team, recognizing the error, and ensures that individual team members value safety as a prime value and do not feel hesitant to bring any such concerns to the table openly and without fear of intimidation.

A team needs to have a built-in transparent escalation path for repeated failures on part of team members to consistently depart from the shared vision. This would be expected to be a rare occurrence in a team where there is mutual respect, good communication, and cohesion toward a shared vision.

## Managing Conflict

Teams often have disagreements within themselves and with external entities. Team members and team leaders need to have tools at their disposal to be able to recognize when a conflict might happen. Early recognition of an evolving conflict helps in making a prompt and fruitful resolution. A culture of open communication helps resolve conflicts within teams. Several strategies for conflict resolution have been proposed.

Recognizing and acknowledging a conflict is critical and an important first step to resolving it. Where possible, the aim should be to achieve a consensus. This also applies to a situation where there is a conflict between a patient and the team. A path to shared decision making initiated by acknowledging that the patient's concerns and his/her right be involved helps resolve most conflicts. Teams should be open and willing to collaborate and expand to include people of interest. For our surgical teams, this often occurs by including the patient in their own treatment team.

## Leadership in the Team

Leaders often define the teams they lead and build. I will illustrate the concept of leadership from the perspective of the chief surgical resident. I consciously leave this to the end of this chapter, as a leader embraces all of the aforementioned tenets and brings them together into a cohesive team.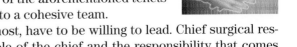

Leaders, first and foremost, have to be willing to lead. Chief surgical residents must embrace the role of the chief and the responsibility that comes with it. The leader helps formulate the team's vision and regularly ensures that the team stays true to it. The leader frequently calls team huddles. For instance, the chief resident calls for "Let's run the list, meet outside the operating room main entrance, 5 minutes." This is especially important in the high-flux environments where team members, patients, and their care plans constantly change.

Leaders have to manage the team's workload and delegate responsibility appropriately. Good leaders are willing and able to recognize when the team is likely to get overwhelmed, step in where required, and mobilize additional support if necessary. Leaders engage the team members and foster their development. Good chief residents provide an excellent educational experience for their juniors and in doing so inspire and motivate them.

An often understated and underrecognized role of the team leader is to manage upstream. We think of team leaders managing the role and responsibilities of their team members; however, it is of equal importance for the team leader to manage the boss. The chief surgical resident with his/her team on a busy surgical service may be caring for patients of upward of 10 attending and faculty surgeons. Each of these surgeons may and usually will have differing expectations on how their patients are managed and how each of them is communicated with. A great part of the chief surgical resident's role as a team leader is to streamline this upstream workflow.

The analogy to rowing upstream is not far from the truth. It helps having the right paddles for each boss. Communicating clearly on expectations as early as possible is critical. It is also important for team leaders to recognize the personality of their attending surgeon and tailor communication appropriately to each. Although it is helpful to get clear guidance on this from the boss upstream, this may not always happen.

## Summary

Building teams within surgery comes with many challenges, chief among which are overcoming hierarchical barriers, managing flux (both the frequent change of the team's members and the rapid turnover of patients and their evolving treatment plans), and aligning the goals of safety for patients and training of surgical residents. Training leaders in surgery with skills to build and lead high-functioning teams would mean embracing these challenges and developing programs within surgical training that build mutual trust and respect, teach effective communication and conflict resolution, and ensure accountability.

# 33 The Relationship to the Nursing Profession

Janine E. Janosky, PhD

PROLOGUE ▶ The tall African American nurse in the minimally invasive suite put her hand on Dr John Flynn's arm. It was a comforting not a coercive touch but firm nevertheless. She took a step away from the others in the room; Flynn followed her, hardly noticing the movement. "You need help," she said in a low voice. She moved closer to the door and, still holding Flynn's eyes, backed through it. He followed her. "I wouldn't say this if I didn't care about you; I wouldn't bother. You have an issue you cannot resolve alone, let me help you."

The program director, the department chair, and John Flynn were a triangle at the small round table. "Look," the program director said, "we won't report to the State or to the Graduate Medical Education office. We will list you as being in good standing here, but you cannot come back next year. We will help you find an opening; worst case scenario you will lose a year." The chair nodded. Flynn swallowed and nodded.

Janine E. Janosky, PhD, is a professor in the Department of Health and Human Services and Dean of the College of Education, Health, and Human Services at the University of Michigan-Dearborn. She has been a champion of interprofessional efforts to improve health care and provider wellness.

There have been, for a century or more, deep and respectful relationships between surgeons and their nurse colleagues. It is fair to say, however, that those were seldom relationships of equality, nor could they often be described as collaborative. This history is more regrettable in light of the surgeon's emphasis on handiwork, an area where the immediacy and relevance of the experience of the nurse may bring clear value. These relationships, characterized by differing positions in a hierarchy, are changing rapidly in the 21st century.

Stronger partnerships with nurses may provide many positive effects on surgeons, in addition to mere "help." Nurses serve as important societal anchors for surgeons. They act as a first line of peer reviewers, giving positive or negative feedback if the appropriate relationship exists. Such orientation and feedback has a stabilizing effect that helps prevent surgeon burnout.

A renewal and strengthening of the relationship between surgeons and nurses has been occurring under the rubric of "interprofessional education." To be sure, other professional groups are often included in the educational exercises described this way. However, the greatest historical tension and the greatest potential gains are from attention to the nurse-surgeon relationships and the most important consequence may be the salutatory impact on patient outcomes.

The lack of alignment between education and practice, the lack of a standardized model of interprofessional education across the education continuum, and significant gaps in the evidence linking interprofessional education to collaborative practice and patient outcomes have been identified as barriers to the maturation of interprofessional education.[1] Part of the problem is that interprofessional education is a complex process with multiple patient, population, and system outcomes.[1] A recent review sponsored by the National Academy of Sciences found a total of 15 articles published between 1999 and 2011 with the methodology that met the stringent criteria for inclusion.[2] A more recent review of the literature that built on the earlier work included literature from January 2011 to July 2014.

One purpose of the reviews was to evaluate the current methods for measuring the impact of interprofessional education on patient outcomes and to describe the challenges of linking interprofessional education interventions with changes in practice and patient outcomes.[2] Outcome mea-
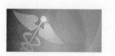
sures of interest included objectively measured patient outcomes and health care process measurements.[2] Subjective self-reported outcomes were also collected, but only if objective measures were also reported. More than 2300 abstracts were reviewed, resulting in 47 additional studies rated on stringent criteria and 15 studies plus the 15 studies from the earlier review.

Among the studies included in this meta-analysis were 6 studies involving a program called "TeamSTEPPS," which has been put forward by the Agency for Healthcare Research and Quality.[3] 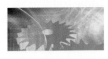 Similarly, 9 studies involved a program called "Crew Research Management," an effort of the Interprofessional Education Collaboratives.[4]

The meta-analyses demonstrated significant improvements in selected patient care outcomes. These included the following:

- Improvements in survival using teams during resuscitations in the intensive care unit
- Improved care quality, frequently reported as practice process changes including adherence to best practices, checklist use, and participation in briefings
- Improvements in hemoglobin A1C, cholesterol, blood pressure, and mobility after stroke
- Decreases in adverse outcomes and improved error reporting and rates
- Improved patient satisfaction
- Improved care efficiency
- Direct reduction in cost

One of the stronger TeamSTEPPS articles reviewed had the following outcomes[5]:

- 94% believed training well organized and content appropriate
- 81% felt more confident about ability to work as an effective team member
- 52% felt confident to train others
- 81% believed training will help their organization improve patient safety
- Trained teams' communication improved significantly when compared with control group

A second trend in the professionalization of nursing has been the formal involvement of Advanced Practice Nurses in Primary Care and the impact on this involvement on Population Health.

In 2008, the Institute of Medicine and the Robert Wood Johnson Foundation (RWJF) collaborated in creating the RWJF initiative on the Future of Nursing with the hypothesis that, without exceptional nursing care and leadership, accessible, high-quality care could not be achieved.[6] Nursing in the United States is the largest sector of the health professions and there are more than 3 million registered nurses.[6] In 2008, there were nearly 400 000 primary care providers of whom 287 000 are physicians, 83 000 nurse practitioners, and 23 000 physician assistants.[7] Although the numbers of nurse practitioners and physician assistants are steadily increasing, the number of medical students and residents entering primary care has declined in recent years.[6] The professionalization of nursing may be expected, therefore, to continue to have an increasing impact on the health of our population.

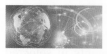

Nursing often involves management of chronic conditions and primary care, including care coordination and transitional care, prevention and wellness, and prevention of adverse events such as hospital-acquired infections.[6] The report and its recommendations on the future of nursing paralleled the near-term challenges identified by the Affordable Care Act in 2010. Health care reform offered an opportunity for nurses to meet the demand for safe, high-quality, patient-centered, and equitable health care services.[6]

Researchers conducted a randomized trial examining primary care outcomes in patients treated by either nurse practitioners or physicians.[8] Patient satisfaction after the initial appointment, health status, satisfaction, physiologic test results 6 months after initial appointment, and service utilization for 1 year after initial appointment were the primary outcome measures.[8] There were no statistically significant differences at 6 months in patients' health status between the groups assigned to nurse practitioners and those assigned to physicians. For patients with diabetes or asthma, there were no statistically significant differences in physiologic measures. Patients with hypertension treated by nurse practitioners had a significantly lower diastolic value. Health services utilization after 6 months or 1 year did not differ significantly by type of provider, although provider attributes of physicians were rated higher in comparison with nurse practitioners.[8]

A review of trials and observational studies published in 2002 noted that patients were more satisfied with nurse practitioner care, had longer consultations from nurse practitioners, and made more investigations in comparison with physicians.[9] A 2010 review echoed these results.[10] When nurses provided care, patient satisfaction with first-contact care for people wanting urgent care was higher and satisfaction with chronic disease management was higher in comparison with doctors.[10] The authors attribute higher satisfaction to the nurses tending to have longer consultations and providing more information to patients.[10] These results were confirmed by other reviews that found quality of care is equivalent whether provided by nurses or physicians.[7,11] The measures included patient satisfaction, self-reported perceived health, functional status, blood pressure, emergency department or urgent care visits, and hospitalization.[11] Better management of lipid levels was found to favor nurse care.[11] Substantial health care savings could be realized by substituting visits to physicians by visits to nurses.[7]

Interdisciplinary care teams met the complex needs of many diabetic patients with modest increases in costs for patients under the care of interdisciplinary teams in comparison with patients treated as usual with improvements in both patient care and clinical outcomes.[12]

Although perspectives of physicians and nurse practitioners differ on the role of nurse practitioners in primary care practice,[13] these data support the conclusion that patients receive equivalent care and, in some cases, achieve better health outcomes. With the potential health care cost savings, primarily because nurse practitioners are paid less than doctors, inclusion of nurse practitioners has the potential to expand access to health care for those who have limited access without increasing the cost of medical care. Expansion of the health care workforce with additional capacity to treat patients would have an impact on population health through management of chronic disease, increased patient-centered care, increased equity, and high-quality care.[6]

Driven by concerns about population health, quality and safety of health care, and health care costs,[14] interprofessional collaborative practice has been recognized as an innovative strategy to increase the health workforce, enhance safety, enrich quality of care, and improve health outcomes.[15] The Institute of Medicine suggested a renewed focus on interprofessional practice to reform health professions education to improve the quality and safety of health care and to increase access for groups and populations that were treated disparately.[1] Many health systems are fragmented and unable to manage unmet health needs.[15] The basis for interprofessional practice lies in educating future practitioners in interprofessional and collaborative learning experiences.[16]

The rise of the nursing profession to a position of equality with other health care professions offers great potential for the surgeon. The relationship has always been intense but has also been one of inequality. Notwithstanding this, surgeons and nurses have often become life partners. Practically speaking, however, for a surgeon to give attention to this relationship, to consciously build it, and to place value on it will produce great rewards. Patients will experience improved hospital outcomes. The Advanced Practice Nurse may choose a career in postoperative care, thereby providing great partnership to the surgeon. Moreover, good, sound, and mutually supportive relationships with the nursing profession can provide personal strength and stability, thus promoting surgeon well-being and preventing dysphoria.

# References

1. Institute of Medicine. *Measuring the Impact of Interprofessional Education on Collaborative Practice and Patient Outcomes.* Washington, DC: The National Academies Press; 2015.
2. Brashers V, Phillips E, Malpass J, Owen J. Appendix A: Review: measuring the impact of Interprofessional Education (IPE) on collaborative practice and patient outcomes. In: Committee on Measuring the Impact of Interprofessional Education on Collaborative Practice and Patient Outcomes, Board on Global Health, Institute of Medicine, eds. *Measuring the Impact of Interprofessional Education on Collaborative Practice and Patient Outcomes.* Washington, DC: National Academy of Sciences, 2015:67–133.
3. Agency for Healthcare Research and Quality. TeamSTEPPS (Team Strategies and Tools to Enhance Performance and Patient Safety). Available from: https://www.ahrq.gov/teamstepps/index.html. Accessed 26 January 2017.

4. SaferHealthcare. *Effecting Positive Behavioral and Cultural Change...Crew Resource Management.* Available from: http://www.saferhealthcare.com/crew-resource-management/crew-resource-management-healthcare/. Accessed 26 January 2017.

5. Weaver SJ, Rosen MA, DiazGranados D, et al. Does teamwork improve performance in the operating room? A multilevel evaluation. *Jt Comm J Qual Patient Saf.* 2010;36(3):133–142.

6. Institute of Medicine. *The Future of Nursing: Leading Change, Advancing Health.* Washington, DC: The National Academies Press; 2011.

7. Naylor MD, Kurtzman ET. The role of nurse practitioners in reinventing primary care. *Health Aff.* May 1, 2010;29(5):893–899.

8. Mundinger MO, Kane RL, Lenz ER, et al. Primary care outcomes in patients treated by nurse practitioners or physicians: a randomized trial. *JAMA.* 2000;283(1):59–68.

9. Horrocks S, Anderson E, Salisbury C. Systematic review of whether nurse practitioners working in primary care can provide equivalent care to doctors. *BMJ.* 2002;324(7341):819–823.

10. Laurant M, Reeves D, Hermens R, Braspenning J, Grol R, Sibbald B. Substitution of doctors by nurses in primary care. *Cochrane Database Syst Rev.* 2005;(2).

11. Newhouse RP, Stanik-Hutt J, White KM, et al. Advanced practice nurse outcomes 1990–2008: a systematic review. *Nurs Econ.* 2011;29(5):230–250.

12. Willens D, Cripps R, Wilson A, Wolff K, Rothman R. Interdisciplinary team care for diabetic patients by primary care physicians, advanced practice nurses, and clinical pharmacists. *Clin Diabetes.* 2011;29(2):60–68.

13. Donelan K, DesRoches CM, Dittus RS, Buerhaus P. Perspectives of physicians and nurse practitioners on primary care practice. *N Engl J Med.* 2013;368(20):1898–1906.

14. Institute for Healthcare Improvement. *IHI Triple Aim Initiative.* Available from: http://www.ihi.org/engage/initiatives/tripleaim/pages/default.aspx. Accessed 25 January 2017.

15. World Health Organization. *Framework for Action on Interprofessional Education and Collaborative Practice.* Geneva, Switzerland: World Health Organization; 2010.

16. Interprofessional Education Collaborative. *Core Competencies for Interprofessional Collaborative Practice: 2016 Update.* Washington, DC: Interprofessional Education Collaborative; 2016.

# 34 The Surgeon as Consultant

Roland T. Skeel, MD

PROLOGUE ▶ Today is the era of specialization and subspecialization of health care. Multiple disciplines are almost invariably involved in reduced care of any complexity. Although this is true in both outpatient and inpatient settings, modern inpatient care requires teamwork, most frequently by multiple specialists.

The complex postoperative patient will frequently demand the expertise of the cardiologist, nephrologist, and anesthesiologist. Relevant to our purposes here the surgeon is also called as a consultant, often to the emergency department or intensive care unit. Furthermore, many new outpatient diagnoses prompt a surgical consultation.

The most complex interpersonal and communication issues involve the triangle of patient, referring physician, and surgical consultant. In almost every case, the patient and the referring physician have a preexisting relationship; often but not always this relationship should persist long after the surgeon's consultation. To interfere with this preexisting relationship is among the most damaging acts to which a surgeon may be tempted. Similarly, for other consultants to undermine the surgeon-patient relationship is almost always damaging. The wise consultant seeks to reinforce the preexisting patient-referring physician relationship and to be vigilant to avoid intrusion into it.

Dr Roland T. Skeel is an oncologist with extensive experience in the field. He has, therefore, acted as a consultant to surgeons and to primary care physicians. He has moreover asked for surgical consultation on many thousand occasions. In this chapter, he gives practical advice for the surgeon's performance of the consultative work and also for the careful handling of the relationship the patient may have with the referring physician.

Dr Roland T. Skeel is a professor of medicine at The University of Toledo College of Medicine.

## Ethical Precepts of Surgical Consultation

The intention to provide the best possible care for the patient and family should be the primary reason that consultations are obtained in medicine and surgery. This intention has as its ethical basis the principles of *beneficence* and *respect for persons*. Beneficence carries with it the secondary corollary, "*Primum non nocere*" or "do no harm," which has evolved from the Hippocratic Oath injunction "to abstain from doing harm." As discussed in the earlier chapter, *respect for persons* carries with it the obligation to do our 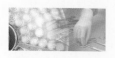 best to promote the *autonomy* of patients who might be affected by our actions. On occasion, the principle of *justice* may also come into play, as the consultant works to provide all patients with an equal opportunity to benefit from the best expertise available to manage their health problems. Finally, when physicians are faced by situations of mass casualties on a battlefield or in an emergency room when triage is imperative, the principle of *distributive justice* becomes a harsh reality.

## Expectations

Clarification of expectations is important to obtain and provide the most helpful surgical consultation. Expectations may differ widely among the requesting physician, the consulting surgeon, and the patient and the patient's family. For that reason it is appropriate, if it has not been explicit, for the consulting surgeon to ask the requesting physician "What is the question you have for me?" or "Is there something specific you would like me to do?" This can be helpful in preventing the consulting surgeon from overstepping the bounds of expectation or from heading in a direction in which neither the requesting physician nor the patient would have interest. Although the majority of consultations probably occur following some kind of written request, particularly now that an electronic medical record is being used extensively, unless the basis for the consultation is straightforward, it is often helpful if there is a personal call from the physician requesting the consultation to the consulting surgeon. This provides an opportunity to give background about the patient's medical and psychosocial condition as well as informing the surgeon regarding the current problem for which the consultation is desired and what expectations might be for the consultation. This is really no different from the increased value of a radiologic or pathologic evaluation when the physician interpreting the images or histologic material has a greater degree of background knowledge about the clinical history.

I, as a medical oncologist, was asked to see a patient whose recent skin biopsy was reported to show Langerhans cell histiocytosis, a malignant condition with dire prognosis. The dermatopathologist rendered his diagnosis based on what was seen on the slides, including supportive immunohistochemical stains. I thought it was important to obtain a second review of the pathology slides. In the meanwhile, the dermatologist and dermatopathologist learned more about the clinical history and both expressed doubt that this was in fact Langerhans cell histiocytosis rather than reactive change. The second opinion pathologist, who also had been informed of the clinical history, agreed that this was most consistent with reactive change. As a consequence, the patient was saved from having an extensive systemic evaluation with computerized tomography (CT) scans or rebiopsy. An important feature to notice in this scenario is that the first pathologist, on learning more about the history, had no reluctance to call me on the phone and say, "I think I was wrong." This is a characteristic of an ethical consultant, the willingness to volunteer that his opinion or decision was wrong. Honesty such as this increases trust and reinforces the belief that the consultant is committed to the best interests of the patient and not moved by personal hubris.

Related to the issue of expectations is the question of how much the consulting surgeon, or any other consultant, should tell the patient. There are at least 3 categories that may be desired: (1) transmitting of information only, (2) providing an interpretation of what the information means, and (3) rendering an opinion about what should be done.

Unless the requesting physician has indicated to the consultant that the patient or patient's family do not wish the patient to know the diagnosis or other information, there is rarely a problem with transmitting information about the findings in the record or on the physical examination, or with providing an interpretation of what the information means. In the circumstance that either the patient or patient's family have given instructions or a request, sometimes a demand, that the patient is not to be informed about clinical findings, particularly if there might be a dire diagnosis such as cancer, there must be a clear understanding among all those involved regarding what will or will not be told to the patient. This raises critical ethical issues regarding the principle of *respect for persons, autonomy,* and *truth telling.*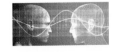

Although, in most circumstances, it is generally the practice in the United States to provide patients with the facts about their disease, there can be issues regarding the patient's cultural and ethnic background, psychologic stability, cognitive function, or comorbid conditions that could modify the usual practice. Although it is most often deemed appropriate for patients and families to be fully informed about their diagnosis and its implications, it is important to be sensitive to cultural, ethnic, or other issues and consider carefully the wishes of the patient and the family *not to know*. It is most important, however, to be clear before the consultation regarding this expectation to avoid embarrassment or a very disturbed patient and family.

In contrast to disclosure and interpretation of facts, it is not always so straightforward that the surgical consultant should provide the patient and patient's family an opinion regarding recommended management before discussing it with the requesting physician. There are 2 fundamental issues to be considered. First, the reason that the surgical consultation that has been obtained has the dual purpose of helping the requesting physician care for his/her patient as well as providing the best possible care for the patient. Therefore, it is respectful of the requesting physician to inform the patient in a timely way of the consultant's recommendations and to discuss the reasons for its basis. Of course, it is often not feasible or even appropriate to separate out informing the patient about the surgeon's opinion on the diagnosis and the appropriate management of the problem. What to do about an acute abdomen does not warrant deferring a recommendation to the patient.

Secondly, when various physicians provide varying opinions to the patient or the family, they can be confused, distressed, and concerned that the physicians are not speaking with each other. Patients generally should not be placed in a position of having to choose between the recommendations given by more than one physician, as they rarely have the medical or technical expertise to make a fully informed decision. It is often not easy, however, for the surgical consultant to avoid giving an opinion about management, because patients and patient families believe, rightly, that the consultation is not just about them but for them, and that they have a right to know what the opinion of the consultant is. After all, the referring physician has asked the surgical consultant to evaluate and recommend, and once there has been a relationship established between the consultant and the patient, the surgeon consultant has an obligation to do so. When the options for management are multiple or complex, the dilemma of how much to tell the patient and family at the first meeting can often be avoided if the consultant simply states that he/she has an idea of what will be the best, but wish to discuss it first with the referring physician to be sure that they both are on the same page. This does take extra time at the outset of a consultation but can end resulting both in a better consultation and time

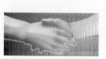

saved in the long run. As noted above, at other times this is not an issue, because the requesting physician has already asked the surgical consultant to "see the patient, give him your opinion, and do whatever you believe would be in the patient's best interest." Occasions may arise when the referring physician wants to have the surgeon and other consultant(s) each discuss proposed procedures, such as surgery vs radiation therapy for localized prostate cancer. This is only appropriate when there is therapeutic equipoise between the procedures and is completely in accord with the wishes of the requesting physician. Such discussion must be deemed beneficial for the patient or the patient has expressed a wish to hear from each specialty to consider himself/herself which among the potential options fit best with the needs.

A particularly difficult dilemma, which rarely arises, is a situation where the consultant believes that there has been major mismanagement of the patient, serious unprofessional behavior, or overt malpractice on the part of the referring physician. The question then arises regarding with whom this should be discussed or to whom this should be reported and how to 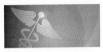 deal both with the referring physician and the patient. I think it is important at the outset to begin with the notion that no physician intends to do wrong to his/her patients. This is not to argue that we do not sometimes observe sloppy or bad habits and serious errors of omission or commission. It is important not to make up excuses for or gloss over such a bad behavior or bad medical practice. Resolution of such a situation usually will involve presenting the situation to a group of peers who can evaluate the facts based on records and interviews with the physicians involved, and often with the patient or patient's family. It then becomes the responsibility of the group of peers to reach a recommendation or decision about how to remedy the problem. The ethical concepts of respect for persons, beneficence, and justice each have something to say on how to best manage difficult scenarios such as these.

## Why Surgical Consults Are Requested

Although at first blush it might seem intuitive that a surgical consult would be obtained because the requesting physician believes that surgical intervention may be required, however, this is not necessarily the case. There are at least 3 reasons that a surgical consultation is obtained: The requesting physician or the family wish to have an opinion from the surgeon regarding (1) whether or not there might be a surgical option for the management of the patient's current problems, (2) what that surgical option might be, and (3) what the potential benefits and risks might be of the surgical option.

Of course, in some circumstances the basis for the consult is fairly simple, such as when a patient presents with evidence of acute appendicitis by history and physical examination, with or without radiologic evidence. When the emergency room physician or primary care physician calls the surgeon in instances such as this, it usually is already clear that an operation is the most appropriate treatment. In most circumstances, it is clear that the potential benefits outweigh the risks of the procedure. Even in this situation there can be different opinions, however, such as whether to use an open or a laparoscopic approach. In that circumstance the surgeon should discuss the options with both the patient/patient's family and the referring physician.

In other circumstances the reason for the consultation and the questions being considered can be more complex. For example, consider the case of a 62-year-old woman who has had a diagnosis of endometrial cancer, metastatic to lymph nodes adjacent to the duodenum. Because the cancer has eroded into the duodenum, the patient previously has developed severe anemia. Prior management of this problem has included duodenal biopsy 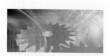 during upper endoscopy, followed by a surgical procedure to bypass the area of bleeding. This was then followed by radiation to the periduodenal mass, which had been to be unresectable. The patient did well following radiation, but a follow-up CT scan 6 months later demonstrated an enlarging mass. The patient was then started on cytotoxic chemotherapy, which she tolerated well, but a follow-up CT scan demonstrated air within the mass adjacent to the duodenum and the descending aorta. A second CT scan with water-soluble contrast confirmed that there was a sinus tract from the duodenum into the mass.

A new surgical consultation was obtained to determine whether there was a surgical option for the management of this new problem, what the surgical option might be, and potential benefits and risks of undertaking an operation or of not undertaking an operation. In this circumstance, the surgeon reviewed the history of previous surgery, if any, on the aorta. After review, the surgeon advised that the probability of the cancer eroding into the aorta was quite low, and the likelihood of benefit for the patient with this incurable cancer would not warrant the risk of an operation to try to close the sinus tract or resect the mass.

The venue at which consultations take place can be quite varied. Classically, we think of a consult taking place in a hospital or office setting by a consultant who has the opportunity to review the patient's record, to review laboratory and imaging studies, to interview the patient, and to do his/her own physical examination. However, this is not the only circumstance in which consultations occur.

One common venue for an indirect, although formal, consultation is through tumor boards. Here there is an opportunity for a brief presentation of the patient's history and examination by one of the physicians, a review of laboratory and radiologic or other imaging, a presentation of pathologic findings including genetic or other molecular information, and discussion among multiple physician specialties, nurses, social workers, chaplains, and others regarding options for patient care. Although determinations by the "tumor board" should never be a substitute for decisions by the patient's primary physicians, the tumor board can be helpful in delineating options and in providing support and insight to the primary physician, which will aid in making difficult decisions. For example, following a tumor board discussion, the primary physician may decide that a surgical procedure is likely to benefit the patient and therefore make a referral to a surgeon for formal consultation and the expected procedure. On the other hand, if during the tumor board presentation it appears evident that the patient's cancer is not operable or that the comorbid conditions are such that the patient would not likely benefit from a surgical procedure, then the formal consultation with the surgeon could be avoided without harm to the patient.

A third type of consultation is the "curbside consult." This occurs when the requesting physician stops the surgeon in the hall and says, "Hey, Bill, I've got a question for you." The requesting physician then gives a brief history and perhaps physical findings or other information and then says, "What do you think?" Although there is real risk that insufficient information has been transmitted, this can be a quick and helpful way to determine whether or not additional evaluation may be needed.

In addition to the 3 expectations from a surgical consultation discussed at the beginning of this section, there are times when the surgeon appropriately will say, "I think you need to see a different surgical consultant" either because he/she is skilled in a special technique or has a greater degree of expertise in the patient's particular problem. An example of this was in a 77-year-old man who had a squamous cell carcinoma involving the gingival ridge that had eroded into the bone and would require a bone free flap graft following resection of the carcinoma. Such a procedure requires coordination between a head and neck surgeon and a plastic surgeon, together with ancillary specialties of speech and nutrition therapy. The surgeon who recognizes the limitations of his/her own abilities or those of her colleagues or of the facilities available might then obtain a secondary consultation with other surgeons at his/her own or another institution to provide the patient with the greatest degree of expertise and probability of control of the disease.

## Other Practical Aspects of the Surgical Consultation

We have already referred to the importance of delineating the reason for the consultation and the questions the requestor wishes the consulting surgeon to address. Depending on the complexity of the issue at hand, the question for the consultant and the expectations could be transmitted in writing perhaps in the electronic medical record, by a phone call, or in personal discussion. As noted, it is usually helpful to provide a background concerning the patient's medical, psychosocial, and family situation or any special considerations such as what may be told to the patient under what circumstances.

One aspect important to the value of a consultation that often is assumed, but not explicitly asked of the patient, is what his/her goals might be. Sometimes this discussion can start with the question, "What can I do for you?" The consultant should not be content with a response such as, "I want to get better!" but should delve more fully into issues related to expec- 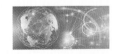 tations and wishes for quality of life and longevity, asking questions about how much risk the patient might be willing to take for a given probability of improvement. The trade-off satisfactory to the patient will not necessarily be what the surgical consultant might have assumed, and learning about patient goals is extremely important. For example, relatively short-term goals might be to see a grandchild born or a daughter getting married. Other patients may have longer-term goals, such to live as long as their own parents did. Not infrequently, older patients or those who have seen relatives suffer following surgery or other treatments are adamant that quality of life is more important than longevity. Only recently, a man in his 50s with metastatic lung cancer declared in no uncertain terms that he would not put his family through the stress of chemotherapy that his wife had experienced 5 years previously. Without knowing of this goal, our approach to his therapy would have been discordant with his wishes, and ultimately not in his best interests, and not respectful of his right to *autonomy*. Clarification of goals can not only help the surgical consultant to make more appropriate recommendations, but may also allow him/her to let the patient know if the goals are realistic from the surgical perspective.

Most referring physicians are interested not only in the primary opinion of the surgical consultant, but also in hearing about options for management and the risks and benefits of those options. The same is true for patients and their families who may have very fixed opinions regarding whether or not 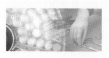 they wish to have additional diagnostic evaluations or therapy. This is particularly relevant to surgical procedures, where some patients are enthusiastic about having a procedure done regardless of the risks, whereas other patients are reluctant to have procedures done even if they are reassured that the potential benefits far outweigh the risks. A classic example is when the patient does not wish to have a cancer operation because he/she has heard that exposure to air would make the cancer spread faster. This will provide the consultant with an opportunity to reassure the patient, in understandable terms, regarding the source of this enduring myth (finding widespread metastatic cancer at laparotomy in the days before CT and positron emission tomography/computed tomography [PET/CT] scanning), and to educate the patient regarding potential benefits and risks of any indicated operation. It should be emphasized that the findings and recommendations must be explained in terms that the patient can understand. This often takes time and in many situations is benefited by the surgical consultant drawing pictures to demonstrate the problem to be addressed and the proposed surgical solution.

The altruistic surgeon will also let the referring physician and the patient know when they require the assistance or expertise of another surgical or nonsurgical colleague to provide the best care for the patient. It is always critical that the surgeon's ego not impede his/her ability to make this decision when deemed appropriate. Such a decision demonstrates his/her commitment to respect the patient's interests and his/her desire to provide the most beneficial care.

When more than one physician is involved in the care of a patient, it is important to have a clear delineation of responsibilities in the sharing of care. At times this may be divided according to the patient's problems, such as heart failure being the responsibility of the internist or cardiologist and perioperative management or wound care remaining the responsibility of the surgical team. It is critical, however, for the patient and patient's family to have a clear idea of to whom they can go to clarify issues and to express concerns. Often this is the primary care physician, but it could well be the surgical consultant at some point during the patient's management. This avoids a common concern that patients have of "I don't know who my doctor is," particularly in the era of inpatient management by hospitalists who do not have a long-term relationship with patients. At a minimum, the patient and the patient's family should know who is responsible for which aspects of the patient care, and during hospitalization, who is the leader of the team.

Finally, it is critical that there not only be verbal discussion of the recommendations but also be written documentation of the consultant's opinion and plans. Often, it is beneficial not only to document in the medical record and talk personally with the referring physician, but also to send a personal letter to him/her, which delineates the findings and recommendations. Such written documentation provides a historical record, which can be used by all in the subsequent care of the patient and may also serve as a reminder for the surgical consultant of findings and recommendations when the patient returns weeks or years later.

# 35 Regret and Apology

Mark R. Bonnell, MD

PROLOGUE ▶ Apologies are not easy, comprised as they are by equal portions of humility and candor. Apology stands opposite to hubris. Human beings possess an uncanny ability to detect real humility and real candor.

The active work of building and maintaining the surgeon-patient relationship is, in significant part, the obligation of the surgeon. Its pursuit constitutes, therefore, an ethical choice. The relationship is best thought of as a therapeutic one, and like all therapeutic relationships, it cannot exist without trust. Furthermore, a single-minded goal of improving patient compliance may not be shared by the patient, particularly those who are careful to guard their autonomy.

Behaviors that are perceived by the patient to be haughty or condescending damage the relationship. Behaviors perceived to be respectful and candid strengthen the relationship. When things go wrong, as they inevitably sometimes do in an active practice of surgery, a humble acknowledgment of responsibility and an expression of real regret can preserve and even deepen the relationship with a patient.

Moreover, acceptance of responsibility is good for the surgeon, whether it occurs with peers or in a more formal setting such as the mortality and morbidity conference. For the surgeon, apology is a pathway to healing and creates a milieu for real personal growth.

Dr Mark R. Bonnell is a cardiac surgeon who was trained at the University of Michigan as this program was being developed. He has, however, come independently to recognize the power of apology in human affairs. He is an associate professor in the Department of Surgery at The University of Toledo College of Medicine.

## Perspective

Surgeons, in the manner of Hippocrates, are taught to be empathetic captains of our patients' ships. This curriculum and charge, however, conflicts with the hidden curriculum and the current system, which discourages empathy in many ways, including an important manifestation of empathy, the practice of apologizing. Medicine has had an awkward relationship 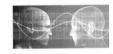 with apology for generations, given the collision of so many things to be sorry about and the mea culpa implications of an apology from a litigation standpoint. Many physicians learn not to apologize in medicine that apology suggests culpability and liability and is to be avoided at all costs. Personally, I was fortunate to be in the company of mentors who advised that honesty, transparency, and empathy even in the form of an apology made one a better doctor, engendered a stronger relationship with patients, and prevented litigation rather than inviting it. To me, it also simply "felt" like the right thing to do. It is beyond the scope of this chapter to argue about the foundations of morals and my gut feeling that apologizing was correct and moral. I leave that to Kant, Hume, Nietzsche, and the like. It is certainly more than coincidence that during these formative years of my medical education, I was at the University of Michigan where a new philosophy of medical malpractice was blossoming, which adopted these same principles and which in hindsight had emanated from the same mentors who influenced me. Adopting this style of practice produced a result exactly as predicted by my mentors. I enjoy close relationships with my patients, openly honor their profound trust, and, at the time of this writing, have not been sued. In a field born of illness and tragedy, we physicians should be stewards of empathy and apology rather the antitheses. Ever-growing technology, automation, and digital medicine provide tremendous opportunity from a quality and safety perspective going forward; it will be a long time, however, before we can automate empathy and compassion. Thus, if medicine is to remain the profession in which we take *care* of people, we as a medical culture will need to carry the torch of empathy with apology as its most genuine manifestation.

## Origin and Development

In modern times, apology is associated with empathy, remorse, or regret. Historically, however, an apology had no link to empathy. Our modern association of the phrases "I'm sorry" and "I apologize" has created this illusion. 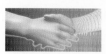 Neither the Merriam-Webster nor the Oxford Dictionaries implies a link between apology and empathy. Plato's Apology for Socrates (399 BC) was Plato's account of Socrates' own defense while he was on trial for charges of "corrupting the youth" and his particular actions—primarily, getting the youth to think. The first known link between apology and regret or "I'm sorry" is attributed to Shakespeare and appears in "Richard III" act II, scene VII when Gloucester says to Buckingham, "My lord, there needs no such apology...." The important association or implication of "I'm sorry" is the link of apology, in any verbal form, to empathy and honesty. How "apology" and any form of empathetic response historically became linked is unclear and could well be the subject of an entire chapter. It is this link of empathy to one's apology that is more important than the form of expression itself. "I'm sorry," for instance, can also be expressed insincerely and even with sarcastic overtones. It is clear that what our patients desire, and what Hippocrates advocated is a sincere, honest, and empathetic sentiment from doctors to their patients in whatever language the current vernacular requires. It is easy to see, however, how the lines between empathy, apology, culpability, and liability become blurred, which sets up an irreducible tension between the empathic care of patients and the status quo as it applies to malpractice and liability. This link to empathy is not lost on the business sector. Mark Murphy, the CEO of Leadership IQ and a New York Times best-selling author, has written a column advocating for "I'm sorry" rather than "I apologize," arguing that the latter is insincere and avoids responsibility. He continues in his column to say that "sorry" communicates empathy and "makes you sound like a human being because it conveys sincerity and immediately reduces customers' anger." Organizations that have implemented processes such as this generally suffer fewer lawsuits. Again, the lines of apology and culpability are blurred by Mr Murphy's statement that "sorry" somehow absolves one of responsibility. Lawyers have likewise wrestled with this, and although nearly 40 states have "apology laws" that aim to define whether statements of apology are admissible as evidence implying responsibility, these laws are highly variable in their interpretation and execution. Richard Boothman, JD, and his fundamental change in malpractice philosophy at the University of Michigan have demonstrated that patients are much more interested in honest acknowledgment and empathy rather than liability and that adopting this approach may lessen the otherwise irreducible tension experienced by practicing physicians.[1]

In March 2002, the University of Michigan health care system fundamentally changed its approach to medical malpractice claims. This was a departure from the traditional "deny and defend" approach that had been and continues to be practiced by most health care entities. This approach of deny and defend was born and indeed continues to be fed and thrive on fears, which include the following:

1. A natural aversion to confronting angry people.
2. Concerns that disclosure might invite a claim that otherwise would not be asserted.
3. Anxiety that the discussion will compromise courtroom defenses later.
4. Fear that the conversation may lead to loss of malpractice insurance or higher premiums.

Given its loathing of litigation, it is ironic that the "deny and defend" strategy remains the dominant response by hospitals and health care providers during the settlement of malpractice claims. Furthermore, the "deny and defend" strategy is incredibly inefficient and costly, both financially and emotionally. There is research to suggest that as few as 2% of medical errors ever receive a lawyer's attention.[2] For every dollar spent on compensation, 54 cents goes to administrative expenses, and nearly 40% of cases do not involve any errors. Patients frequently have fairly noble intentions when pursuing litigation. In a study by Charles Vincent et al, it was found that the common reasons for many lawsuits were to have unanswered questions answered, find accountability, and ensure that the same mistake would not be made with another patient. Nearly 40% of the respondents in the study said that an explanation and an apology would have made a difference in their decision to pursue litigation.[3] With this in mind, the University of Michigan instituted a program to achieve a systematic and principled response to unanticipated patient outcomes and, at the same time, route patient complaints to groups dedicated to clinical quality improvement or peer review. This program was based on 3 principles:

1. Compensate quickly and fairly when unreasonable medical care causes injury.
2. Defend medically reasonable care vigorously.
3. Reduce patient injuries (and therefore claims) by learning from patients' experiences.

This fostered a culture of consistency and predictability for patients, medical staff, lawyers, and courts. Figure 35.1 illustrates the University of Michigan Claims Management Model.

Although many predicted that an open and honest disclosure system would result in a flood of litigation, the results have shown that claims fell from 136 in 1999 to 61 claims in 2006. These data are also unadjusted for increases in clinical activity over the same period.

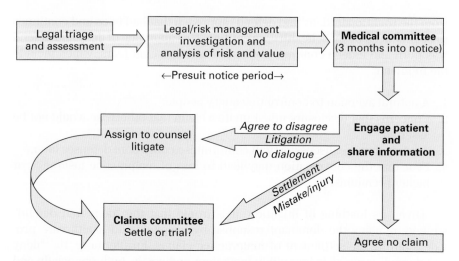

FIGURE 35.1 **University of Michigan Claims Management Model.** (Boothman RC, et al. A Better Approach to Medical Malpractice Claims? *Journal of Health and Life Sciences Law.* 2009;2(2).)

The University of Michigan was also able to reduce processing time from an average of 20.3 months to about 8 months, and the average litigation cost was decreased by more than 50%. To date, the University of Michigan experience has shown that there are ethical and financial benefits to disclosure and transparency when applied to malpractice. This new approach to malpractice gave physicians freedom to express sincere apology, and therefore empathy, and gave patients the honest and empathetic acknowledgment they sought. The common ground is empathy. The derivation of human empathy is a subject beyond the scope of this chapter. A brief exploration of the origins of empathy, what erodes it, and what cultivates it is pertinent to this discussion of apology and how it may help us recapture a commitment to empathic care.[1]

The important link is that apology is associated intimately with empathy. Studies have shown that empathy is associated with increased "moral" behavior. Certainly the foundations of morality can be argued, but most would agree that the fundamental pillars include reciprocity and fairness as well as empathy and compassion. There is abundant and credible evidence that empathy and its building blocks are demonstrable in animals.[4] In fact, empathy has its roots in far more primitive forms of animal behavior such as synchrony as exhibited by schooling fish and in humans as the phenomenon of yawn contagion.[5,6] There are, in fact, human studies showing increased capacity for empathy associated with a more robust yawn contagion reaction.[7] Frans de Waal[8] has shown in animal studies of empathy that it is possible to demonstrate reciprocity and recognition of fairness in primates and elephants.[9–11] Is a dog really sorry when it looks at you with that "guilty face," with its tail between its legs and your destroyed new Nikes at its feet? The so-called apology bow demonstrated by dogs is a gesture of submission,[12] which is more akin to shame than guilt. The dog's behavior of hanging its head and putting its tail between its legs to look submissive is consistent with feelings experienced by humans who feel shame accompanied by a sense of shrinking or "being small" and by a sense of worthlessness and powerlessness. The dog's posture in this case is sadly likened to a resident or medical student who has been likewise shunned in our system of medical and, especially, surgical education. Shame corresponds with attempts to deny, hide, and escape the situation ("deny and defend"). Physiologic research has shown shame to induce elevated levels of proinflammatory cytokines and cortisol levels. There is also a strong link between shame and anger and antisocial behavior. This anger tends to be expressed in more volatile, intense, and destructive ways and can lead to a dangerous spiral. Shame also leads to a decreased capacity for empathy and, furthermore, more frequent instances of substance abuse, relationship turmoil, and suicide. Physiologically, shame is manifested in higher systemic vascular resistance and heart rate leading to increasing risk of cardiovascular disease. A study in HIV patients showed an association with declining T cell counts and that shame may have negative immunologic effect in people with otherwise intact immunity.[13]

Guilt, on the other hand, is an adaptive emotion that may prompt reparative actions, confession, and apology. Guilt creates greater other-oriented empathy and leads to more constructive intentions and decreases hostile and illicit behaviors. There is a close association in the setting of wrongdoing between guilt and shame. It has been shown that "shame-fused guilt" removes any of the positive or constructive aspects of guilt. "The advantages of guilt are lost when a person's guilt experience is magnified and generalized to the self."[13] This shame-fused guilt offers little opportunity for redemption and is likely at the core of the painful self-castigation and rumination well described in the clinical literature. There is an important association with culpability as well, and significant problems arise when people develop an exaggerated sense of responsibility for events or outcomes well beyond their control. Sound familiar? Our surgical culture is to accept blame for everything. For example, as a transplant surgeon, I empathize deeply with those involved with the Duke transplant ABO incompatibility scandal of 2003 when a 17-year-old girl with O blood type received a heart-lung transplant from an ABO type A donor, resulting in acute rejection and death of the organs and patient. This was by and large a systems issue, but at the end of the day the transplant surgeon took the fall.[14] A similar incident here at the University of Toledo Medical Center captured national attention in 2012 when a kidney from a living-related donor was thrown away in the garbage.[15] In this case, the University of Toledo Medical Center took immediate action to sincerely apologize to the family, offer compensation, and complete a thorough quality improvement investigation. 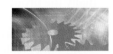 Personally, as a cardiac surgeon, I have made the agonizingly long walk from the operating room to the waiting room to tell a family that their loved one "died on the table." My approach in these cases has included sincere apology acknowledging that I am truly sorry for their loss and grief and regret that

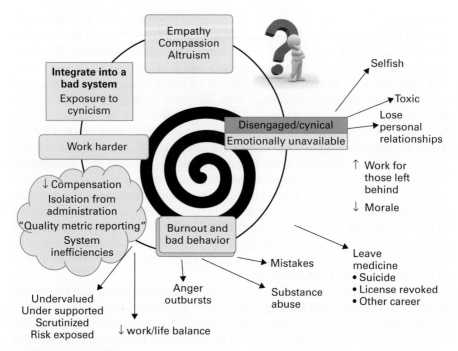

FIGURE 35.2 **The spiral.**

my skill and technology were inadequate to avoid a mortal outcome. I have, in some cases, wept with my patients and their families. Ironically, in almost every case I remember, the family reached out to comfort me as much as themselves: an expression that is immensely gracious and humbling.

We are taught, especially in surgery, to be the captain of the ship, accepting all responsibilities without respect to complexity in an evermore complex system that sometimes fails us along the way. What is more, we are trained within a system that uses shame to motivate and promotes self-castigation (think about the last mortality and morbidity conference). Is it any wonder that we adopted a "deny and defend" approach to medical malpractice? Is it a surprise that physicians now demonstrate the highest professional suicide rate, experience burnout at record levels, and have higher than average rates of divorce (see Figure 35.2)? We should be ashamed of ourselves, which is actually the problem. We must move beyond our inner dog and overcome our instinctive shame and evolve to a more productive and healthy emotion of guilt in its pure form.

Our concern for others at a human level, therefore, has deep evolutionary behavioral roots. Empathy increases our concern for others, promotes helping the distressed, and inhibits aggressive and harmful behavior. It also promotes health in the empathizer. In addition, it is a powerful driving force. Sir William Stokes said in his address to Meath Hospital in Dublin in 1894

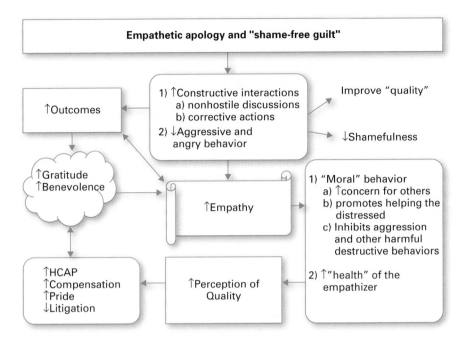

FIGURE 35.3 **Pragmatic impact of empathy in health care.**

when referring to the accomplishments of many of the greats of medicine and surgery, "...the best part of whose knowledge was gained by their sympathy with human suffering...the impassioned expression on the face of science."[16] Indeed, empathy and feelings associated with it are what drove many of us into this field. It continues to empower many of us to proceed, and the loss of empathy as a whole is what, I believe, has driven much of the negativity we find in our profession today. Figure 35.3 proposes what an infusion of empathy and an excision of shame could affect in our practice environment.

Apology may, or may not, be linked with empathy, but it is clear that in our present society, the expectation is that apology will carry empathy and when it does not, it is perceived as being insincere, patronizing, and dehumanizing.[17] It is clear from human psychology research and animal behavioral science that empathy and the "healthy" guilt that may be associated with it drive resolution and constructive reparation; it promotes health and deters aggression and anger. It is, likewise, clear that shame spoils the lot, reducing our capacity for empathy and inspiring antisocial behavior and physical health concerns. We, as surgeons, have been raised in a system that uses shame as a corrective force, and we are furthermore asked to accept full responsibility, morally and legally, for a complex and often dysfunctional system over which we have little control. The spiral illustrated in

Figure 35.2 is a predictable outcome of the current system. The notion of "apology" in surgery and medicine is inextricably linked to empathy, which defines the expectation of patients and should, therefore, define our practice. The malpractice reform spearheaded by Boothman at the University of Michigan demonstrates how we can break the chain connecting bad outcomes to shame and connect them instead to honest admission and healthy guilt and promote an empathic response. While this paradigm shift in malpractice philosophy is remarkable, it is equally remarkable that there has been little acceptance of this new practice after nearly 2 decades of demonstrable success morally and financially. The success of this program should empower us surgeons to honestly and sincerely apologize to our patients and inspire us to create more acceptance of empathy into our individual practices and practice environments as a whole. Apology may help rekindle the joy of patient care and make us better doctors.

# References

1. Boothman RC, Blackwell AC, Campbell Jr DA, Commiskey E, Anderson S. A better approach to medical malpractice claims? The University of Michigan experience. *J Health Life Sci Law*. January 2009;2(2):125–159.
2. Studdert DM, et al. Disclosure of medical injury to patients: an improbable risk management strategy. *Health Aff (Millwood)*. 2007 Jan-Feb;26(1):215–226.
3. Vincent C, Phillips A, Young M. Why do people sue doctors? A study of patients and relatives taking legal action. *Lancet*. 1994;343:1609–1613.
4. Sapolsky RM. B*ehave: The Biology of Humans at Our Best and Worst*. New York: Penguin Press; 2017. 796 pp. *Science*. June 23, 2017;356(6344):1239. doi:10.1126/science.aan4208.
5. Campbell MW, Carter JD, Proctor D, Eisenberg ML, de Waal FB. Computer animations stimulate contagious yawning in chimpanzees. *Proc Biol Sci*. December 7, 2009;276(1676):4255–4259. doi:10.1098/rspb.2009.1087.
6. de Waal F. Moral behavior in animals. TED Talk; 2011 November at TEDxPeachtree.
7. Campbell MW, de Waal FB. Methodological problems in the study of contagious yawning. *Front Neurol Neurosci*. 2010;28:120–127. doi:10.1159/000307090.
8. Brosnan SF, De Waal FB. Monkeys reject unequal pay. *Nature*. September 18, 2003;425(6955):297–299.
9. Suchak M, de Waal FB. Monkeys benefit from reciprocity without the cognitive burden. *Proc Natl Acad Sci U S A*. September 18, 2012;109(38):15191–15196.
10. Plotnik JM, Lair R, Suphachoksahakun W, de Waal FB. Elephants know when they need a helping trunk in cooperative task. *Proc Natl Acad Sci U S A*. March 22, 2011;108(12):5116–5121. doi:10.1073/pnas.1101765108.
11. Conniff R. *The Ape in the Corner Office: How to Make Friends, Win Fights and Work Smarter by Understanding Human Nature*. Crown Business Press; April 2005.
12. Lents NH. The guilty dog look and other borrowed signals. *Psychol Today*. April 2017; Online Publication.
13. Tangney J, et al. Moral emotions and moral behavior. *Ann Rev Psychol*. 2007;58:345–372.

14. Campion EW. A death at Duke. *N Engl J Med.* March 20, 2003;348:1083–1084. doi:10.1056/NEJMp 030033.

15. CNN Online Report August 2012.

16. Sir William Stokes. *The Ethics of Operative Surgery. Dubl J Med Sci.* Oxford University; November 1894.

17. Robbennolt JK. Apologies and medical error. *Clin Orthop Relat Res.* February 2009;467(2):376–382.

# 36

# End-of-Life Decisions in the Perioperative Period

Lloyd A. Jacobs, MD

PROLOGUE ▶ The work of a surgeon is unique. No other discipline works in the difficult medium of blood and flesh. No other discipline works as close to the dividing line between death and life. No other discipline can claim the authority of his/her experience as can the surgeon.

The uniqueness of the surgeon's work is often concentrated in the perioperative period: before, during, and after an operation performed with the surgeon's own fallible hands.

The principle of a patient's autonomy is clear, in the absence of infancy or dementia. A patient's right to self-determination seems absolute, and a patient's decision to forgo resuscitation or other procedures is a legitimate exercise of autonomy. However, a decision to do that raises specific difficulties in the perioperative period when complications may be easily corrected and success rates for resuscitation are far greater than those on a general surgical unit or in the community. As almost always, communication failures are often at the crux of things.

New and appropriate emphasis has been given to decisions in the postoperative period. Decisions during this phase of a surgical episode are of an entirely different order from those required during the preoperative or intraoperative period. Specifically difficult are decisions about end-of-life issues during that period.

Silber and colleagues called attention in 1992 to the importance of "rescue" from the impact of complications occurring in this phase.[1] They and subsequent investigators have provided evidence that decisions made or not made during this period may be a driving factor in determining quality-of-care metrics for both hospitals and surgeons.[2] Moreover, multiple studies have shown evidence that management of complications during this period is an important driver of the overall cost of a surgical episode.[3] These discussions have heightened the awareness of the critical nature of decision making during this period.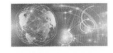

Self-aware surgeons recognize that this phase is one of maximal stress for a number of reasons. First, as has already been alluded to, increased oversight of this period, including great pressure to shorten postoperative length of stay, requires decisions be made in a compressed time frame or under unfamiliar conditions including during telephone conversations. Moreover, great improvements in intensive care unit care, interventional radiology and dialysis and respiratory care, while salutatory, have greatly increased the sheer number of decisions to be made.

The surgeon experiences significant loss of control during this phase. This is the period during which the surgeon is most constrained to share decisions with the internist, the anesthesiologist, or the house staff and nursing staff. In addition, although mutual support from these trusted colleagues may reduce surgeon stress, the sharing also contributes to a sense of loss of control. Late complications frequently present to the emergency department of the hospital where the operation was performed or, more disconcertingly, to an outside hospital. These events often occur at unpredictable hours and occasionally under dire circumstances.

Moreover, it is at this time when the surgeon must wait: wait for flatus, for restored oxygenation, or for mental clarity. More foreboding is the waiting for fever, or wound dehiscence, or renal failure. Waiting has an almost metaphysical aspect, and this period requires a mind-set that differs fundamentally from that of the preoperative and intraoperative periods where the surgeon is largely in control. Waiting for that which may or may not occur is unsettling as the play "Waiting for Godot"[4] implies and may contribute to surgeon "burnout."[5] Individual surgeons display various coping strategies during this period, which unfortunately include early morning rounding or leaving the postoperative care largely to the nurses or to the house staff or the intensive care unit staff.

It is hypothesized, however, that, increasingly, the surgeon "sets up" himself/herself, the patient, and the patient's family for further difficulties if the necessity for end-of-life considerations arise during this period. This "setting up," or creation of unrealistic expectations, occurs during the discussions with the patient or his/her family concerning the initial operation. This is particularly conspicuous when the patient is very old or frail or the patient's condition is perceived preoperatively to be nearly futile. In these settings, the surgeon often shares his/her hesitancy with the patient or his/her family but then creates the expectation that: "if we do operate we must go all the way" in dealing with postoperative complications as they 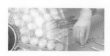 may unfold. By creating these expectations the surgeon ensures that if the patient dies during the postoperative period that he/she himself/herself will be frustrated and may experience regret. The family will, of course, be disappointed and may experience buyer's remorse. The house staff and nursing staff will feel that expectations were not met and the patient, of course, will be dead.

A number of disconcerting thoughts arise concerning this tendency to insist on responding to every step in an avalanche of complications; the response often even includes cardiopulmonary resuscitation at the moment of death. Could this tendency relate to hubris on the part of the surgeon? Could it relate to a fear of failure or to fear of criticism from colleagues at a morbidity and mortality conference? More likely, can this tendency be related to a failure to see the patient's life in broad context, and to strive to provide a "good death"[6] as part of the surgeon's commitment?

A special instance of this situation arises when a patient who has a long-standing do not resuscitate (DNR) order needs and consents to an operation intercurrent to his/her progressive and progressing disease. An example might be a perforated viscous in a patient with advanced metastatic colon cancer. Should the preexisting DNR order be canceled? Does or should the institution have a policy requiring cancelation or continuance of the DNR specification? Is the surgeon or anesthesiologist justified in refusing intra-operative care unless the order is canceled? Several points should be made.

Several national organizations recommend a "required reconsideration" at this juncture. Clearly, a clarifying conversation with the patient and the patient's surrogate is implied in this. The ethics are clear; most believe that the patient's right to autonomy is absolute; the surgeon's right to decline to care for the patient is relative and depends on the urgency of the situation.

Most problems in this career are problems of communication, not problems of rights or values. Of particular note should be the surgeon's ego investment in the outcome of operation and the great difficulty this involvement brings to the appropriateness of "letting go." "You won't die on my watch" is the underlying emotion.

The discussion regarding postoperative care is highly reminiscent of "the slippery slope" argument, which in its extreme form suggests that a single puff of marijuana smoke will begin an inevitable train of events, which will cause the smoker to end as a hopeless heroin addict. The central notion is that there is no reasonable stopping place. The surgeon seems similarly to believe that once begun there is no reasonable place during the postoperative phase to change the goals of care from survival to the goal of a "good death." Douglas Walton has put the situation as follows[7]:

> *"The slippery slope argument...is used as a tactic to try to suggest that you will be locked into a sequence of consequences with no turning back, once you have made the initial step."*

> *"But most arguments...are more like staircases than slippery slopes—at each step we can decide whether we want to go further down or not."*

Surgeons must develop a sense of this staircase quality of the unfolding of events during the postoperative period and recognize that there are many decision points along the way.

The business notion of "sunk costs" may be helpful here. Operations and other therapies now past are "sunk," and gone and should not be counted as weighing on the decisions of today. Careful observations of surgeons' behavior suggests that they are more willing to reoperate on patients whose initial operation was by another surgeon or at a different hospital when "sunk" costs do not seem to be a personal investment about to be abandoned.

End-of-life decisions are difficult in any case.[8] End-of-life decisions during the postoperative period present additional difficulties characterized by a sense of investment and ownership and loss of control. These difficulties are often exacerbated by the surgeon himself/herself who may set the expectation of "going all the way." Thoughtful, self-aware judgment is required.

# References

1. Silber JH, Williams SV, Krakauer H, Schwartz S. Hospital and patient characteristics associated with death after surgery: a study of adverse occurrence and failure to rescue. *Med Care.* 1992;30(7):615–629.
2. Ghaferi AA, Birkmeyer JD, Dimick JB. Complications, failure to rescue, and mortality with major inpatient surgery in medicare patients. *Ann Surg.* 2009;250(6):1029–1034.
3. Abraham CR, Werter CR, Ata A, et al. Predictors of hospital readmission after bariatric surgery. *J Am Coll Surg.* 2015;221(1):220–227.
4. Beckett S. *Waiting for Godot.* New York: Grove Press, Inc.; 1954.
5. Balch CM, Freischlag JA, Shanafelt TD. Stress and burnout among surgeons: understanding and managing the syndrome and avoiding the adverse consequences. *Arch Surg.* 2009;144(4):371–376.
6. Hinshaw DB. *Suffering and the Nature of Healing.* Yonkers: St. Vladimir's Seminary Press; 2013.
7. Walton D. *Slippery Slope Arguments.* Oxford: Clarendon Press; 1992:29.
8. Entire issue devoted to death, dying, and end of life. *JAMA.* 2016;315:227–260.

# 37 Medical Litigation

James M. Tuschman, JD
Coleen C. Wening, MBA, JD

**PROLOGUE** ▶ Among the most difficult and stressful experiences of a life in surgery or medicine is the all too common experience of being the defendant in a lawsuit. No other process has a similar power to undermine one's sense of well-being; no other process instills feelings of doubt and guilt with more force. Still, the writers of this chapter correctly point out that nearly every surgeon will encounter this experience sometime in his/her career. If, in fact, knowledge is power, the purpose of including this detailed analysis of the process is to provide knowledge that may serve as prophylaxis to the surgeon, against the despair and self-doubt often precipitated by this experience. The more you know, the less the pain!

There are, we have emphasized elsewhere, an infinite number of tellings of any operation or even of any prognosis for a complex disease state. There are similarly an infinite number of tellings of an event or events that precipitated a lawsuit. A lawsuit invariably evokes defensiveness and a tendency to revise one's recollection. The surgeon must choose from the infinite tellings, a narrative that is not self-deprecating, not defensive, but that has the verisimilitude of truth. Once that telling is chosen, it must be adhered to carefully. Moreover, it goes without saying, or should, that this is a mental exercise and that no evidence may be tampered with. Doing so only invites detection and then increases stress and anxiety.

**308**

Mr James M. Tuschman is the combination of both a scholar and an experienced practical attorney. He has experienced the medical malpractice arena from both the plaintiff's and the defendant's perspective. His breadth and authority are therefore unusual. He is a 1966 graduate of the Ohio State University College of Law. He has served as a medical malpractice trial lawyer for 50 years, representing doctors and hospitals, as well as patients. He currently lectures in Legal Specialties at The University of Toledo. Mr Tuschman has been recognized in *Best Lawyers in America* in addition to many other publications. He is a member of the International Society for Barristers and the National Trial Lawyers Association.

Ms Coleen C. Wening is a recent Juris Doctor graduate from the University of Toledo College of Law. Her concentration is in Health Law. Ms Wening also holds an MBA from the University of Toledo and a BA from the University of Cincinnati. She has worked as a health care administrator for almost 25 years at both large, integrated health networks and independent medical organizations.

Surgeons have an obligation to their individual patients and society at large. These duties may conflict.

The duty to the individual patient is entailed in the famous aphorism "Do no harm." Although the origin of the phrase is complex, it is among the most widely held statements of obligation of surgeons and physicians in general. Reference is made to the avoidance of harm in the oldest documents of medical ethics including the Hippocratic Oath, which in one translation states: "I will keep them from harm...."

When, however, a patient has incurred harm, or believes he/she has, as a result of the act(s) of a surgeon, the surgeon's embeddedness in a society becomes paramount. Every jurisdiction, historically and geographically, has had laws dealing with such occurrences. The following paragraphs attempt to distill those laws as they currently exist in the United States to a compendium with which every surgeon should be familiar.

In 1995, baby girl Alys was born premature at just 26 weeks' gestation. Despite weighing less than 2 pounds, she was surprisingly well developed and healthy, thriving after the birth without a ventilator. However, because of the common preemie condition of patent ductus arteriosus, a surgery was needed to close the arterial duct to allow Alys to oxygenate her blood through her own lungs. The cardiothoracic surgeon assigned to her case had not performed this procedure for more than 5 years and never on an infant. He tried unsuccessfully for 2 hours to find the duct and damaged Alys's phrenic nerve in the process. The baby was placed on a ventilator, as she was unable 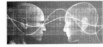 to breathe on her own because of the loss of control over her diaphragm. Aggressive respiration treatment resulted in the damage of lung tissue and the brain. The baby was eventually transferred to a children's hospital where a second duct closure surgery—performed by a qualified pediatric surgeon—was successful. However, a nurse at this facility misplaced an arterial line in Alys's left arm, which led to a loss of blood flow. In addition to not discovering the condition for 10 days, the attending neonatologists delayed the administration of therapeutic medications for an additional 4 days because they were awaiting another specialist's consultation. Drug therapy was unsuccessful and Alys's left arm was amputated 1 week later. Additionally, the baby is permanently and "profoundly retarded, unable to speak, fed through a tube, and wheelchair-bound and receives oxygen 24 hours a day." A Philadelphia jury found Alys's condition was not a result of her premature birth, as defendant physicians and hospitals argued, but instead was the result of their medical negligence. In what may amount to the highest verdict in medical malpractice litigation history, the plaintiff was awarded $100 million.[1]

## Introduction

Medical malpractice law provides a remedy for patients to recover compensation for harms resulting from substandard treatment. In 2008 alone, medical malpractice litigation cost $10 billion in damages, legal fees, and administrative costs.[2] Physicians practicing "defensive medicine" to avoid lawsuits added $45.6 billion to annual health care spending.[2] Considering there were more than 2.36 million recorded medical errors in 2008 alone, malpractice lawsuits are an unavoidable fact of life for all physicians, for which they must have a basic understanding and preparation.[3] The issue affects nonsurgeons and surgeons alike because the likelihood of doctors being sued at least once in their career is between 75% and 99%, respectively.[4] The latter face increased risk of multiple malpractice suits because of the invasive nature of their work, complications related to anesthesia and infection, and the seriousness of the conditions they treat.

Notwithstanding the direct association to their professional activities, doctors must also contend with changing attitudes regarding legal action grounded in untoward medical results. Contrasted with previous generations, patients today, like Americans generally, are more litigious. Unfortunately, doctors are often perceived by patients and their families as overpaid deep pockets, charging too much for health care, and driving up patient personal costs.

At the same time, the modern version of health care delivery makes it probable that physicians will be found "guilty by association" at some point in their 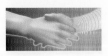 careers. The concept behind Patient-Centered Medical Homes and Medicare Accountable Care Organizations, which place a focus on collaboration among a patient's team of physicians and health care facilities, means doctors will be grouped together in any joint-defendant negligence claim. It is an historical perception that many preliminary malpractice tactics—which practitioners consider nuisance measures—are fact-finding missions to identify who out of these multiple parties are primarily responsible for a patient's illness or injury. Thus, many physicians believe they are also forced to unjustifiably defend their treatment to have their names removed from these complaints.

Finally, today's physician-patient relationship possesses little to no personal connection that might otherwise prevent the filing of a suit. For their part, patients tend to shop around for services from multiple providers, are more likely to leave physicians who deliver poor customer service rather than remain with those who provide great medical care, insist on inexpen-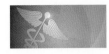sive treatment options such as over-the-phone prescription medication maintenance, and use the Internet for self-diagnosis. But when negligent medical treatment does occur, they rightfully want answers. Unfortunately, some doctors are poor communicators without any discernible "bedside manner." They are taught to avoid speaking to patients and family members when things go wrong, because either they do not know what to say or they do not want to incriminate themselves. Patients sometimes get their answers, as well as the advice to sue, unofficially from hospital registered nurses (RNs) who are very familiar with incompetent care and treatment.

## An Action in Tort

As a special subcategory of tort law, a discussion of medical malpractice begins with the basic elements of negligence. Tort law comprises state statutes and the common law—decisions passed down by courts through case law—therefore, specific rules and judgments will vary from state to state. Regardless, all states place the burden of proof in tort cases on the plaintiff to establish the prima facie elements of duty, breach, causation, and damage.[5] Legally, failure by the plaintiff to prove even one of these elements will render the lawsuit insufficient. Additionally, the level of proof needed in tort cases is "a preponderance of the evidence." This means the plaintiff must prove it is more likely than not the defendant's negligence caused their damages. Understandably, this standard is much lower and easier to achieve than the "beyond a reasonable doubt" burden required in criminal cases.

## Medical Malpractice

Medical malpractice specifically refers to professional negligence by a health care provider in which the treatment supplied was substandard and caused harm, injury, or death to a patient.[6] In most cases, the medical malpractice is unintentional and involves a medical error in diagnosis, medication dosage, health management, treatment, or aftercare. The injury can be either physical or emotional in nature, or both.

Clearly, medical malpractice does not exist every time there is a negative or bad outcome, especially if it is an anticipated, reasonably known risk discussed in advance between the patient and the physician. Negligent conduct can include direct care provided by the doctor in the form of either an affirmative act performed in error (commission) or a failure to treat when necessary (omission). Vicarious liability, also known as agent or employer 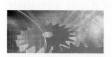 liability, also exists in the provider's supervision of others, such as RNs and personal office staff, who act in a careless or negligent manner. Therefore, health care employers are ultimately responsible for whom they hire and supervise, usually regardless of whether the employee follows direct orders or acts on his/her own.

## Expert Witnesses

Medical malpractice claims are distinguishable from traditional negligence lawsuits, such as those involving automobile accidents, primarily because most states require a malpractice complaint be filed with an expert medical witness's certification that the plaintiff's claims have merit. Thereafter, the four tort elements come into play, usually necessitating the testimony of an expert medical witness or witnesses during discovery or trial to establish their existence and comply with the burden of proof. Two exceptions to this litigation strategy exist: (1) when a provider commits gross negligence, such as operating under the influence of alcohol or drugs, or (2) when the medical treatment is so common, or the negligence is so obvious, a lay juror could conduct an adequate evaluation without assistance, such as when a surgeon leaves a foreign object in a patient's body. In these situations, no expert witness is required.

Malpractice litigation often becomes a "battle of the experts." Because expert testimony is generally required for the plaintiff patient to prove his/her case initially by means of the affidavit of merit, it is also a necessary tactic of the defense to use its own expert. Often, multiple experts are needed to prove and defend each of the separate malpractice elements. The result is a jury that must weigh complicated facts—hopefully made more comprehensible by the experts—in determining which party is more believable or convincing. The decision can at times turn on the expert's qualifications, a threshold issue established before his/her substantive testimony.

The court's responsibility in any litigation is to maintain the legal rules of trial. As such, it establishes the witness's legal qualification as a medical expert. Qualification is the same regardless of who the witness is testifying for. Individual state rules of evidence (usually adopted from the federal rules) require that (1) the testimony is being offered as expert testimony[7]; (2) knowledge, skill, experience, training, or education qualifies the expert; and (3) the testimony will assist the trier of fact in coming to his/her decision.

Concentrating primarily on the second element, there are very few concrete principles to guide this process. It is generally recommended that the expert witnesses be board-certified, even if the defendant physician is not, because this proves an exceptional level of knowledge, skill, experience, training, or education. Some states go further and require first-hand experience with the standard of care and practice in the same subspecialty as the defendant. However, a majority of states consider knowledge, skill, experience, training, or education under the "totality of the circumstances," an approach based on the specific issues of each case. In other words, there is no quantitative measure—such as medical school attended, specialty, amount of time in practice, number of books or articles written on the topic, status as a university professor, or volume of the same procedures performed—to tell a judge at what point a witness crosses the line from a mere professional colleague to an expert in his/her field. Instead, the court collectively weighs all information given and determines if the witness establishes his/her status as an expert.

Consider again the recommendation that an expert be board-certified. Depending on the circumstances of the case, he/she may not need to be certified in the same specialty in which the defendant doctor practices. For example, if the duty, breach, and injury are all based on the failure of a primary care physician (PCP) to order a particular diagnostic test, and the specialist witness is also well versed in the general standards of use for that test, he/she need not be certified in internal medicine. The reverse is also permissible in that a general practitioner may be qualified to testify as to the care provided by a specialist as long as the specific treatment is something both provide. The basic test is as follows: "(1) What procedure(s) is the source of the malpractice claim; (2) whether this procedure(s) is common to both specialties; (3) what experience the purported expert has with this specific procedure(s); and (4) whether the standard of care applicable to the procedure(s) is common to both specialties." Thus, it is also not required for the expert to practice in the same specialty as the defendant or specifically in the areas of radiology or pathology, depending on the type of test. Instead, the witness might specialize in the condition the patient was ultimately diagnosed with and can speak to the symptoms of the disease, the appropriateness of ordering the test, accuracy of the test, and the rate of success when the condition is diagnosed and treated early. Conversely, a PCP cannot be qualified as an expert for or against a neurosurgeon when the issue is the performance of a specific surgical procedure. Overall, the expert and defendant should share a common knowledge and practical experience with the treatment at issue, and the standard of care is the same for both practitioners despite their different professional roles.

At a minimum, the expert must be licensed or practicing in any state within the United States. However, some states strictly require experts be either licensed or licensed and practicing in the state or community in which the incident occurred. If not current at the time of trial, courts may at least demand that licensing and practice coincide with the date of the incident. The purpose of these conditions is to establish the expert's knowledge of 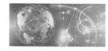 the standard of care as of the date of the injury, which is most likely to be present when continuing education and professional experiences are up-to-date.

Finally, other limitations wholly unrelated to a witness's qualifications as an expert may preclude a party from serving as such. "Commonality of coverage" by the same medical malpractice carrier is one area to raise concern.[8] A majority of jurisdictions will allow the use of a "substantial connection" test to attack the witness's credibility. This is accomplished through the introduction of insurance evidence typically prohibited in tort actions. The issue is whether an expert witness can remain neutral if he/she shares the same liability carrier as the defendant. Some states have interpreted the introduction of such evidence as an automatic bar to the witness's testimony.[8]

## The Surgeon as an Expert Witness

Surgeons may find serving as an expert witness to be interesting, intellectually stimulating, and even financially beneficial. However, potential expert witnesses should be aware that their testimony can and usually is scrutinized by the attorneys and experts on the "other side" of the litigation. In fact, this scrutiny may subject the expert witness to eventual disciplinary sanctions from professional organizations and state medical boards. (Testimony is given under oath and must be accurate, honest, and informed.)

Again, the specific duty of the expert witness in medical malpractice cases is to explain to the judge and jury what the defendant physician did 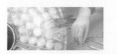 or should have done, and whether that act of omission or commission complied with the applicable standard of care for circumstances that are identical or similar to those that are the subject matter of the case. This testimony is based on a review of the relevant medical records and perhaps depositions and other discovery information and then providing an opinion on the quality of care, treatment, and medical management offered by the defendant physician in the case. Additionally, scientifically valid expert testimony not only assists the deliberations in a case but also establishes the applicable standard of care and provides the critical linkage on causation (deviation from the standard of care that directly and proximately causes the patient's injury or death).

The American legal system is adversarial, allowing each side of a lawsuit to present the opinions of an expert witness. However, surgeons should agree to participate as an expert and to testify only in cases that they believe to have strong merits, whether in support of the plaintiff patient or the defendant doctor. Those who serve as experts should not spend disproportionate amounts of time testifying in multiple cases. Rather, they should try to be available to serve only as a minor component of their professional activities. In other words, physicians who make being an expert witness a full-time job can eventually lose their credibility, regardless of which side uses them. Accordingly, the ethical guidelines, set forth below, should be followed by physicians who serve as expert witnesses in medical malpractice cases:

- Hold a current, valid, and unrestricted license to practice medicine in the state where he/she is practicing;
- Be certified by the specialty board in his/her specialty or subspecialty;
- Qualified by experience and possess demonstrated competence in the subject and issue in the case at hand;
- Familiarity with the subject matter of the case at the time of the alleged occurrence giving rise to the claim;
- Testimony that is honest, impartial, and complete;
- Readily available with a clear objective;
- Based on personal experience, specific clinical or surgical references, or generally accepted opinion in the field of specialty that is the subject of the case;
- Compensation that is reasonable and commensurate with the time and effort given to preparation in the matter; and
- Cognizant that transcripts of one's expert testimony are public records that can be subject to independent peer review.

## Jury's Role

The role of the jury is to be the ultimate "trier of fact." As such, it is responsible for applying the expert testimony to the facts of the case. As a matter of law, expert witnesses are only permitted to provide opinion testimony. They are prohibited from making any decisive statements or legal conclusions about the facts of the case that could influence the jury's final decision. In other words, the expert may not "take the verdict away from" the jury. Instead, expert witnesses are permitted to refer to facts "consistent with" either standard or substandard care, as well as whether the alleged breach "caused" the plaintiff's injuries. The jury then determines the degree of liability for all defendants—as well as for the plaintiff if he/she is found to have negligently contributed to his/her own medical condition—and the amount of damages to be awarded.

## Duty Owed to the Patient

The defendant doctor must first be identified as a party who owed a duty of care to the plaintiff patient at the time treatment was or should have been rendered. At its most basic level, the duty is created with the formation of the doctor-patient relationship. At the same time, some specific duties, such 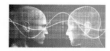 as providing informed consent and maintaining confidentiality, are inherent to the association.

## Doctor-Patient Relationship

Primarily, it is the formation and continuation of the doctor-patient relationship that creates the practitioner's duty. Any process by which a doctor examines, diagnoses, or treats a patient creates a duty to provide appropriate care, treatment, and medical management to the patient. This includes agreement by the doctor to provide an initial service even if he/she has not yet done so. For example, allowing a patient to schedule a future office appointment may create the expectation a relationship exists. Depending on the scope, a consultation by a specialist may or may not create a relationship: a mere discussion between colleagues does not, whereas a physical examination by a specialist does. At the same time, although there is typically no legal requirement for physicians to accept new patients, doctors should verify their obligations under any separate contracts with facilities and insurance companies.

Of specific relevance to surgeons are limitations on the scope of treatment. Surgeons often see patients only on an immediate pre-, peri-, and postoperative basis, thus deferring long-term care to PCPs and other specialists. Doctors may dictate the appropriate scope of the relationship if the limitations are communicated to the patient in advance. Therefore, the cardiovascular surgeon who does not routinely prescribe maintenance blood pressure and blood-thinning medications must timely notify the cardiac bypass patient that these should be obtained from, and monitored by, a different professional.

The physician's duty to treat continues for as long as the patient's condition lasts, or until the relationship has been severed by either the doctor or the patient. There are numerous reasons a practitioner may act to terminate the relationship. These include the innocuous (physician relocation or retirement) and the adverse (lack of patient compliance with the recommended treatment plan to their own detriment, failure to follow established practice policies, failure to pay a bill, general absence of a mutually beneficial relationship). To prevent abandonment of patients, individual states dictate the procedure by which separation must occur. Statutes addressing this issue typically dictate the type and duration of the required follow-up care, as well as the manner,

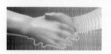 timing, and minimum content of the patient notification, such as information instructing the patient on obtaining a copy of his/her medical record for subsequent physicians. To avoid future liability, practitioners may also opt to formalize their own termination by the patient—especially when received verbally—by sending a confirmation letter containing the required information.

## Informed Consent

Always inherent in the doctor-patient relationship is the duty to provide informed consent. Two affirmative acts on the part of the doctor will exemplify full compliance with this duty. First, the "rule of self-determination" requires the physician to provide reasonably sufficient information to the patient for the latter to make an informed decision as to the treatment options. Second, the physician is obligated to obtain prior agreement from the patient before performing any nonemergent, invasive, or experimental treatments, or diagnostic tests.

For informed consent to be valid, it must include information describing for the patient—in terms he/she can understand—the nature of the condition, the likely treatment options, the benefits and reasonably known risks (subject to interpretation by experts) of each option or options discussed, including delay of treatment, and the best recommendation[9]; many statutes refer to 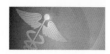 these as the "risks, perils, options, and hazards." It is left up to the provider in his/her interactions with the patient to determine the level of detail and the amount of discussion required. Some patients may be more informed and have a faster understanding, whereas others may take longer to process the information they have received. Overall, surgeons should personalize the discussion with each patient to learn their individual goals and to address which treatment option or options are most likely to provide or hinder the desired outcome. For example, an orthopedic surgeon performing knee replacement surgery on a 45-year-old long-distance runner must discuss any risks that could result in long-term reliance by the patient on a cane—a conversation wholly different from one held with an 85-year-old sedentary great-grandmother currently confined to a wheelchair. Whenever possible the discussion and consent must also disclose any subsequent action deemed necessary by the physician. Hence, a gynecologist removing a uterine cyst should have discussed with the patient in advance the possibility of a partial or full hysterectomy while still under anesthesia. There are exceptions for emergency situations and consent can be implied (in some jurisdictions) when a reasonable person would have requested and allowed the same treatment.

A patient's detrimental reliance on the informed consent is the cornerstone of many medical malpractice cases. Regardless of how detailed the discussion becomes, all data given to patients must be truthful and realistic. Whether it is provided in terms of success or failure rates, this information often forms the basis of a patient's reliance on the outcome of the treatment. If a patient chooses a particular option because the surgeon claims to have performed 5000 procedures with a 95% success rate, the doctor must be prepared to defend such a claim in court. The facts strongly favor the patient who can show his/her injury or illness was a result of risks he/she was not made aware of and he/she would have forgone the treatment had he/she been adequately informed. Some states also require the patient to demonstrate that most reasonable persons in the same or similar situation would also have rejected the treatment.

Informed consent is the responsibility of the medical health care provider (always a physician), and the conversation must be timely memorialized, along with the signed form, in the patient's medical record. Informed consent expires and a new consent must be obtained, therefore, if surgery is rescheduled for some reason. For example, a consent signed over 6 months before surgery will be too old to stand up in court. Also, a replacement surgeon is prohibited from performing a procedure under the original informed consent that does not list his/her name. At the same time, properly obtained 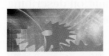 consent means a patient has had the opportunity to discuss his/her questions and concerns directly with their health care professional. Instead, busy surgeons often mistakenly delegate this responsibility to office staff who simply read the document to the patient word for word or place it in front of the patient for automatic signature. In some cases, surgery is scheduled over the phone and the consent is included in a packet mailed to the patient who brings it to the hospital on the day of surgery. Only later, out of the patient's presence, does the physician sign the document as a simple matter of chart completion. Unfortunately, while such shortcuts are efficient for the surgeon, it is not properly obtained "informed" consent. A physician's ability to defend a malpractice lawsuit grounded in lack of consent could turn on the adequacy of this process. Bottom line, the medical doctor must be the one to disclose and discuss the risk information with the patient.

Finally, the lack of valid informed consent is its own cause of action against a provider. In other words, a patient may bring a legal claim against a doctor for the lack of informed consent just as he/she could for wrongful death, loss of consortium, negligent infliction of emotional distress (NIED), and so on. As such, states provide patients with 3 possible remedies under which to sue: medical malpractice, the absence of informed consent, and the intentional tort of battery. Under the theory of medical malpractice, a patient may claim that a surgeon's fraudulent misrepresentation of information relating to the potential success of the treatment caused them to elect the procedure. When the lack of consent is claimed, it is the conduct of performing the unauthorized procedure that creates the tort. Otherwise, the patient may claim intentional battery based on unauthorized contact by the doctor against the body of the patient. Professional liability insurance typically expressly denies coverage of such "intentional acts," such as performing unauthorized procedures.

## Confidentiality

Physicians also have a fundamental duty of confidentiality, which, when breached, is another permissible basis for a malpractice claim by a patient. The general rule of physician-patient confidentiality means that the physician may not make an unauthorized disclosure of a patient's medical information. When records are requested by third parties, the duty extends the doctor's responsibility to notify the patient if any requests lack an appropriate release. Under the law of torts, the patient must show that an unauthorized disclosure caused him/her damage, although the injury need not be physical or economic.

There are exceptions to this duty that can be broadly characterized as medical necessity and legal obligation. Some disclosures are essential to the relationship, including continuity of care through referrals and operational requirements such as government reporting and billing. However, doctors and other health care workers are barred from accessing medical records of patients in whose care they take no part. This is of greater concern for computer-based systems holding large amounts of data accessible by many uninvolved parties.

Rules of evidence recognize the physician-patient privilege related to confidentiality in legal proceedings, unless the practitioner is properly compelled to disclose the information, such as by a subpoena. In complying with subpoenas, the doctor has no responsibility to verify the document's validity before the release of records, if the information was released in good faith and he/she had no actual knowledge of a defect. At the same time, a patient automatically waives his/her right to privacy—and the authorization requirement—when he/she sues the practitioner or another third party over an issue related directly to the care received. For example, a suit for medical malpractice against a physician or for product liability against a medical device manufacturer automatically waives the privilege, enabling the medical record to be used by the defense in discovery and testimony. Finally, states statutorily require physicians to disclose certain information as a matter of "public policy." This includes information about patients treated for communicable diseases who are a danger to the public and for injuries suggestive of involvement in a crime, such as gunshot wounds.

Like the formation and termination of the doctor-patient relationship, the duty of confidentiality is largely regulated by the state law dictating the ownership and care of records, content of the release, acceptable timing of compliance, and appropriate charges. The Health Insurance Portability and Accountability Act of 1996 also regulates access to, and privacy of, health records on a federal level. It, however, does not provide a private right of action for a patient to sue a provider or facility for breach of confidentiality. Rather, it exposes the breaching party to federal sanctions and fines on a per incident level.

## Deviation From Duty (Breach of the Standard of Care)

In a nutshell, the medical standard of care is the type and amount of skill and attention that a prudent, similarly trained health care professional, in the same or similar medical community, would have provided to the patient. Like traditional tort actions, the objective standard of care applied is that of "a reasonable person under the same circumstances." In the case of medical malpractice, 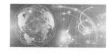 that reasonable person is another physician. This results in a higher professional standard because of the practitioner's degree of knowledge, skill, experience, and care, generally equating to the customary standard of the medical community for the provider's specialty and level of expertise. The basic question is as follows: What are the accepted practices surrounding the medical procedure or course of treatment that led to the alleged medical negligence? An expert medical witness in the same or similar specialty as the defendant almost always provides the answer. Consequently, the standard for doctors is different from that of nurses, surgeons from that of PCPs, and cardiothoracic surgeons from that of gastroenterologists. The standard of care is further specified on a case-by-case basis as reflective of the customs and procedures used when particular medical conditions are present, such as comparisons of cataract surgeries between different ophthalmologists.

## Standard of Care

It is the plaintiff's medical expert who provides the key evidence—through detailed and often quite complex testimony—painstakingly walking the jury through the plaintiff's condition, the appropriate course of treatment or diagnosis methodology, and exactly what the doctor did (or did not do) at each stage of care. After qualification, the expert is called on to testify as to the accepted standard of care for the case being tried. However, his/her testimony is not automatically accepted as the standard of care simply because of this "qualified" status. Instead, the standard of care is also subject to verification:

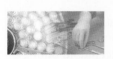 The expert will also be called on to prove the justification for his/her position based on legal rules related to scientific and technical evidence. First, it must have been, or can be, tested. Second, testing must include appropriate controls. Third, there must be a known rate of error. Fourth, it must be subject to peer review through duplicity and publication. Fifth and finally, the related scientific community must generally accept it. The information is often introduced with medical treatises and other published documents, such as those describing clinical practice guidelines and evidence-based medicine, as exhibits. Clinical practice guidelines are premised on the notion that both medical professionals and patients are human and that misunderstandings, errors, and injuries are inevitable without systems and checklists. In addition, the concept of evidence-based medicine is extracted from rigorous clinical studies.

## Defining "Community Standard"

State courts differ on what is meant by the "medical community" as applied to the duty analysis; therefore, 2 basic versions exist. Most states adopt the customs and practices of the national community of providers practicing in the same medical field or area of specialty. Custom is defined as a significant group of physicians in the area or specialty performing in the same way. The remainder of states forming the minority apply the modified community standard, determined by a like community, similar in geographic size, population, urban and rural areas, industry, and available health care services. (Courts have abandoned the concept of the strict "locality" rule, which invokes the customs and practices in the same community where the care was received. The reason is to avoid potential collusion among doctors in improperly protecting or targeting one of their colleagues.) Hence, the very important role of the expert witness is obvious: He/she weighs the actions of the defendant physician against those of similar providers treating the same condition and identifies any deviation from the accepted community standard.

Health care professionals are only liable for harm or injuries resulting from deviations in the quality of care a competent doctor would normally provide in the same or similar circumstances and that resulted in harm or injury to the patient. Direct nonconformity with the preferred treatment plan of the expert medical witness is not automatically indicative of a breach of duty. Again, the test is an objective one; that the expert must testify the defendant's approach was a deviation from the customs and procedures of the medical community "as a whole." Where multiple treatment options are accepted as valid, no breach exists when a physician uses one of them.

## Discovery

Once the duty of care has been identified, a plaintiff must show that the defendant breached his/her duty through conduct that fell below the applicable standard of care. This is an evidentiary process for which plaintiffs have the primary burden. As such, direct evidence of the conduct is the best way to show breach of the standard of care. This includes evidence from both the medical records and various eyewitness testimony of events.

Because the medical industry is one of the only professions that creates a daily diary of the care, treatment, and medical management given by the treating professional, Exhibit 1 in every malpractice case is always the plaintiff patient's medical record(s). Depending on the provider, the medical record can serve as either a shield against liability or a sword used against them. To avoid the latter, doctors must maintain an accurate, logical, detailed, and legible medical record. Failures here can and usually will result in an impaired defense of the case, or an outright loss. Cases can also turn on the failure to implement the plan of action and treatment that was recorded, thereby causing harm to the patient. Conversely, if something is not recorded, it typically cannot be defended in court; therefore, the record should document the full decision-making process, including test results and pertinent patient history, that contributed to the choice of a specific treatment plan. Furthermore, the record must also comprise any discussions related to informed consent not included on the signed form. Above all, because many health care 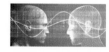 providers enter observations, orders, progress notes, treatment protocols, and the like, it is important that there be a consistency in these notations. Contradictory entries can lead to infighting among health providers and provide supporting evidence for the plaintiff's case that substandard care took place.

Timely documentation in the patient chart means *at the time of treatment*, not when the records are subpoenaed for discovery. At the same time, the medical record must be unaltered and truthful. Once notification of a claim is made, the paper chart should be sequestered under lock and key or the electronic file should have additional levels of password security added. Cases can actually turn on evidence that the health care provider modified the record after being advised of a pending lawsuit. A case in point is *Freeman v. Fisher*.[10] Patient Mary Freeman was taking the blood-thinning medication Coumadin. Five weeks after seeing her physician for a routine PT-INR test, she suffered a massive stroke resulting in severe and permanent neurologic damage. She spent the remainder of her life, about 2.5 years, in a nursing home. While Mary was still in the hospital, her husband Charles stopped by the medical office and retrieved a copy of her records. On filing their claim against the physician for medical malpractice, another set of records was obtained. It was obvious by comparison that the office notes had been supplemented at some point between the two requests: The original records failed to notate any change in the patient's Coumadin dosage at her last office visit, but the second set indicated it had been reduced with a new prescription and the change discussed with the patient. At deposition, the doctor denied altering his records, but when presented with the two different versions, he revised his initial statement. Instead, he stated he must not have charted on the day of the office visit and updated the file at a later point in time. Again, he claimed—and the file indicated—to have written a new prescription for Coumadin based on a reduction to the dosage (the pills Mary had on hand could not have been used for this purpose) and explained the change to the patient. Instead, there was a record at the Freeman's regular pharmacy that Mary's prescription from a previous visit had been refilled. The doctor had not changed the prescription per his deposition testimony and the patient had continued to take the original dose, causing dangerously high PT-INR levels. The lawsuit was settled in favor of the Freemans for a substantial monetary award under court seal.

## Res ipsa loquitur

Sometimes, direct evidence is not available and a patient must depend on circumstantial evidence and the legal doctrine of res ipsa loquitur ("the facts speak for themselves"). Basically, this means the evidence, while not iden-

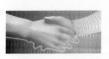

tifying the specific acts or conduct, could not otherwise have occurred unless negligence was present. Commonly used by surgical patients who were not conscious when the alleged injury occurred, there is either an inference or presumption of negligence with 3 required elements. First, in the absence of negligence, the accident would not ordinarily have occurred. It does not require all possible causes of an injury or illness be eliminated, just that the physician's negligence is the most probable cause. Second, the defendant had exclusive control of the "instrumentality" that caused the illness or injury. Exclusive control does not limit responsibility to a single entity. Instead, multiple parties may share control of the instrumentality and thus the responsibility for the breach. Third, the patient did not act in a way that contributed to the negative result. This is protection for the physician who relies on 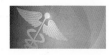 information from the patient to his/her own detriment in treatment decisions.

Again, states treat res ipsa loquitur differently. Most states adopt the inference standard. They will find for the defendant doctor if he/she presents any evidence that it is unlikely his/her conduct was negligent. A minority of states place a higher burden on the physician to defend a res ipsa claim by creating a rebuttable presumption of negligence. In other words, the burden of proof shifts to the defendant, and a lack of sufficient evidence on the part of the practitioner will lead to a verdict in favor of the patient.

Consider the case of a patient who dies of sepsis after a hernia operation. At autopsy, a latex sponge was found left in the peritoneum. There is no direct evidence it was left during the most recent surgery; however, assuming no other possibility, there is also no evidence pointing to who in the operating room actually left it behind. Adding to the complexity, the patient had an allergy to latex of which he was aware but he failed to inform medical personnel. Leaving any foreign object behind during surgery is an example of action that would not occur except for negligence. At the same time, without proof as to the identity of the negligent party, multiple persons present in the operating room may be found individually or jointly responsible for this conduct. This includes the nurse who passes instruments to the surgeon and is responsible for verifying everything is returned, the resident who closed the incision, and the surgeon himself/herself. Finally, there is responsibility on the part of the patient to notify his surgeon and hospital personnel he is allergic to latex and his failure to do so could have contributed to the extent of his infection. Who prevails is a jury determination.

## Negligence Per Se

The theory of negligence per se automatically combines and proves the previously discussed elements of duty and breach, making it extremely plaintiff-friendly. The theory is premised on the existence of a law or statute that is broken: The law creates the duty and the violation of the law creates the breach. In most states, when a defendant has broken the law, the plaintiff then needs to prove only the additional elements of causation and damages. (Some states only permit negligence per se as evidence of the element of breach.) Thus, automatically jumping 2 of the 4 tort law hurdles can be very helpful to a plaintiff.

For the purposes of permitting use of the per se rule, there is a test to determine if a particular statute is applicable to the circumstances of the case. Overall, the actions of the defendant physician must be of the "class 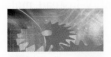 of harm" or the plaintiff patient of the "class of person" the statute was meant to address. Therefore, the statute must clearly define the required standard of contact, the standard must be intended to prevent the type of harm that occurred, the plaintiff is a member of the class of persons the statute was designed to address, and the violation must be a proximate cause of the harm.

For example, in the context of medical malpractice, it would be a violation of the state medical board to administer anesthesia while under the influence of alcohol or drugs. (As a general rule, an intoxicated person owes the same level of care as a sober person unless the intoxication is involuntary.) Any failure by the surgeon to recognize his/her colleague's incapacitation or to report it to through the appropriate channels is also a violation. Thus, such an incident could constitute negligence per se by both parties.

The law does permit a defendant to provide excuses for his/her violation, of which there are five categories.[11] First, violation was reasonable because of the actor's incapacity. Second, the actor neither knew nor should have known of the occasion for compliance. Third, the actor was unable to comply with the statute after reasonable diligence or care. Fourth, an emergency confronted the actor not due to his/her own misconduct. Fifth, compliance involved a greater risk of harm to the actor or others. Even if a provider can use an excuse to show his/her actions are not negligence per se, the patient plaintiff may still move forward with his/her lawsuit based on the traditional *prima facie* approach to medical malpractice this chapter primarily addresses.

## Causation

The third tort element of medical malpractice is causation, both actual and proximate. Each has its own tests that must be shown by the plaintiff in support of his/her claim. Once actual cause is proven, the plaintiff must show how proximate that cause was to the harm.

First, patients must prove that the provider of services directly caused their harm. The primary test used by courts is the "but-for" rule: But for the defendant's conduct, the patient's illness, injury, or death would not have occurred. This test is also applied in the reverse: If there had been no negligence, would the injury have still materialized? If the answer is "yes," then there is no direct causation. For example, a patient has surgery and spontaneously aborts her pregnancy. Had the patient known she was pregnant, the surgeon who failed to inquire into the possibility of this condition would be negligent. However, if the patient did not know she was pregnant and was not able to reveal it even if asked, the doctor is not negligent because the loss of the pregnancy would have occurred regardless.[12]

Second, plaintiffs must show what is known as "proximate" cause. This theory is best explained as a review of the closeness or remoteness of the doctor's actions to the patient's injury, illness, or death. In other words, the closer the proximity, the more likely the physician will be found to have caused the patient's harm. Conversely, a practitioner may be found not liable if his/her actions were "sufficiently removed," even if he/she set in motion the events causing plaintiff's harm. Here, the facts are examined based on three questions: (1) Was the harm caused by the doctor's negligence reasonably foreseeable, (2) was the harm caused by the physician within the scope of the risks created by his negligent behavior, or (3) is the practitioner's liability limited to either the types of injuries or the classes of persons risked by his/her negligence? These questions primarily address how predictive or probable the results were. An affirmative answer to any of these questions will prove the existence of proximate cause. Therefore, the more foreseeable a chain of events and harms, the more likely proximate cause will be found.

There are permissible defenses to causality. Overall, the goal of the defense attorney is to show that the chain of causality was broken or some superseding cause or causes led to the patient's harm. However, not every circumstance will be relevant or even permitted. For example, suicide by the patient in wrongful death cases is treated differently depending on the cause of action. In a traditional tort action, it breaks the chain of causality. The result is that the original or alleged tortfeasor is not the proximate cause of the person's death and the elements are not met. However, medical malpractice is an exception to this general rule. If a patient ultimately commits suicide because of the harm or harms caused by a physician, the latter may still be found negligent for damages related to the original injuries and the patient's death.

Challenges to proving the cause also exist when plaintiffs suffer injury at the hands of multiple parties, also known as tortfeasors. For example, when the conduct of any one of multiple persons can realistically result in the same harm, or when the conduct of each of them combine to cause the injury in a manner that cannot be assigned, all may be found factually responsible. However, if a subsequent party only exacerbates a harm already present when he/she met up with the plaintiff, the defendant is only liable for the additional illness or injury. Consider the case of a young child who presents to an urban emergency room (ER) with a closed skull fracture and subsequently 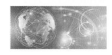 spends 5 weeks in the hospital. Accidently hit in the forehead with a golf club, the patient was sent home with stitches. The ER physician failed to order an X-ray that would have revealed the fracture and ultimately led to immediate surgery. Instead, by the time the patient returned to the ER the next day with symptoms of a concussion, infection had developed. Eventually, she also contracted a second staph infection from a nurse responsible for changing her dressings. Corrective surgery had to be delayed multiple times and the patient was at risk of additional serious injury, requiring constant supervision while hospitalized. In this situation, even though the individual who swung the golf club was the direct cause of the injury and was responsible for the initial ER treatment and subsequent surgery, the ER physician and hospital could be found negligent in causing the infections that resulted in 4 weeks of additional hospital expense, pain and suffering, and future treatments for the recurring blood condition. Essentially, the latter is an intervening cause.

The ultimate conclusion of a discussion of causation is that even though a provider may be found directly responsible for harm to a patient, he/she may still be found not liable if the direct cause was unforeseeable and sufficiently removed from the injury, illness, or death.

## Damages/Death

A successful tort claim requires actual harm to the person in the form of injury, illness, or death. A lack of damage or harm means no tort exists. This is true even if the provider acted negligently by owing a duty and breaching it. Therefore, if a doctor dismisses a patient from his/her practice without following the appropriate protocols—such as failing to provide a 30-day notice—the 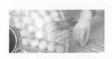 patient will not have a medical malpractice claim if he/she did not go without needed medical services during that time. (Note, this will not necessarily protect the professional from disciplinary action on the part of the state medical board if the patient makes a complaint.)

Injury and illness are very broad concepts and can range from temporary, curable conditions to permanent impairments. Primarily, they are physical, tangible disorders that are patent or otherwise easy to prove. Both include physical harms requiring additional corrective treatment or surgery as well as conditions that cannot be repaired, such as the loss of a limb due to mistaken amputation or the failure to appropriately treat an underlying condition before it reaches a critical stage. This latter theory of harm is known as loss of opportunity and equates to the difference between diagnosis, treatment, and recovery that would have occurred under an acceptable standard of care and what occurred under negligent care. For example, a provider may be found negligent for the percentage of lost opportunity when, timely diagnosed, the patient had a 75% chance of survival but instead was not diagnosed until there was a 25% chance of survival.

Injury or illness may also include psychologic or mental conditions. NIED is permitted in most jurisdictions as a separate, stand-alone cause of action for medical malpractice. The duty is found in the provider's responsibility to protect a patient's emotional well-being. A majority of states only require a plaintiff to show behavioral changes or differences. Otherwise, a minority of states are divided as to whether a claim of physical harm or contact must accompany NIED or whether NIED must be proven with a physical manifestation of stress. Stated another way, to show negligence, either a physical harm caused the NIED or NIED caused a physical harm. In California, for example, doctors are held liable for emotional stress caused by negligent misdiagnosis. A minority of states analyze emotional harm using the same negligence test used for physical injuries.

In the case of patient injury, loss of consortium may also be brought by family members. Again, the family member is the plaintiff and he/she must prove a complete loss of companionship for a definite period. Typically, spouses may recover for social and sexual companionship and parents may recover for the companionship of a minor child only. Children are unable to recover for the loss of a parent's companionship.

When death is the injury, states recognize and permit 2 types of legal action, either wrongful death or survivor. Two major differences exist between the 2: Who is eligible to file the claim and what types of damages are available. In a wrongful death action, the patient's estate files suit on behalf of any beneficiaries the patient supported financially. The primary type of recovery is loss of support. Some states also allow loss of consortium, punitive damages, lost guidance and nurture for minors, and costs for funeral and burial services. Conversely, survivor actions are brought in the patient's name by the spouse, child, parent, or another state-recognized relationship of the patient. The claimant is eligible to bring the same negligence action the patient would have had. As such, the damages belong to the patient and recovery extends to predeath medical expenses, lost earnings, and pain and suffering.

Finally, most states also recognize wrongful conception/pregnancy and wrongful birth claims. Gynecologists and urologists who perform sterilization procedures should take note; physicians can be found liable for damages related to the creation of an unwanted pregnancy or the lifetime support—including college—of the resulting child. However, in most states, liability will only be assigned if the child was born with physical or mental disabilities that result in extraordinary support expenses.

---

## Recovery and Settlement

Refer again to the case of Baby Alys. How did the Pennsylvania jury decide $100 million was appropriate reimbursement for the injuries caused by defendants' negligence? By the time the case made it to trial, Alys was around 5 years old. Her birth mother—who was 17 years old when Alys was born—had given her up for adoption 3 years earlier. Her adoptive parents had likely already incurred millions of dollars in medical and other related expenses. For example, in addition to Alys's bills for the hospitals, doctors, surgeries, and ancil- 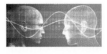 lary medical services that started when she was born, her mother and father had to spend more money to get her home. They needed to either retrofit where they lived or buy a new home to accommodate her wheelchair, oxygen, and hospital-grade crib and beds. They needed to buy a handicap-rated van to transport her back and forth to doctor visits, rehab, and family and social events. Because Alys requires full-time care, they have probably had to hire home care nurses on a permanent basis. And, it is very possible her mother or father also had to leave a job or career to stay home with her and to coordinate her care. But what of Alys's future needs? It is probable she will require additional surgeries to maintain her feeding tubes. Alys's inability to walk, breathe on her own, and the like means she is more susceptible to pneumonia and other complications. As she grows, her wheelchair and bed will need to be replaced. As she gains weight, additional equipment will be needed to move her. Her chronic conditions are bound to become worse over time and millions of dollars more will be spent on her care. Finally, Alys will never go to school—except perhaps to special public programs for brief social interaction—nor will she ever get married or financially support herself. Alys is very likely to die before her parents and they will be required to pay for her funeral. For determination of the compensatory damages, the testimony of an expert or experts, such as economists and life planners, would have been needed to paint a picture for the jury of the financial equivalents of all of these circumstances. Even the already incurred expenses would have been under scrutiny for their reasonableness and relatedness to Alys's injuries. At the same time, the plaintiff's attorney would have requested punitive damages in an amount necessary to send a message to the defendants—and other medical professionals—regarding their negligence. To accomplish this, the attorney would have used expert testimony to illustrate the difference between Alys's anticipated medical condition at the time of her birth (related to her premature status) and what has resulted from the negligence of the medical providers. At the same time, he/she would have presented a "Day in the Life" video to the jury proving exactly what Alys and her parents experience daily and then convert it into long-term financial and emotional perspectives for the period of her life expectancy.[13]

## Recovery

Medical malpractice lawsuits allow plaintiffs to seek many types of damages. The primary recovery for negligent tort claims is compensatory damages. These awards are designed to make them economically whole by putting them back in the position they were in before the injury. This is accomplished 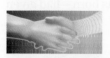 by using compensatory damages to reimburse a patient or family for identifiable and calculatable economic losses related to past and future medical expenses, costs associated with providing ongoing handicap accommodations, and loss of future earnings. Previously incurred expenses for which actual bills exist require no calculation. On the other hand, future expenses are less concrete and require the assistance of skilled economists and life planners. In addition to estimating the costs of the future care and needs of the plaintiff, rates of economic growth and inflation also need to be included in the calculation. Many life factors are also taken into consideration including the plaintiff's age and life expectancy, pre- and postinjury earning capacities, level of previous activity, and dependence on the injured by other members of the family. Noneconomic compensation is also available for actual physical injury, disfigurement, pain and suffering, and emotional distresses such as the loss of enjoyment of life. These are not tangible; they cannot and are not reflected on a bill or receipt. It is often up to a jury to determine how 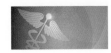 much these injuries are worth (some state statutes include actuarial charts that place exact values on specific limbs both for injury/loss of use and amputation). Finally, punitive damages are awarded when a defendant's conduct is wanton and reckless. Even though states cap these latter damages by statute, they typically reflect the highest costs to defendants. Punitive damages are designed to send a message because they take into consideration the overall unconscionability of the defendant's actions. The more catastrophic the injury, the higher the damages and the possibility of a structured settlement (payments made over a time). In 2009, the average inpatient malpractice award was $362 965 while the average outpatient award was $290 111.[14]

## Jury Trial

The decision to move forward with a jury trial, versus settling a case, is one of legal strategy. It must be made with adequate consultation and understanding between the defendant and his/her attorney. Depending on the facts of the case and the characteristics of the parties, jury trials can be a gamble between multiple resolutions. First, juries may negatively view defendant physicians as cocky, overconfident, conceited, and void of concern regarding the consequences of their actions. Juries will award damages to plaintiffs just to send a message to the defendant or defendants. On the other hand, plaintiffs are just as much at risk of losing in a jury trial. Juries may see plaintiffs as contributorily negligent for their injuries. Or, plaintiff claims may be viewed by juries as frivolous actions meant to harass a provider or to go after deep pockets. Finally, juries may sometimes compromise with their verdict. They will find the physician negligent but may only award the plaintiff a nominal, or the statutorily-capped, amount. Lower awards occur because modern juries are hesitant to award large verdicts because of jealousy of the plaintiff or the belief a large award will increase their own health care costs.

A jury verdict is not the final word, however. Both parties have the right to appeal the decision even if the verdict was in their favor. For example, some jurisdictions permit a winning plaintiff to request additions, also known as additur, to the awarded amount. At the same time, most states allow the losing defendant to make a request of remittitur for the purpose of reducing the judgment. A losing party may also appeal the final verdict outright.

## Settlement

Approximately 93% of medical malpractice claims end in settlement.[15] Although one or both parties may think they are giving up the opportunity for their "day in court" to tell their story, settlement reduces the risks associated 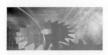 with a jury trial. However, it also means that a defendant provider must accept the consequences associated with an adverse malpractice decision and appropriately report it. Consultation with the attorney helps to weigh the risks and benefits of a settlement against the possible results of a jury trial. This decision may also require the input of the insurance carrier and a medical corporation.

## Comparative and Joint and Several Liability

Back to Alys. In addition to the total damage award of $100 million, the jury had to decide the issue of comparative negligence. This means it had to calculate what percentage of fault to assign to each defendant. In this case, it assigned 90% ($90 million) to the first hospital and the cardiothoracic surgeon, and 10% ($10 million) to the children's hospital and the neonatologists. Although these amounts were definitely meant to send a message—and they probably succeeded—the likelihood Alys actually received anything close to this amount is low for many reasons, but primarily because of coverage limits on medical malpractice insurance and the ability of the defendants to pay. Instead, there was probably a substantial settlement that will remain under seal. However, the final amount will still be divided and paid based on a 90/10 assignment of comparative fault.[13]

Although no physician welcomes any medical malpractice judgment, regardless of the amount, those joined with other defendants may consider 10% liability to be a lucky escape. Unfortunately, this can create a false sense of security when viewed in light of the doctrine of joint and several liability. This doctrine basically equates to the theory that any defendant to a group action could be required to pay a judgment in full. They then must further use the court system to obtain reimbursement from their codefendants.Therefore, the larger, better-insured urban children's hospital found to be only 10% negligent could be forced to pay 100% of the awarded judgment to the plaintiff while also expending additional time, effort, and legal expense to obtain reimbursement from the smaller, possibly lesser-insured community hospital for its 90% share of the liability.

## Defenses

In addition to defending or countering medical custom—a theory unique to medical malpractice negligence—tort law also provides physicians defending themselves against malpractice claims with options that might reduce or terminate liability. These are called "affirmative defenses" because they place the burden of proof on the defendant doctor. In other words, the plaintiff with the burden of proof regarding the practitioner's liability does not have the initial burden of proving the insufficiency of any proffered defenses, although they will be ready to argue against them. Some defenses, such as statute of limitations, are procedural, while others, such as assumption of the risk, are substantive.

## Procedural

Procedural defenses are most often found in state statutes. As such, plaintiffs and jurors may view them as strictly technical, creating "outs" or excuses for a physician who is otherwise negligent. In addition to statutes of limitations, Good Samaritan statutes and contractual clauses of waiver of liability and arbitration are examples of procedural defenses.

Statutes of limitations are both straightforward and complicated. Regulated by statute, as the name suggests, they vary from state to state; however, most require that medical malpractice claims be filed within 2 or 3 years of the injury or harm.[16] They also permit an extension to the statute of limitations by providing that notification of intent to file be made to the potential defendant. For example, in Ohio, the statute of limitations may be extended by 6 months when the plaintiff patient provides what is known as a "180-Day Letter" of notification to the physician, as long as it is sent before the statutory time runs out.[17] This letter can also serve the dual purpose of requesting medical records for an attorney or expert to review. What is not always clear is when the statute of limitations begins to run. This is due to a plaintiff not being able to pinpoint the actual date of their injury. When this occurs, courts will apply the "knew or should have known" standard for timing. The effect of this is to toll or delay the statute of limitations so that it begins at the point in time when a reasonable person knew or should have known of their injury as well as the actual and proximate causes of it. Thus, a patient whose symptoms do not begin until after the traditional statute of limitations has expired may still be able to bring a negligence lawsuit against his/her health care provider(s). Another extension available to minors should be of particular concern to pediatric surgeons. When an injury to a minor occurs, the clock on the statute of limitations does not begin until the patient reaches the statutory age of majority, usually 18 years.

Good Samaritan statutes can protect medical personnel who provide emergency care in good faith. The most common scenario is when the services needed to treat the emergency are not within the scope of education, training, or experience of the render- 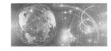 ing provider, but they are given as the best effort to assist the individual in need. This includes services provided either outside or inside of the hospital environment. For example, a physician who fails to prevent a customer in a restaurant from choking is equally protected from liability in that death as an ER physician called to assist in the maternity ward during a crisis when the mother dies after delivery.[18] States are split as to whether the demonstration of gross negligence—such as preventing a more qualified individual from rendering care—bars the use of the Good Samaritan defense.

Although rare, written agreements can exist between providers and patients for medical services. These are mostly used in situations of cash-based elective surgeries and other procedures, voluntary experimental treatments, and the use of medical devices. These contracts are distinguishable from informed consent and insurance assignment agreements in that they likely include traditional arbitration and waiver of liability clauses. These clauses limit the parties' ability to litigate damages. Arbitration clauses control the forum and methods by which claims can be resolved by removing them from the courts, and waivers of liability completely indemnify the physician or device company against liability. Although these clauses may provide protection against patient lawsuits, physicians and medical organizations 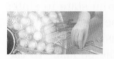 need to remain mindful of the positions patients are in as unsophisticated contracting parties. Form contracts that provide no recourse for customization or alteration by patients, including the ability to consult with an attorney before signing, are known as adhesion contracts and will not always hold up under court scrutiny. In these situations, courts have the option of voiding the entire contract or only voiding those sections and clauses found to be in violation of traditional contract rules.

## Substantive

Substantive defenses have been established over time by tort law. They are determined on a case-by-case basis and are highly dependent on the facts. Unlike the procedural defenses above, however, substantive defenses serve to reduce the physician's liability by showing that the patient had some level of knowledge and control over the events that led to his/her illness, injury, or death. In addition to assumption of the risk, other substantive defenses include contributory negligence and superseding causes.

Assumption of the risk is the theory that patients understand the hazards related to their medical treatment and knowingly accept them anyway. Although the assumption may be implied by the patient's actions—such as pursuing consultation, scheduling treatment, and presenting on the day of the procedure—there is a requirement that the patient have actual knowledge, provided by the clinician, of the reasonably known risks. The patient must make a personal determination that the risks associated with the treatment are rare enough or are outweighed by the potential benefits. This burden is most likely met by obtaining a valid informed consent, which will provide a higher level of information by expressing it in a written document. Although assumption of the risk is not an available defense in emergency situations, it may be used when an authorized representative makes the decision on behalf of an incapacitated patient, which is the additional fact the clinician must prove. Surgeons must bear in mind, however, that patients cannot prospectively agree to negligent care. This means their consent is based on the assumption of the risk reasonable in the absence of negligence. For instance, an ear, nose, and throat physician cannot rely on an informed consent listing hoarseness as a possible side effect for polyp removal when it occurred because the doctor cut the larynx in error.

Additionally, a patient's lack of compliance with physician advice or recommendations could result in contributory negligence. In some cases, this will absolutely absolve the physician of liability, whereas in others, it may only reduce it. For example, the patient who aspirates during surgery and dies could be found wholly contributorily negligent because he/she did not follow *nil per os* or nothing by mouth orders and did not admit to having eaten for fear the procedure would be canceled. On the other hand, the physician or hospital could be found partially negligent for failing to provide the patient with a full explanation of the risks of eating before receiving anesthesia. Test results are another area ripe for the contributory negligence defense. Patients often neglect to obtain needed blood and diagnostic testing recommended and ordered by their physicians. However, this patient behavior is not an absolute defense for the physician; failure of the doctor to adequately explain why a particular test is important, or to follow up on missing results, could create liability if the patient experiences damages due to delay of treatment.

Finally, as previously discussed in relation to proximate cause, a superseding event that worsens an initial injury caused by the defendant practitioner may erase professional liability altogether. The additional event must have been unforeseeable. For example, a cardiologist in a rural community performs a cardiac catheterization during which he nicks a major vessel. Unable to make the repair himself, the physician arranges for an immediate transfer by ambulance to an urban trauma center 50 miles away. En route, a semitruck pulls out in front of the ambulance and causes a collision, throwing the patient out of the vehicle and killing him instantly. Because the accident was unforeseeable, the injury caused by the doctor during the medical procedure could be outweighed by the events of the accident that caused the patient's death. If foreseeability was present, the event is considered "intervening" and will not protect the defendant physician.

## The Effects of a Malpractice Claim/Award

Regardless of whether defendant doctors ultimately prevail, malpractice claims have serious, long-term professional consequences. Primarily, physicians have a duty to report all malpractice claims made, including those 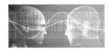 pending or resolved. In addition to notifying the National Practitioner Data

Bank, the centralized authority that tracks and certifies physicians, doctors are also obligated to disclose the status of all claims to facilities where they have or are requesting privileges and to insurance companies with which they have participation agreements. Any failure to report could constitute material misrepresentation by the practitioner and place his/her medical license and privileges at risk.

A minimum amount of coverage—higher for surgeons because of the increased risk of their specialties—is required by facilities, health insurance companies, and other professional contracts. But claims, settlements, and jury awards influence liability coverage. As with private insurance, medical malpractice premiums increase based on claims history: A high volume of claims may result in higher premiums or a loss of coverage. And when the coverage is not enough to fully pay plaintiffs' awards, the provider becomes personally liable for the difference.

Medical malpractice also creates noneconomic losses for the health care industry. Providers who practice in areas with high costs for liability coverage may consciously avoid riskier treatments or procedures, or they may change specialties. Thus, some very qualified surgeons will not be available to provide care for patients who need it.

## Defendant Trial Strategy

Defense of a malpractice lawsuit requires a high level of strategy. Serious decisions must be made to determine what direction the defense will take. As discussed above, for example, will an attempt at settlement be immediate, or will the case make it to a jury? Thought must also be given to addressing witnesses in a way that does not victimize or psychologically "reinjure" the patient. More of these vital considerations are discussed below.

The most important step for any defendant physician is choosing the right lawyer, even though in many cases the liability insurance carrier assigns the attorney, leaving the defendant without a lot of input. Under these circumstances, the physician needs to make sure he/she has a good rapport with the assigned representation. If such a relationship does not exist, the doctor should not hesitate to inform the insurance company and to make alternate arrangements as soon as possible to avoid jeopardizing the case. Regardless of on whom the responsibility of hiring the lawyer falls, the defendant can and should assist in verifying his/her level of expertise. Primarily, a malpractice 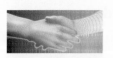 defense attorney must be well versed in medicine on his/her own and should not have to ask the physician client to explain medical conditions or procedures. Similar to a patient looking for an experienced surgeon, a malpractice attorney should have a minimum amount of knowledge, experience, and success in his/her field to create confidence in his/her client. In addition to having some medical knowledge in his/her own right, a competent attorney will also be proficient in modern trial practices. Specifically, the use of technology and models—in the form of computerized simulations—can go a long way in making complicated medical explanations easier for a jury to understand. At the same time, focus groups may help the defense in determining how a jury is likely to render its verdict.

Once the lawyer has been identified, the defendant physician must regularly meet and work with him/her. In other words, it is vital that the doctor participate in his/her own defense. Again, the lawyer-client relationship very much parallels the doctor-patient relationship: The attorney provides the 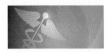 expert advice and facilitates the process while the client determines the focus and direction of the case. Failing to participate ties the attorney's hands and only makes the defense more difficult.

The defendant practitioner can also assist the attorney by researching expert witnesses, including those he/she will use in defending his/her own case and those the plaintiff plans to introduce. It is important to anticipate all the strengths and weaknesses in any expert witness's background that can help or hinder a case. Luckily, the Internet has decreased the figurative size of the medical community, and information on providers and educators likely to serve as expert witnesses is easily obtainable. Also, the witness's reputation in the medical community by those who attended the same institutions or worked with them may prove invaluable.

Whether the surgeon is acting as an expert, testifying as a witness to events for or against a colleague, or appearing on his/her own behalf, there are guidelines medical professionals need to follow. First, as stated earlier, the standard of proof is a "reasonable degree of medical probability." This means the outcome was more likely than not. An expert witness need only show the negative result was or was not probable, but for the negligence, which is numerically equivalent to 51% or more. Second, all witnesses need to make medicine understandable. Doctors must resist using obscure and technical medical terms and instead must explain conditions and procedures in layperson's terms. As soon as a witness talks above a juror's level of understanding, he/she will lose his/her attention and sympathy. Third, additional ways to avoid alienating a jury is to be professional, appear humble, and cooperate with the attorney conducting the questioning. Fourth, the witness needs to address the "why" factor. Jurors want to be given another plausible explanation for why the patient appears in the current physical condition—in a wheelchair, missing a limb, disfigured, and so forth—or is deceased, if the defendant or defendants are not responsible.

Finally, most medical malpractice attorneys prefer the concept of a joint defense. When a plaintiff names multiple defendants such as physicians, facilities, and corporations, using the same lawyer to coordinate the defense can have positive results. As long as the interests of the parties are not in overt conflict—where proving one party's lack of liability directly implicates the liability of a codefendant—the same attorney can be used for the group. Otherwise, the plaintiff's strategy will be to "divide and conquer" by playing the defendants against each other.

# Conclusion

Although most physicians will be unable to avoid a malpractice claim altogether, they can take preemptive action to successfully defend one. Proactive physicians will be well informed about the claim process and how their actions could satisfy the required elements, will follow procedures to maintain compliance with best practices, will remain current as to accepted medical guidelines and standards of care, will be adequately insured, will notify their malpractice insurance carrier immediately on receipt of notification of any claims made, and will commit to meet and work with their attorney in their own defense. Physicians should also document any potential claims—before they are made—based on unusual events or results; if the practitioner is part of a larger organization, this usually means reporting the circumstances to a centralized risk department.

Finally, some medical malpractice attorneys may suggest that an honest and sincere apology can go a long way toward deflecting a lawsuit. Patients and family members who are given answers and are able to see the human, humble side of the physician who is capable of making a mistake but also accepting of responsibility, may be less likely to sue.

# References

1. The National Law Journal, *A Premature Baby Wins $100 Million in Court; Big Gets Bigger; Verdicts: The Big Numbers of 2000; Medical Malpractice.* Vol. 23 (February 19, 2001); see also *Albright v. Cavarocchi*, Phil. Co. CCP No. 97-09-3379, 2000 Nat. Jury Verdict Review LEXIS 2184 (October 20, 2000).
2. Mello MM, et al. National Costs of the Medical Liability System, *Health Aff.* 2010; 29(9):1569–1577. Available from: http://content.healthaffairs.org/content/29/9/1569.full.
3. Jill Van De Bos, et al. The $17 billion problem: the annual cost of measurable medical errors, *Health Aff.* 2011;30(4):596–603. Available from: http://content.healthaffairs.org/content/30/4/596.full.
4. Jena AB, et al. Malpractice risk according to physician specialty. *N Engl J Med.* 2011;365:629. ("Among physicians in low-risk specialties, 36% were projected to face their first claim by the age of 45 years, as compared with 88% of physicians in high-risk specialties. By the age of 65 years, 75% of physicians in low-risk specialties and 99% of those in high-risk specialties were projected to face a claim.").
5. The elements are discussed in more detail below.
6. While this discussion is directed at physicians, hospitals are also subject to medical malpractice claims. For the seminal case that recognized facilities as providers of medical services and first applied the theories of direct and vicarious liability to them, see *Darling v. Charleston Memorial Community Hospital*, 211 N.E.2d (Ill. 1965).
7. 61 Am Jur 2d Physicians, Surgeons, and Other Healers § 320 (2nd 2015) ("'Testimony,' in the context of the requirement that negligence in a medical malpractice case be established by expert testimony, is defined as evidence that a competent witness under oath or affirmation gives at a trial or in an affidavit or deposition; it may include in-person testimony given at trial, a deposition, or a written affidavit or declaration.").

8. *Hawes v. Chua*, 769 A.2d 797, 810 (D.C.2001) (citing *Davis v. Immediate Med. Services, Inc.*, 80 Ohio St.3d 10, 1997-Ohio-363, 684 N.E.2d 292; 1997. ("The substantial connection analysis looks to whether a witness has 'a sufficient degree of 'connection' with the liability insurance carrier to justify allowing proof of this relationship as a means of attacking the credibility of the witness.'").

9. *Canterbury v. Spence*, 464 F.2d 772, at syllabus (D.C.Cir.1972) ("Physician has duty, as facet of due care, to warn of dangers lurking in proposed treatment and to impart information which patient has every right to expect; reasonable explanation required means generally informing patient in nontechnical terms as to what is at stake, i.e., the therapy alternatives open to him, goals expected or believed to be achieved, and risks which may ensue from particular treatment and no treatment.").

10. *Freemna v. Fisher*, G-4801-CI-200802452, Ohio Common Pleas Court, Lucas County (03/08/2010) (Plaintiff's name misspelled in the online court docket).

11. Restatement (2d) of Torts, §288A, Excuses for violation of a statute.

12. See, eg, *Salinetro v. Nystrom*, 341 So. 2d 1059 (Fla.App.1977).

13. Claudia Ginanni, *Award Compensates 5-Year-Old for Injuries After Birth*, The Legal Intelligencer; October 23, 2000. Available from: http://www.klinespecter.com/sites/www.klinespecter.com/files/Vlasny.pdf.

14. Bishop TF, et al. Paid malpractice claims for adverse events in inpatient and outpatient settings. *JAMA*. June 15, 2011;305(23):2427.

15. David Goguen JD. *National Medical Malpractice Statistics*. Available from: http://www.medicalmalpractice.com/national-medical-malpractice-facts.cfm#.

16. In Ohio and some other states, the statute of limitations is one year from the later of (1) the date of the malpractice, (2) the termination of the doctor-patient relationship, or (3) the date on which the injury was or should have been "reasonably discovered" by the patient.

17. O.R.C. § 2305.113(B)(1).

18. *Hirpa v. IHC Hosp.*, 948 P.2d 785 (1997).

# 38

# E-mail: The EMR

Lloyd A. Jacobs, MD

PROLOGUE ▶ In nearly every survey of practicing surgeons asked to specify factors believed to contribute to burnout, the electronic medical record (EMR) is the first or second. The surgeon is faced with a difficult set of choices: forego the meaningful sustaining work of being present to the patient or give up large blocks of time to the EMR that had previously been devoted to leisure. Expensive workarounds may also be tried. Furthermore, e-mail messages and requests from patients may be intrinsic and inappropriate.

The ubiquity of electronic communication modalities is presenting significant ethical dilemmas to surgeons and to the medical profession at large. There are no quick and easy answers.

The surgeon has an obligation toward the acquisition and handling of patient information. There are many who argue that the memory, accessibility, and the indelible nature of information, which the electronic age has brought, constitute a revolutionary chapter for civilization. Some argue that the mental processes of human beings have been changed. Certainly, the so-called information age has brought new dilemmas to the practice of surgery.

We should begin where we have so often found a beginning: in the Hippocratic writings. The oath addresses the handling of patient information and the obligation to the confidential use and guardianship of it. Historically, surgeons and physicians have been careful of this obligation and, as a general statement, have executed their obligation to confidentiality well.

The Hippocratic Oath avoids a clear delineation of what constitutes confidential material but relies on the generalization: "…that which on no account one must spread abroad…." This, of course, leaves the practicing surgeon and the surgical resident with little guidance as to what must be so treated. Societal context also is of little help: the norms are changing rapidly and new communication strategies are being invented nearly daily. The best way, I believe, to define what fits the Hippocratic category is to remind ourselves of the surgeon's role as the agent of the patient. Under this rubric, the surgeon is obliged to do not what he/she would want himself/herself but what the patient wants or would want. If, therefore, the patient has confidentiality concerns about a cancer diagnosis, the surgeon is obliged to try to meet his/her needs. This is not straightforward, however, in our world of evaluation and management codes and insurance claims. Once again, the surgeon is called on to strive for an unreachable goal.

Some aspects of patient confidentiality are unequivocal: Do not talk in elevators or cafeterias and such are taught to us as medical students. It is the new world of electronic media that confounds, but Facebook, e-mail, Twitter, and Instagram are best seen as merely new and more efficient ways that information may be "spread abroad." Nothing that the patient may deem confidential should be committed to these media without careful thought. Painful lessons are widely known implying that nothing committed to these media is irretrievable to a determined hacker or gossip. There will be a new electronic communication app released next week or next year; the same principles will apply. Mere redaction of identifiers will not suffice. Encryption currently is insufficiently widespread to make these communications foolproof. The surgeon should consciously move from a stance in which he/she judged what should on no account be spread abroad to a posture where the patient's desires are given great weight and usually prevail. The patient must consent to his/her information being supplied to insurers or to similar agencies. Such permission is often included on consent forms in hospitals and in other practice settings, but what is stated above once again sets an unattainable goal for the work-a-day surgeon; the moral act is in the striving not in the perfection.

Dr Elizabeth Rao was already at home when she remembered that she had promised to contact her colleague, a year her junior, who was scheduled to participate in a liver transplant operation the next day. Rao dialed her colleague's cell; no answer. She e-mailed the following message: "Tomorrow's 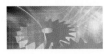 liver has active Hep C. Be careful!" She went out for the evening feeling that she had kept her promise.

Regretfully, the transplanted liver precipitated a hyperacute rejection phenomenon. The patient was listed as an emergency for any available liver, but before one became available she slipped into hepatic coma and then renal failure. She died on the sixth posttransplant day.

The patient's chart, the EMR, and the institution's data banks were all subjected to a review of an unexpected death. Dr Rao was dismayed to find her e-mail in the package for review. Worse, the attending transplant surgeon had entered a chart note almost simultaneously with Rao's e-mail. It said: Hep C inactive, patient a good risk for transplant.

E-mail correspondence is increasingly being used as a communication tool between a patient and his/her surgeon. The surgeon has an obligation to be at least minimally aware of whatever encryption or lack of it exists in any e-mail system he/she uses. The field of cybersecurity is rapidly changing; there is no stability of practice patterns in this area. The patient's needs and desires should be governed. In e-mail correspondence with patients, formal consent may be inadequate: The surgeon should wait for the patient to mention potentially sensitive data or specifically ask permission to transmit such information. The best generalization is to assume that no electronic transmission is immune to hacking and that any electronic transmission may ultimately become public.

Most hospitals and many well-run practices have policies forbidding browsing by employees without a demonstrable "need to know" information in the record. These cases have often involved celebrity patients and mere curiosity on the part of employees. Many such employees have had their employment terminated for cause. It is important to notice that this strict prohibition may also include surgeons and surgical trainees.

Bewildering complexities have accompanied the introduction of governmental incentives for the EMR. Clearly, the availability of prior health information in a near instantaneous way is a great advantage to the surgeon and  the patient in an emergency. The sharing throughout a system of hospitals or other consortia extends this advantage widely. Even in routine settings, the trending of data values or the avoidance of administration of medicines to which a patient is allergic has been facilitated. The price of these advantages is significant, however.

Patients are increasingly reluctant to reveal certain aspects of their medical histories. For example, many patients will not mention or refuse to discuss details of a history of psychiatric illness without assurance that such information will not be entered into the EMR. Such requests pit the surgeon as patient advocate against the rules of his/her hospital, group practice, or even insurers and government agencies. It should be noted that, historically, most psychiatrists have kept separate "personal" notes about their patients.

Many surgeons have resorted to "white lies" under these circumstances, with all the potential pitfalls related to that practice. The surgeon must learn to say, "I'm sorry I cannot do that," or "I need to let you know that I will need to...." Still, we have a deep and venerable commitment to hold confidentially information that patients would not wish to have "spread abroad."

The practice of "white lies" injures the surgeon more than the patient or agency lied to. It "hardens one within and petrifies the feeling."[1] Even more injurious to the surgeon is the impact on his/her productivity and sense of well-being that results from the requirements of the EMR. Thousands of anecdotes speak to this impact. An accomplished pediatric urologist was admitted to a prominent cancer hospital shortly before and somewhat after the implementation of an EMR at that hospital. He speaks of a dramatic change. The thoughtfulness and solicitude of the staff were radically changed, he reports. Eye contact in the examination room is reported to have diminished. A computer screen has, it seems, the power to mesmerize; surgeons are reported to behave distractedly with the examination room device. The surgeon has an obligation to consciously and actively build a relationship with his patients. To understand fully the nature of this relationship requires a brief digression to consider the notion of "presence." The surgeon must be "present" to his patients. The idea is best grasped by avoiding structuralism, which would grant solidity to the concept. Presence is the nonsubstantial, fleeting, but very real center of a person's being; it contributes power to the development of the relationship, and it is the critical ingredient of that which creates the surgeon-patient relationship.

Absence of "presence" and the attendant failure of the development of a relationship are most often attributable to the surgeon's deficiency. Distractions, multiple demands, and health issues contribute to a failure of "presence." And apropos to our train of thought here, obsession with the EMR, concern for coding accuracy, and other documentation issues have the potential to render the surgeon "not present" when in dialogue with the patient. In common parlance, his/her mind is elsewhere.

For those conscientious persons who attempt to do their recording after the patient has gone, many hours are required and tricks of memory create inaccuracies at an alarming rate. As so often throughout this book we have identified a problem that is impossible of solution, immediately at least. Perhaps new apps will ameliorate some of this dilemma.

Patient portals exemplify a special aspect of the EMR. Many patients perceive them to be a boon to their sense of autonomy and control and therefore to their well-being. But recently, Dr Ellen Friedman, an otolaryngologist, injected another note into the discussion. She describes having received an e-mail describing the histology of her own colonoscopic biopsy specimen.[2] Her comments speak less about her need for information or confidentiality and more and eloquently about the anxiety produced by this event and her need for face-to-face communication in such circumstances. She felt the communication to be impersonal, almost brusque and inadequate to her needs for emotional support. Although Friedman's point may often be valid, it 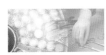 once again points out a difficult trade-off: timeliness of communication and the nature of the communication compete.

The use of white lies is detrimental to the surgeon. The surgeon as a patient may himself/herself experience a distracted caregiver. However, the greatest impact of the EMR on the surgeon is a sense of loss of meaning.

Evidence showing that the EMR increases surgeon stress, renders personal time management more difficult, and contributes to burnout has begun to accumulate. In another chapter the phenomenon of burnout is more fully discussed, and its etiology is related not only to the factors mentioned but also to a sense of meaninglessness derived from ambiguity or absence of ethical norms, particularly when new rules and practice requirements provoke division. A world with a plethora of new rules and an inattention to ethical nuances seems accurately to describe some aspects of the milieu in which modern surgeons are constrained to work. We have emphasized that the "striving for" is that which is of value. In the area of EMRs, it seems difficult to know what it is for which one should strive.

# References

1. Burns R. *Epistle to a Young Friend*; 1786.
2. Friedman EM. A piece of my mind. You've got mail. *JAMA*. 2016;315(21):2275–2276.

# 39 Social Media

Lisa M. Kodadek, MD

PROLOGUE ▶ There is little need in the spring of 2017 to assert that social media have changed our world. The domestic politics of the United States have been changed, probably forever. Wars and rebellions across the world have been influenced by the advent of ubiquitous social media platforms. The workplace has changed. It is no surprise, therefore, that the practice of surgery has also changed, albeit slowly and hesitantly. It has been conjectured that the very mind of humankind is being changed in ways that are difficult to predict.

Still, Dr Lisa M. Kodadek analyzes and predicts with great perspicacity what the impact of this new connectedness will have on the surgeon's day-to-day work and the new ethical dilemmas it will bring. Persons the age of most practicing surgeons today may not be as competent to that task as is Dr Kodadek.

Dr Lisa M. Kodadek is a general surgery resident in the Department of Surgery at Johns Hopkins University School of Medicine.

## Abstract

Social media refers to virtual Internet communities where user-generated interactive content is shared with others through a standard and universally accessible interface. Social media is used by many surgeons for both personal and professional networking; many national surgical organizations and medical institutions maintain a presence on social media to promote their missions. Although this technology confers many benefits, it is important to recognize and protect against potential misuse. The era of social media introduces new challenges, but the traditional ethics of medical professionalism must be upheld and applied to this technology. It is important for surgeons to accept personal responsibility and accountability for the use of social media platforms and to take action to ensure patient privacy is protected and professionalism is maintained online. Furthermore, as the digital communication culture values expediency and brevity, education of medical students and surgical trainees may need to focus more on specific skills such as face-to-face conversation and critical reflective thinking. This chapter will focus on ethical considerations for surgeons who use social media in both personal and professional capacities.

## Introduction

Social media refers to virtual Internet communities where user-generated interactive content (information, photos, videos) is shared with others through a standard universally accessible interface such as a computer or mobile phone.[1] Popular sites for social and professional networking include Facebook, with 1.23 billion daily users,[2] and Twitter, which publishes over 500 million user updates daily ("tweets").[3] A wide array of other social media platforms are available and are used for many different purposes. For example, social media may allow for collaborative online projects (Wikipedia),[4] content sharing (YouTube)[5] as well as blogging and microblogging (Myspace, Tumblr).[6,7] Various social media sites are geared at professionals (LinkedIn)[8] and even, specifically, health science and medical professionals (ResearchGate, Doximity).[9,10] These sites are meant to allow professionals to connect with one another, network with employers and colleagues, and promote and disseminate scientific research. Furthermore, various national organizations use mainstream social media sites such as Twitter to promote their mission, highlight their events, including major national meetings,[11,12] and even host online Twitter Journal Clubs to discuss new scientific research.[13,14] Social media allows individuals, including surgeons, to engage others in a manner once unfathomable. Although social

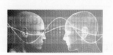

media confers many benefits, and revolutionizes the way we communicate, it is important to recognize and protect against misuse. The basic ethics of medical professionalism must be upheld in the era of social media, and it is important to accept personal responsibility and accountability for the use of these platforms.

## Background

Social media is the hallmark of Web 2.0. The term Web 2.0, coined in 1999, has been used to refer to the second stage of development of the World Wide Web (WWW), which was highlighted by a move from static proof-of-concept Web pages to dynamic user-generated Web content.[1] The WWW is an information space where resources are located by Uniform Resource Locators, 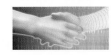 and data communication occurs through an application known as Hypertext Transfer Protocol.[15] The WWW is accessed through the Internet, which is a global system of computer networks that links devices using Transmission Control Protocol and Internet Protocol, collectively known as the Internet Protocol suite.[16] Web 2.0 applications are designed to be either open or closed in terms of accessibility. Open sites, such as Twitter, broadcast information to the general public and are easily accessible by any individual online. Closed sites are only available to certain communities of individuals and require approval to view content, typically after the individual provides evidence of membership in the community. For example, Doximity is a physician-only social network where physicians use their real name and submit their credentials for vetting before they may participate in the network.[10] Some sites, such as Facebook, are both open and closed: Users may customize various privacy settings to allow some content to be broadcast publicly but other content to be broadcast to a limited group of users.

Web 2.0 is possible, in part, because Web site operators, by the United States Telecommunications Act of 1996, are not legally responsible for user-generated content.[17] The user alone faces civil liability for defamatory or illegal content.[18] This poses risk to users because social media collapse a wide range of audiences into a single context; the audience intended or imagined by the user is discrete, but the true audience is unbounded.[19] Social media users routinely underestimate or miscalculate their invisible audience, and users often forget that social media has made the world smaller: There are only 4.74 degrees of separation between any two people on Facebook.[20] The audience is at once bigger than the user intends and also more interconnected with one another than imagined. This presents a problem because we communicate differently based on where we are and with whom we are speaking.

Communication is always about context and the intended audience. With face-to-face conversation, our language, style, and cultural references are based on readily apparent social cues that allow us to regulate the appropriateness of our dialogue. It would seem obvious to many that the way we communicate with patients in the clinic is different from the way we communicate with colleagues in the operating room. Furthermore, our communications with relatives and friends are different from our communications in the workplace. However, the era of social media has created a context where a patient, colleague, and relative—in fact, the entire world—all become part of the same unlimited and invisible audience.[21] Furthermore, communications with this audience are indelible, irrevocable, and infinitely accessible. This new reality and the attendant ethical considerations must give pause to the prudent surgeon.

## Medicine and Social Media

Social media technology is broadly accessible, and its use by health care professionals is very common. A 2011 survey by QuantiaMD determined that

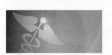 87% of physicians in the United States use social media for personal reasons, and the most common site used by 61% of respondents was Facebook.[22] This survey also determined that 67% of physicians use social media for professional reasons, and the most common sites used were closed online physician communities. Doximity has over 50 000 active physician members online, and the site is used by 9% of physicians in the United States.[23] Social media use in the medical field is very common and serves varied purposes including medical education,[24] discussion of medical research,[13,14] public health,[25] promotion of national medical organizations,[11,12] patient support groups,[26] and patient recruitment for studies.[27] Although health professionals in general tend to adopt novel innovations relatively late, it is important to recognize that social media has become an accepted part of our professional culture.[28,29] The numbers are staggering: In 2011, US hospitals hosted 1068 Facebook accounts, 8154 Twitter accounts, and 575 YouTube channels.[30] Medical institutions have created social media command centers to "monitor and protect the brand in the increasingly important world of social media."[31,32] Social media residency is available to teach health professionals a "strategic plan for using these tools."[33] Some argue that if the health care industry is to remain relevant, it can no longer ignore social media.[29,34]

## Surgeons and Social Media

Surgeons, in particular, tend to be early adopters of innovation. Among physicians, surgeons are the most active users of social media and comprise the largest proportion of physicians who use Twitter.[35] Among the prominent health care organizations worldwide, the American College of Surgeons (ACS) is the most active in terms of presence on social media and posts an average of 3.3 messages on Twitter each day.[36] An ACS survey of members showed that 55% of surgeons use Facebook, 48% use LinkedIn, and 82% view videos on YouTube.[37] Among general surgery program directors (PDs), 68% use Facebook and 40% use Twitter.[38] Social media use is common and increasing among many different surgical disciplines, including vascular,[39] breast,[40] colorectal,[30,41] plastic and reconstructive surgery,[42,43] urology,[28,44] and global surgery.[45]

Many surgeons are enthusiastic about the benefits of social media and routinely encourage trainees to join social media sites for various purposes including networking within an online community, career development, and advancement of surgical science. National surgical organizations, including the ACS, provide step-by-step guides for surgeons to become involved with social media, build a following, and engage the online community.[37,46,47] Surgeons have been instrumental in demonstrating the ways in which social media may be used to build a global community. For example, the #ILookLikeASurgeon campaign on Twitter, started by a general surgery resident, has served to challenge gender stereotypes in the surgical field.[48] This social media campaign has been endorsed by many national surgical organizations and has reached over 75 countries.[49] Surgeons have used social media to build their practice and career.[30,50] One prominent surgeon-blogger has even argued that surgeons have a *moral obligation* to participate in social media to communicate accurate scientific information to the public.[51] Some physicians feel their colleagues who use social media are *better doctors* and may provide better patient care.[30,52] However, there is no evidence to date that a good virtual doctor is a good real doctor, and unsettling is the truth that some physicians criticize their colleagues who are not on social media.[53]

## Maintaining Professionalism Online

The era of social media introduces new challenges to the difficult concept of medical professionalism. Medical professionalism, online or not, is difficult to define, but everyone seems to know what it is.[53] Furthermore, there is a tendency for discussions concerning professionalism and social media to conclude that "professional behavior must evolve to encompass these new forms of media."[54] Online medical professionalism should not be considered a new concept: Professionalism is an old concept and must simply be applied to a new situation. Concepts of medical ethics and professionalism, once established, should be able to be applied universally in any day or era, and for any situation or technology, argues Dr John Weiner: "Whether it is Hippocrates or Osler or Facebook, the guidelines should be the same."[53] Professionalism is the ethical foundation of the surgeon's relationship with patients and contract with society; the advent of social media does not change this central tenet of our practice.

Some national organizations have suggested that the best way for physicians to maintain professionalism in the era of social media is to maintain separate professional and personal identities online. Much attention has been placed on the use of appropriate boundaries on social media platforms. As noted by Lois Snyder with the American College of Physicians, "One way to maintain trust is to maintain boundaries in healthcare. 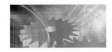 Boundaries are no less important online."[55] A 2013 policy statement from the American College of Physicians and Federation of State Medical Boards offers this position: "The boundaries between professional and social spheres can blur online. Physicians should keep the 2 spheres separate."[56] However, as argued by Dr Matthew DeCamp in a Viewpoint piece published in the *JAMA*, maintaining separate professional and personal identities online is operationally impossible and inconsistent with the concept of professional identity.[57]

Social media exists in a primarily public space; it does not exist in exclusively professional or personal spaces. When attempting to discern whether content should be posted on social media, the question should not be whether the content is *personal* or *professional*, but whether the content is appropriate for a *physician* in a *public space*.[58] Consider the case of surgeons who participate in medical volunteerism abroad and take photographs to capture and share their experiences.[59] Is it appropriate to share these photos on social media sites? The question is not whether these photos are personal or professional. The question is whether these photos are appropriate for a physician to share in a public space. Although the intent of the surgeon is to share an impactful professional experience with others, this type of behavior violates patient privacy and confidentiality.

The difficulty with boundaries and separation of professional and personal identity online has been recognized by other physicians.[59,60] Dr Danielle
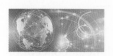
Ofri, who writes for *The New York Times* health blog Well, comments that she keeps all personal information off the Web and limits her online presence to her professional side.[60] She writes, "This means letting go of the fun and casual side of social media, but I think that's simply part of the territory of being a doctor. It's the same reason I don't wear flip flops and shorts to work, much as I'd surely love to. Giving up posting vacation pictures doesn't seem like a particularly high price."[61] Although it seems a simple solution to just keep personal information off the Web, this is not a realistic expectation, especially for young physicians and trainees who have been exposed to social media and the Internet for most of their lives. Furthermore, physicians' personal information, such as address, mortgage, marriage records, and court filings, may be easily obtained online.[61-64]

Surgeons must remember that their presence on social media reflects not only on themselves as individuals but also on the entire surgical profession. Maintaining public trust is crucial to preserve the integrity of the profession. The American Medical Association offers a policy concerning the use of social media in which they caution: "Physicians must recognize that actions online and content posted…can undermine public trust in the medical profession."[65] A recent study showed that 12.2% of surgical residents have unprofessional content on their publicly available Facebook pages, including references to binge alcohol use and sexually explicit content.[66] Another study found that 3% of tweets by self-identified physicians on Twitter were unprofessional, and surgeons comprised the largest subset of physicians in this study when identified by specialty.[35] Among recent graduates from urology residency programs, 13% had clearly unprofessional content on their publicly available social media sites including depictions of intoxication, profanity, and unlawful behavior.[67] Among medical students, use of profanity online, discriminatory language, depiction of intoxication, and sexually suggestive material is common.[68] General surgery PDs have commonly viewed the social media profile of students and residents and have reported taking action based on these findings.[38] Eleven percent of PDs reported lowering the rank of a surgical residency applicant or removing the applicant completely from the rank list because of online behavior. Ten percent of PDs reported formal disciplinary action against a surgical resident for online behavior. The majority of PDs (68%) agreed that online professionalism is important and that residents should receive instruction on the safe use of social media. However, most programs do not have formal didactics or known institutional policies in place. Although unprofessional behavior online is less common among faculty surgeons, one study found that among 758 general surgery faculty identified online, 5% had clearly unprofessional content.[69] Inappropriate language and sexually suggestive material were the most common types of clearly unprofessional content, and all of the faculty identified with such unprofessional content were men.

Although privacy settings are available for users to limit who may view their activity on social media, these settings are not always used and are often misunderstood. Furthermore, the point of social media is to share rather than withhold information. One may surmise that the only way to avoid sharing unprofessional content on social media is to avoid use of social media altogether. However, it is nearly impossible to avoid a "digital identity" as a surgeon because information including education, training, board certification, publications, disciplinary action, and malpractice claims may all be available online.[61] Furthermore, the public may expect their surgeon to have an online presence because "digital connectedness" is expected and even considered a mark of a reputable surgeon.[61] It becomes paramount for surgeons to manage their digital identities and maintain a thoughtful and measured approach to professionalism online.

## Protecting Patient Privacy

Surgeons are ethically and legally obligated to protect the privacy of their patients. Most physicians in the United States swear an oath on graduation from medical school, which highlights their ethical obligations to patients. Nearly all versions of these oaths recognize the importance of patient privacy, for example, "I will respect the privacy of my patients, for their problems are not disclosed to me that the world may know."[70] In contradistinction, the Twitter Privacy Policy reminds users that "What you say on Twitter may be viewed all around the world instantly."[71] We have the privilege of caring

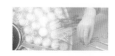

for patients and performing operations, but we do not have the right to share our patients' experiences with the whole world. Social media has created a tempting platform for surgeons to share their experiences, but sharing any information about the clinical care of patients may potentially violate patient privacy and the Health Insurance Portability and Accountability Act (HIPAA). A survey of physicians concerning the use of social media for professional communication noted that the most common concern about interacting with patients online was liability and patient privacy.[22]

Although blatant patient confidentiality breaches seem easy to avoid, they are not nonexistent. A Mayo surgery resident was fired for taking a photo of a patient in the operating room during a cholecystectomy.[55,72] A number of hospital executives were fired after a "surgery selfie" photo was shared on social media showing a group of surgeons posing around an unconscious patient during an operation.[73] A concerned physician wrote a letter to the editor of *The New York Times* after the newspaper reported that a surgeon sent a photo of a patient's amputated extremity to his wife after treating the patient for injuries sustained in a bus crash.[74] The writer commented, "Let's just hope the surgeon or his wife do not post the photo on their Facebook page."[74] Fortunately, these obvious violations are infrequent, but they do serve warning to others that severe disciplinary action and loss of employment may result from inappropriate and unprofessional use of social media.

Unfortunately, less obvious and more insidious violations of patient privacy are commonplace. A multi-institution study of Facebook use by surgical residents at 57 different residency programs showed that 12.2% of users with public profiles had clearly unprofessional content, including HIPAA violations.[66] A single-institution study found that 14% of surgical residents and faculty had content publicly available on Facebook that referenced specific instances of patient care.[75] A 2009 article published in the *JAMA* reported results of a survey conducted among US medical schools concerning medical students and social media.[68] Sixty percent of medical schools participating in the survey had experienced incidences of medical students posting inappropriate content online. Six percent of cases of unprofessional social media content involved patient confidentiality violations.

Although obvious violations of patient privacy may be infrequent, a "gray area" has been identified concerning the ethics of patient storytelling.[76] It is possible for health care professionals to share patient stories on social media in a manner that is technically compliant with the HIPAA, yet it still raises concerns from an ethical standpoint. The motivations 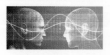 for sharing these stories may be varied and include the provider's or student's desire to reflect on a meaningful experience or seeking social support in the event of a patient death or bad outcome. This type of storytelling, even when patient identifiers are excluded, may still undermine public trust, violate expectations of privacy, or inadvertently identify a patient. This type of sharing presents risk to patients, providers, and the profession. If providers or trainees find themselves with a desire to share patient stories or professional experiences on social media, it may be important to self-reflect on this tendency. What need is being fulfilled by sharing about one's professional life on social media? Are there other outlets for 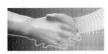 support (eg, small group of colleagues, family, and so forth) that do not potentially threaten patient privacy and the profession? Medical schools and surgical residency programs should address these issues and ensure trainees have a thorough understanding of the potential consequences of their actions online. Some educators believe that posting any kind of patient narrative on social media, even when technically HIPAA compliant and done in a respectful manner, is always inappropriate.[77,78]

## Communication in the Era of Social Media

As surgeons, our ability to communicate with patients and colleagues is central to our professional lives. Conversation allows us to be present, listen, and experience the joy of being heard and understood. Conversation allows us the capacity to develop empathy, form and maintain therapeutic relationships with our patients, and teach more junior colleagues. Social media has fundamentally changed the way we communicate as humans. Sherry Turkle, in her book entitled *Reclaiming Conversation: The Power of Talk in a Digital Age*, explores the consequences of social media and the new digital communication culture.[79] As a society, our passion for technology is manifested by our frequent use of social media platforms to form bonds with others. However, this same technology tempts us away from face-to-face conversation and leaves many young people bereft of important communication skills. Conversation, of course, is the most human—and humanizing—thing we do, Turkle argues. As surgeons, we must protect the sanctity of patient-doctor communication by educating medical students and residents to properly converse with their patients. Furthermore, as digital communication culture values expediency and brevity, education of medical students and surgical trainees may need to focus more on specific skills such as critical reflective thinking. Social media and the Internet allow access to knowledge, but they cannot teach someone to think critically.[53] Only a traditional relationship between the attending physician and student or trainee can allow for the transfer of knowledge, skills, and mentorship necessary to allow an individual to develop experience and wisdom. Some argue that a physician cannot gain true knowledge from reading a live Twitter feed such as a journal club[13,14]; true knowledge is gained from reading a paper, engaging in lengthy discussion, and allowing time for reflection and true dialogue.

Patients need their surgeons to be able to communicate in real-time, face-to-face, with neither the aid nor constraint of social media platforms. In the social media era, young people would rather text on their phone than talk to one another; they would sooner create a 280-character message ("tweet") for an anonymous audience than turn to the person next to them and hold 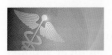 a real conversation. This flight from conversation may ultimately threaten the fundamental interaction central to medicine: communication between the doctor and patient. Many young surgeons would prefer to use tests and laboratories to make a diagnosis rather than actually talking to a patient. Talking to patients may be difficult and requires skills that many young surgeons may not have fully developed. This reliance on data as opposed to discussion and the tendency for surgeons to stare at computer screens rather than engage patients threaten the sustainability of the therapeutic relationship. As Paul Kalanithi stated in his posthumously published memoir *When Breath Becomes Air*, "When there's no place for the scalpel, words are the surgeon's only tool."[80] We must ensure that surgical residents and young surgeons have every tool necessary to provide the highest level of care possible to all patients.

## Accepting Personal Responsibility

It is important for surgeons to accept personal responsibility and accountability for use of social media platforms and to take action to ensure patient privacy is protected and professionalism is maintained online. Numerous studies have demonstrated that unprofessional behavior online is relatively common among medical students, surgical residents, and faculty surgeons.[66–69] Most physicians do not exhibit inappropriate behavior when interacting off-line, which highlights the point that many health professionals do not respect the Internet and social media sites as a *public space*. A false sense of anonymity or privacy may contribute to this behavior. Surgeons must be cautious as the Internet is capable of "many-to-many" communication and the spread of information may be rapid and beyond any user's control.[57] It is critically important to remember that actions online may lead to serious consequences for individuals, and the content posted may undermine public trust in the surgical profession. We must teach our medical students and trainees about the importance of professionalism in all domains including both public and private spaces. We as surgeons must think critically about our actions and reflect on our motivations for sharing content online. Finally, we must exercise measured restraint and avoid posting any material on social media about patient care. Our patients expect utmost confidentiality, and they deserve no less. The relationship between surgeon and patient is what we have trained so long to enjoy, and it is far too sacred a thing to share with the entire world.

# References

1. DiNucci D. Fragmented future. Available from: http://darcyd.com/fragmented_future.pdf. Accessed April 19, 2017.
2. Facebook, Inc. Facebook Investor Relations. Facebook reports fourth quarter and full year 2016 results. Available from: https://investor.fb.com/investor-news/press-release-details/2017/Facebook-Reports-Fourth-Quarter-and-Full-Year-2016-Results/default.aspx. Accessed April 19, 2017.
3. Twitter, Inc. Twitter Milestones. Available from: https://about.twitter.com/company/press/milestones. Accessed April 19, 2017.
4. Wikipedia. The free encyclopedia. Available from: https://www.wikipedia.org/. Accessed April 24, 2017.
5. YouTube. Available from: https://www.youtube.com/. Accessed April 24, 2017.
6. Myspace. Available from: https://myspace.com/. Accessed April 24, 2017.
7. Tumblr, Inc. Available from: https://www.tumblr.com/. Accessed April 24, 2017.
8. LinkedIn. Available from: https://www.linkedin.com/. Accessed April 24, 2017.
9. ResearchGate. Available from: https://www.researchgate.net/. Accessed April 24, 2017.
10. Doximity. Available from: https://www.doximity.com/. Accessed April 24, 2017.
11. Cochran A, Kao LS, Gusani NJ, Suliburk JW, Nwomeh BC. Use of Twitter to document the 2013 Academic Surgical Congress. *J Surg Res*. 2014;190(1):36–40.
12. Attai DJ, Radford DM, Cowher MS. Tweeting the meeting: Twitter use at The American Society of Breast Surgeons Annual Meeting 2013–2016. *Ann Surg Oncol*. 2016;23:3418–3422.
13. Eastern Association for the Surgery of Trauma Twitter Journal Club. Available from: https://www.east.org/education/publications/twitter-east-journal-club. Accessed April 24, 2017.
14. Surgical Outcomes Club Twitter Journal Club. Available from: http://www.surgicaloutcomesclub.com/twitter-journal-club. Accessed April 24, 2017.
15. Hypertext Transfer Protocol. Wikipedia. Available from: https://en.wikipedia.org/wiki/Hypertext_Transfer_Protocol. Accessed April 26, 2017.
16. Internet Protocol Suite. Wikipedia. Available from: https://en.wikipedia.org/wiki/Internet_protocol_suite. Accessed April 26, 2017.
17. Public Law 104-104th Congress. Telecommunications Act of 1996. Available from: http://www.gpo.gov/fdsys/pkg/STATUTE-110/pdf/STATUTE-110-Pg56.pdf. Accessed April 24, 2017.
18. Stewart DR. *Social Media and the Law: A Guidebook for Communication Students and Professionals*. New York, NY: Taylor & Francis; 2013.
19. Marwick AE, Boyd D. I tweet honestly, I tweet passionately: Twitter users, context collapse, and the imagined audience. *New Media Soc*. 2010;13(1):114–133.
20. Markoff J, Sengupta S. *Separating you and me? 4.74 degrees. The New York Times*; November 21, 2011. Available from: http://www.nytimes.com/2011/11/22/technology/between-you-and-me-4-74-degrees.html?_r=2&scp=1&sq=4.74&st=cse. Accessed April 24, 2017.
21. Kodadek LM. First-place essay—con: the writing is on the (Facebook) wall: the threat posed by social media. *Bull Am Coll Surg*. November 2015;100(11):21–23.
22. Modahl M, Tompsett L, Moorhead T. Doctors, patients & social media. Available from: http://www.quantiamd.com/q-qcp/doctorspatientsocialmedia.pdf. Accessed April 24, 2017.

23. FierceHealthIT. Available from: http://www.fiercehealthit.com/press-releases/50000-physicians-now-doximity-medical-network#ixzz1zyc1bcbb. Accessed April 26, 2017.

24. Cheston C, Flickering T, Chisolm M. Social media use in medical education: a systemic review. *Acad Med.* 2013;88:893–901.

25. Chew C, Eysenbach G. Pandemics in the age of Twitter: content analysis of Tweets during the 2009 H1N1 outbreak. *PLoS One.* 2010;5:e14118.

26. Bender JL, Jimenez-Marroquin MC, Jadad AR. Seeking support on Facebook: a content analysis of breast cancer groups. *J Med Internet Res.* 2013;13:e16.

27. Ramo D, Prochaska J. Broad reach and targeted recruitment using Facebook for an online survey of young adult substance use. *J Med Internet Res.* 2012;14:e28.

28. Borgmann H, Woelm J, Nelson K, et al. Strategy of robotic surgeons to exert public influence through Twitter. *Int J Med Robot Comput Assist Surg.* 2016;13(1). doi:10.1002/rcs.1739.

29. Trinh QD. Why I care about social media—and why you should too. *BJU Int.* 2013;112:1–2.

30. Margolin DA. Social media and the surgeon. *Clin Colon Rectal Surg.* 2013;26:36–38.

31. Social Media Command Center Monitors and Protects. Johns Hopkins Medicine. Available from: http://www.hopkinsmedicine.org/news/articles/social-media-command-center-monitors-and-protects. Accessed April 25, 2017.

32. Case Study: Creating a Social Media "Command Center." eHealthare Strategy & Trends. Available from: http://ehealthcarestrategy.com/healthcare-marketing-social-media-command-center/. Accessed April 25, 2017.

33. Social Media Residency. Mayo Clinic social media network. Available from: https://socialmedia.mayoclinic.org/social-media-residency/. Accessed April 26, 2017.

34. Why the Healthcare Industry Can No Longer Ignore Social Media. Now Marketing Group. Available from: https://nowmarketinggroup.com/why-the-healthcare-industry-can-no-longer-ignore-social-media/. Accessed April 26, 2017.

35. Chretien KC, Azar J, Kind T. Research letter: physicians on Twitter. *JAMA.* 2011;305(6):566–568.

36. Ralston MR, O'Neill S, Wigmore SJ, Harrison EM. An exploration of the use of social media by surgical colleagues. *Int J Surg.* 2014;12(12):1420–1427.

37. Yamout SZ, Glick ZA, Lind DS, Monson RA, Glick PL. Using social media to enhance surgeon and patient education and communication. *Bull Am Coll Surg.* 2011;96(7):7–15.

38. Langenfeld SJ, Vargo DJ, Schenarts PJ. Balancing privacy and professionalism: a survey of general surgery program directors on social media and surgical education. *J Surg Educ.* 2016;73(6):e28–e32.

39. Cochrane AR, McDonald JJ, Brady RRW. Social media use among United Kingdom vascular surgeons: a cross-sectional study. *Ann Vasc Surg.* 2016;33:252–257.

40. Ekatah GE, Walker SG, McDonald JJ, Dixon JM, Brady RRW. Contemporary social media engagement by breast surgeons. *Breast.* 2016;30:172–174.

41. McDonald JJ, Bisset C, Coleman MG, Speake D, Brady RRW. Contemporary use of social media by consultant colorectal surgeons. *Colorectal Dis.* 2014;17:165e71.

42. Mabvuure NT, Rodrigues J, Klimach S, Nduka C. A cross-sectional study of the presence of United Kingdom (UK) plastic surgeons on social media. *J Plast Reconstr Aesthet Surg.* 2014;67(3):362e7.

43. Camp SM, Mills II DC. The marriage of plastic surgery and social media: a relationship to last a lifetime. *Aesthet Surg J.* 2012;32(3):349–351.

44. Matta R, Doiron C, Leveridge MJ. The dramatic increase in social media in urology. *J Urol.* 2014;192(2):494–498.
45. Leow JJ, Pozo ME, Groen RS, Kushner AL. Social media in low resource settings: a role for Twitter and Facebook in global surgery? *Surgery.* 2012;151(6): 767–769.
46. Ferrada P, Suliburk JW, Bryczkowski SB, et al. The surgeon and social media: Twitter as a tool for practicing surgeon. *Bull Am Coll Surg.* 2016;101(6):19–24.
47. #HELP! Social Media for the Surgeon: Getting Started, Building a Following, and Building a Community—Podcast #55. Traumacast. Eastern Association for the Surgery of Trauma. Available from: https://www.east.org/education/online/traumacasts/detail/81/help-social-media-for-the-surgeon-getting-started-building-a-following-and-building-a-community. Accessed April 25, 2017.
48. Rimmer A. Female surgeons use Twitter to challenge stereotypes. *BMJ Careers.* Available from: http://careers.bmj.com/careers/advice/Female_surgeons_use_Twitter_to_challenge_stereotypes. Accessed April 24, 2017.
49. #ILookLikeASurgeon Update. Association of Women Surgeons. Available from: https://www.womensurgeons.org/ilooklikeasurgeon-update/. Accessed April 25, 2017.
50. Find an Expert. Christian Daniel Jones, MD, MS. Johns Hopkins Medicine. Available from: http://www.hopkinsmedicine.org/profiles/results/directory/profile/10003148/christian-jones. Accessed April 26, 2017.
51. Logghe H. #ILookLikeASurgeon: with a moral obligation to tweet? Allies for Health Blog. Available from: http://alliesforhealth.blogspot.com/2017/02/ilooklikeasurgeon-with-moral-obligation.html. Accessed April 25, 2017.
52. Mandrola J. Doctors and social media: It's time to embrace change. MedCity News. Available from: http://medcitynews.com/2014/02/doctors-social-media-time-embrace-change/. Accessed April 25, 2017.
53. Weiner J. A personal reflection on social media in medicine: I stand, no wiser than before. *Int Rev Psychiatry.* 2015;27(2):155–160.
54. Mansfield SJ, Morrison SG, Stephens HO, et al. Social media and the medical profession. *Med J Aust.* 2011;194(12):642–646.
55. Snyder L. Online professionalism: social media, social contracts, trust, and medicine. *J Clin Ethics.* 2011;22(2):173–175.
56. Farnan JM, Snyder Sulmasy L, Worster BK, et al. Online medical professionalism: patient and public relationships: policy statement from the American College of Physicians and the Federation of State Medical Boards. *Ann Intern Med.* 2013;158(8):620–627.
57. DeCamp M, Koenig TW, Chisolm MS. Social media and physicians' online identity crisis. *JAMA.* 2013;310(6):581–582.
58. Devon KM. Status update: whose photo is that? *JAMA.* 2013;309(18):1901–1902.
59. Farnan JM, Arora VM. Blurring boundaries and online opportunities. *J Clin Ethics.* 2011;22(2):183–186.
60. Ofri D. Should your doctor be on Facebook? *The New York Times.* Available from: https://well.blogs.nytimes.com/2011/04/28/should-your-doctor-be-on-facebook/?_r=0. Accessed April 26, 2017.
61. Azu MC, Lilley EJ, Kolli AH. Social media, surgeons, and the internet: an era or an error? *Am Surg.* 2012;78:555–558.
62. Gorrindo T, Groves JE. Web searching for information about physicians. *JAMA.* 2008;300:213–215.

63. Thompson LA, Dawson K, Ferdig R, et al. The intersection of online social networking with medical professionalism. *J Gen Intern Med.* 2008;23:954–957.

64. Mostaghmim A, Crotty BH, Landon BE. The availability and nature of physician information on the internet. *J Gen Intern Med.* 2010;25:1152–1156.

65. American Medical Association. Opinion 9.124. Professionalism in the use of social media. Available from: http://www.ama-assn.org/ama/pub/physician-resources/medical-ethics/code-medical-ethics/opinion9124.page?. Accessed October 10, 2015.

66. Langenfeld SJ, Cook G, Sudbeck C, Luers T, Schenarts PJ. An assessment of unprofessional behavior among surgical residents on Facebook: a warning of the dangers of social media. *J Surg Educ.* 2014;71(6):e28–32.

67. Koo K, Ficko Z, Gormley EA. Unprofessional content on Facebook accounts of US urology residency graduates. *BJU Int.* 2017;119(6):955–960.

68. Chretien KC, Greysen SR, Chretien JP, Kind T. Online posting of unprofessional content by medical students. *JAMA.* 2009;302(12):1309–1315.

69. Langenfeld SJ, Sudbeck C, Luers T, Adamson P, Cook G, Schenarts PJ. The glass houses of attending surgeons: an assessment of unprofessional behavior on Facebook among practicing surgeons. *J Surg Educ.* 2015;72(6):e280–e285.

70. Dickstein E, Erlen J, Erlen JA. Ethical principles contained in currently professed medical oaths. *Acad Med.* 1991;66:622–624.

71. Twitter, Inc. Twitter privacy policy. Available from: https://twitter.com/privacy?lang=en. Accessed April 26, 2017.

72. BBC News. US 'penis photo doctor' loses job. Available from: http://news.bbc.co.uk/2/hi/7155170.stm. Accessed April 26, 2017.

73. Ng N. Chinese doctors punished for so-called 'surgery selfies.' CNN News. Available from: http://www.cnn.com/2014/12/23/world/asia/china-doctor-selfies/. Accessed April 26, 2017.

74. Kulberg AG. "The Bronx Bus Crash" (letter). *The New York Times.* http://www.nytimes.com/2011/03/15/opinion/l15bronx.html. Accessed April 26, 2017.

75. Landman MP, Shelton J, Kauffmann RM, Dattilo JB. Guidelines for maintaining a professional compass in the era of social networking. *J Surg Educ.* 2010;67(6):381–386.

76. Wells DM, Lehavot K, Isaac ML. Sounding off on social media: the ethics of patient storytelling in the modern era. *Acad Med.* 2015;90:1015–1019.

77. Chretien KC, Farnan JM, Greysen SR, Kind T. To friend or not to friend? Social networking and faculty perceptions of online professionalism. *Acad Med.* 2011;86:1545–1550.

78. Kind T, Greysen SR, Chretien KC. Pediatric clerkship directors' social networking use and perceptions of online professionalism. *Acad Pediatr.* 2012;12:142–148.

79. Turkle S. *Reclaiming Conversation: The Power of Talk in a Digital Age.* New York, NY: Penguin Press; 2015.

80. Kalanithi P. *When Breath Becomes Air.* New York, NY: Random House; 2016.

# 40 Ethical Obligations to the Patient Versus the Profession

James C. Stanley, MD

PROLOGUE ▶ Frequently, throughout this book, the surgeon is called on to choose between a societal imperative and the welfare of his/her individual patient. It may bear repeating that the societal imperative is often a utilitarian ethic, whereas the commitment of loyalty to an individual patient is a deontological ethic derived from the authority of our discipline. The tension encountered is most often with a hospital, an accountable care organization, or an insurer; Dr Stanley describes in detail the anguish which occurs among surgeons themselves, engaged as it were, in what may seem to be a battle for turf, but which is in reality a deep commitment to the welfare of humankind.

Dr James C. Stanley is professor emeritus of surgery at the University of Michigan Medical School.

In another time eons and eons ago, life evolved from the generation of organic compounds in a primordial sea of simple elements. And that took time. As evolution progressed, so did the survival skills and sophistication of all advanced life on the earth. Not every species survived. Similarly, specialization in medicine has evolved from one generation to another generation. These changes in medicine have not always been pain-free or peaceful. And not all fields of medicine have survived.

An accounting of the events surrounding vascular surgery's survival in its effort to treat the sick (the patient) and become recognized as an independent specialty by the American Board of Medical Specialists (ABMS; the profession) is a story of conflicting ethics. The involved parties included individual surgeons believing it was the core of their nature to provide society with the best care versus organizations bound by duty to follow their time-honored rules regardless of the outcome. Both groups claimed an ethical basis for their actions.

Vascular surgery is demanding with little margin for operative errors. The specialty, as we know it, was conceived nearly 75 years ago. It began by surgeons doing something in the operating room because it made sense even when no one had ever written or talked about it. The discipline passed through its adolescence in the 1970s, a time when a disproportionate number of operating room failures became apparent because of inexperienced surgeons. This was attributable, in part, to insufficient training of surgeons in general surgery residencies and inadequate numbers of surgeons trained in vascular surgery fellowships. This combination of 2 failings posed an ethical dilemma in surgical circles and became the impetus for some to demand additional training for those desiring to practice vascular surgery. That was the beginning of vascular surgery's move toward independence as a surgical specialty.

To understand the underpinnings of this, one needs to recognize the importance of professional behavior defined by egos and dollars, and that 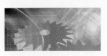 requires a certain degree of insight to recognize that some medical organizations place the welfare of physicians above the care of patients. That is an unnerving thought that questions the objectives of many professional organizations. Vascular surgeons found themselves decades ago in such an environment.

The vascular surgery community's repeated attempts over a number of decades had been unsuccessful in convincing the American Board of Surgery (ABS) to establish a certificate-granting training program beyond the general surgery residency. Then in the early 1980s the 2 national vascular societies, the Society for Vascular Surgery (SVS) and the North American Chapter of the International Society for Cardiovascular Surgery (NA-ISCVS), created an independent group of their own, charged to evaluate and approve North American vascular surgery fellowships.

In response to vascular surgery's moving ahead with a formal educational agenda of its own, the ABS in 1982 reacted by creating a certificate of "Special Qualifications in General Vascular Surgery." The certificate quickly became controversial. The word "special" was offensive to practicing surgeons, especially those in the private sector. The ABS appeared to want the certificate to be in the hands of a limited number of vascular surgeons…who, in order to sit for the examination to be certified, had to have documented credentials in educating trainees and publishing papers or had to be affiliated with learned surgical organizations. None of the latter had to do with direct patient care or clinical competence, which was the normal measure for issuing board certification in most ABMS specialties. The first certifying examination was given to 14 sitting directors of the ABS, including some who had not undertaken any vascular surgery procedures in years.

It was an uncomfortable situation that favored the privileged and elite. It certainly did not favor training more vascular surgeons but instead seemed centered on academic credentials unrelated to the competent care of patients having vascular disease. Years later, the certificate became practice oriented and was retitled "Added Qualifications in Vascular Surgery," but the surgical community's distrust of the ABS persisted.

Continued concern expressed by the vascular surgery community that less well-trained general surgeons were performing vascular surgery beyond the scope of their residency training led the ABS to double down on its belief that vascular surgery was an "essential pillar" of the general surgeon's residency experience. Subsequently, the ABS set high expectations for the number of arterial reconstructive procedures that each resident in training should complete. General surgery residency programs that did not provide this experience were at jeopardy to be placed on probation by the residency review committee for surgery (RRC-S). The mandated numerical standard initially proposed was 44 major arterial procedures per graduating general surgery resident. Furthermore, these vascular operations were to be provided the general surgery trainee before becoming available to train the vascular surgery fellow. That resulted in insufficient numbers of vascular operations to train vascular trainees in nearly a quarter of the nation's existing vascular surgery fellowships.

The resulting shortfall in conventional vascular operations available to train vascular surgery residents became worse as endovascular, catheter-based procedures supplanted many of the open arterial reconstructions, reducing the number of conventional vascular operations even further. Many questioned why the ABS wanted to continue to train more general surgeons to do vascular surgery, when they were not doing it as well as vascular surgeons. Ill-placed favoritism to train general surgeons appeared to be the answer.

Conflict between the vascular community and the ABS continued to smolder for more than a decade. Then in June 1996 Frank Veith's SVS presidential address "Charles Darwin and Vascular Surgery"[1] became a call for vascular surgery to change its paradigm of training and practice, by separating itself from the general surgery community. Interest in independence for vascular surgery had become a subject of conversation, and in September 1996, this author and Robert Smith III, as the sitting presidents of the SVS and NA-ISCVS, respectively, oversaw the incorporation of the American Board of Vascular Surgery (ABVS). The founding directors of the ABVS encompassed the Executive Councils of the 2 national vascular surgery societies. Better patient care by better training became their mantra.

The quest for independence intensified a year later when a manifesto was published regarding the rationale for the establishment of the ABVS.[2] The handwritten signatures of all 22 executive officers of the SVS, the NA-ISCVS, and the Association of Program Directors in Vascular Surgery (APDVS) were included in the publication. Although it was a factual statement and 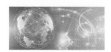 not meant to be inflammatory, it was perceived to be a threat to the tradition of organized medicine and to the ABS in particular.

The manifesto was followed by this author's presidential address before the June 1997 SVS annual meeting entitled "The American Board of Vascular Surgery."[3] This written document was a direct challenge to the existing attitude and utterances of the ABS. A lot of posturing was going on, but pursuing board approval by the ABMS would prove a daunting task.

The ABMS, the parent body governing specialty care in North America, as its published objective, has to maintain and improve the quality of medical care by helping boards develop and utilize professional and educational standards for evaluating and certifying physician specialists. However, in its daily dealing with requests to recognize new and evolving specialties, an inherent bias exhibited in their rules and regulations spoke against any real change within the existing ABMS board structure.

The movement toward vascular surgery having its own independent responsibility for determining the best means of training and certifying its surgeons was to better the care of patients with vascular disease. Thus, at first glance, it would seem that the ABVS and ABMS were on the same page. However, the ABVS objectives evolved from 2 issues: (1) Were sufficient numbers of qualified surgeons going to exist to care for patients with vascular diseases in the next millennium? and (2) Will they provide high-quality care? The ABVS believed that the ABMS actions prevented an affirmative response to either of these questions.

In regard to the first issue, there was an obvious need for more surgeons to care for vascular patients in the future, given the predicted greater than 70% increase of individuals most at risk for vascular disease from 2010 to 2030, those being older than 65 years. However, in 1996 because of the large number of vascular cases mandated by the RRC-S to train general surgeons first, there remained insufficient operative cases to train additional vascular surgeons at many institutions. This was a contentious issue. Many complex procedures done solely by general surgeons were never assigned a similar quota number and that made the ABS mandated quota for vascular surgery cases appear discriminatory.

Although society would likely have fared better with more vascular surgeons, it was clear that fellowships in vascular surgery would only detract from the general surgery trainee's ability to meet their own quota. And failure to meet the quota was a red flag to RRC-S reviewers in their evaluations of general surgery residencies. It was under that shadow that vascular training programs at many institutions fell into disfavor. This occurred despite published data demonstrating that most general surgeons did not utilize their

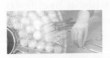 residency's experiences in vascular surgery to care for patients with vascular disease during their subsequent careers. Nevertheless, the ABS remained steadfast in its position that general surgeons at the completion of their residencies must be well trained in vascular surgical procedures. The ABVS perceived this to be a squandering of training material that could and should have been used to train vascular surgeons.

High-quality care was a secondary issue. Medical ethics support the tenet: Do the greatest good for the greatest number—sort of a distributive justice claim that is a reasonable concept regarding global efforts, but one that may fall short when individual lives are at stake. Just think about it… First, assign values to surgical outcomes of #1 to #100, with #1 being death, #2 to 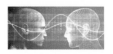 #10 being loss of a limb, a stroke, loss of a kidney, and so forth, and #100 being life without any postoperative residual. Then apply these metrics to a hundred patients. Poor results in such an analysis may go unrecognized even with a modest number of #1 to #10 outcomes. The moral question was how many poor outcomes are acceptable. Most learned and ethical individuals would say "none" if those complications were avoidable.

Such a question about quality care became public in the mid-1990s when numerous articles documented outcomes that were not as good as expected when vascular procedures were performed by those whose training was limited to a general surgery residency. The ABVS strongly opposed the importance of distributive justice as the reason to train more general surgeons to perform vascular surgery, given their poor outcomes compared with those of fully trained vascular surgeons. Abdominal aortic aneurysm repair and carotid endarterectomy were 2 clear examples of this issue. Indications for these procedures were reasonably well defined, and many general surgeons believed they had the requisite skills to perform these procedures. Nevertheless, those who performed fewer of these operations had much poorer outcomes compared with those who performed these procedures regularly, and the latter were predominantly vascular surgeons, not general surgeons.

An evolving 2-class system of patient care existed in the 1990s, and the potential deficit in the workforce to care for patients with vascular disease seemed inevitable unless a change in training and certification occurred. The ABS was perpetuating a system that was producing inadequately trained physicians to undertake vascular surgery. That bordered on self-serving protectionism at best.

The discrepancy in vascular surgery care became newsworthy in an article entitled "The Surgery Your Doctor Should Not Perform" in *The Wall Street Journal*.[4] The author was Thomas M. Burton, a senior medical writer for the Journal, who received a Pulitzer Prize for this and 5 other articles in a series about vascular diseases. He unequivocally stated the case that vascular surgeons, not general surgeons, should be the doctor chosen to perform abdominal aortic aneurysm surgery. The previously uninformed public was being awakened.

The cliché "jack of all trades, but master of none" may be an acceptable label for someone doing menial labor, but it is unacceptable when a defenseless anesthetized patient's life or limb is put at risk by an untrained or inexperienced surgeon. At issue is the right treatment for the right disease at the right time in the right patient…by the right physician. Choices by a surgeon are often difficult to reverse. After all the asleep patient in the operating room is in no position to ask that the surgeon makes a different choice; at that point 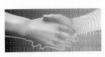 they cannot negotiate with the one wielding the scalpel. Correct choices are made by most surgeons every day. And it is not an obscure thought that right choices are what medical organizations such as the ABMS and ABS should be expected to make. Organizations making the wrong choices and ignoring the patient are not tenable in contemporary times.

The ethical imperatives experienced by surgeons when confronted with broader issues of health care can be imposing, and without a moral compass during such encounters, many become withdrawn, refusing to take a position on difficult issues while performing their defined duties in a quiet and civil manner. However, given the fact that lives may be at stake, their silence can mask what is, by all measures, an unethical stance. Saying nothing and not speaking up may be deleterious to patients. Ethical failures were repeated by many surgical leaders during the times the vascular surgery community became engaged in its struggle to have the ABVS recognized as an independent ABMS board.

The vascular surgery community was deeply divided between those who supported the ABVS and rejected being considered a subspecialty of general surgery and those favoring staying under the umbrella of the ABS. A brief review of the happenings during those times is appropriate to clearly define the ethical steps and missteps behind the independence movement.

During the 5 years following the incorporation of the ABVS, its directors reaffirmed their belief in what was good and right regarding the care of patients with vascular disease. However, given the ensuing tension between the ABVS and ABS, many vascular surgeons struggled with their own positions and were loath to even enter into discussions on the independence topic. More often than not, they tried to avoid incurring criticism from surgical leaders who considered general surgery to be too important to be fragmented by vascular surgery's exit. In those days the importance of beneficence to patients in the long-term seemed completely dissociated from the security or short-term personal gains available to the practicing surgeon.

In 2002 the ABVS finally petitioned the ABMS to become a specialty distinct from general surgery and submitted their proposal to the Liaison Committee for Specialty Boards (LCSB). The criteria to become such a board were tightly prescribed in the ABMS rules. The ABVS considered its application to include specific documentation as to how vascular surgery met each of the ABMS criteria required to become a certifying board.

On December 18, 2002, the ABVS and ABS representatives presented their briefs before the LCSB. The initial presentation by the ABVS was undertaken in the presence of the ABS presenters. After the ABVS representatives spoke they were asked to depart the hearing. The ABS then presented their opposing perspective to the LCSB in the absence of ABVS representatives. The ABVS was provided no chance to address the ABS objections to their becoming a separate ABMS board, yet an unchallenged opportunity did exist for the ABS to counter the ABVS presentation. By any measure, the atmosphere created by the LCSB was not one of neutrality or what others would have considered even-handed at weighing the issues.

The ABVS received notice in a letter 2 days later, December 20, 2002, that their application was rejected on a "global basis," but that an appeal or reapplication could be made within 6 months. The ABVS immediately asked to be informed of the specific reasons for the rejection to determine the appropriateness or inappropriateness of an appeal or reapplication. The response on December 30, 2002, rebuffed the ABVS again without any details regarding the very criteria by which it was to have been judged…and had allegedly not met, stating that the rejection was based "on a totality of criteria." It was highly unlikely that the ABVS proposal could have failed on every count, given the rather simple "fill-in-the-blank" bits of information required to satisfy many of the required criteria. This was disturbing and caused the ABVS to question the integrity of the process.

In 2003 the ABVS made a similar inquiry to the American Medical Association (AMA), one of the organizations responsible for appointing members to the LCSB. Their response was unsettling: "No vote was taken on each of the individual criteria…and… Therefore, no formal record exists of which of the criteria formed the basis for the denial… Due to this, there is no way to provide you with the information that you request." It was almost surreal to realize that the LCSB had no formal records relating to the basis for the rejection at a meeting whose sole purpose was hearing the ABVS proposal to become an ABMS board.

Shortly thereafter, in the fall of 2003, a group of leaders from the major organizations involved in what had become a very divisive climate met in Philadelphia at the ABS offices. The topic of discussion was an alternative to an independent ABVS…an ABS sponsored primary certificate in vascular surgery that could be gained by trainees independent of their having to first complete a general surgery residency. This represented a step toward what the ABVS had wished to achieve at the start in 1996. Nevertheless, ABS ownership of training and an unwillingness to transfer authority for training to others was apparent as the specifics of the primary certificate were developed.

During the process of preparing the primary certificate proposal, the ABS executive director was asked if the ABS initiative to establish the primary certificate in vascular surgery failed for any number of political reasons at the RRC-S or ABMS level, would the ABS then support an ABVS application to the ABMS? His response and that of the existing ABS chair was that such support "would not occur," in that they already had a subspecialty certificate in vascular surgery, that training in the basic techniques of vascular surgery was critical to many areas of general surgery and they must be assured that this 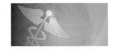 training would be maintained. This clearly reflected the ABS interest in prioritizing certification in general surgery over that of vascular surgery. Although the primary certificate could be viewed as a step toward independence, it was actually dependent on continued approval of the ABS directors who were dominated by general surgeons. Because of this, the ABVS proceeded in its appeal to become an ABMS board.

It is noteworthy that the ABVS deferred a 2003 appeal of their rejection by the LCSB to become an ABMS board. This was done to give the ABS primary certificate proposal an opportunity to move forward. However, it became evident that the primary certificate would not be a stepping-stone toward an independent board, and in February 2005, the ABVS appeared before an appeal panel, appointed by the ABMS and Committee on Medical Education of the AMA. The meeting was tightly prescribed by rules, among which was a statement that the proceedings were not to be transcribed or recorded in any manner, and it was a condition of appearing at the hearing that this rule would be honored. No explanation for this rule was given, but it did not foster a sense of confidence among the ABVS presenters that they might be given an unbiased judgment from the panel. The presentations of the ABVS and ABS were given and an opportunity for rebuttal was afforded the ABVS. Nevertheless, the appeal was rejected and the proposal 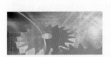 to become an ABMS board was not accepted. The basis for the decision was that the ABS had already established training and certification in vascular surgery; witness the subspecialty certificate "Added Qualifications in Vascular Surgery." That conclusion had not been anticipated, and it had never been given earlier as a reason to reject the ABVS proposal.

Shortly after failing the appeal, the ABVS-ABS conflict became public with a lengthy article entitled "Vascular Surgeons Bang on the Specialists' Door" authored by Reed Abelson.[5] Her work quoted a number of individuals and the issues were well stated. David Meltzer, a physician and economist at the University of Chicago, stated "Physicians are a bunch of monopolists who control entry into their profession in all sorts of ways" and William Gay, executive director of the American Board of Thoracic Surgery, acknowledged that doctors making rulings on board issues can be described as "a good old boys' club." Philipp Lippe, executive medical director of the American Academy of Pain Medicine, who saw his specialty fail to gain ABMS recognition, described the decision making: "It's a closed process behind closed doors." The position of the ABS was aptly stated by their executive director when commenting on their subspecialty "Added Qualification in Vascular Surgery" certificate: "We're not particularly interested in giving that up." Monopolists, old boys, and closed doors do not give one a great sense of transparent ethical behavior by the ABMS. But all of that aside, the ABVS vice-chair, Frank Veith, was quoted in Abelson's article as saying "We're never going to go away, because our cause is just." This commitment was secure.

Individual vascular surgeons are a unique group with personal obligations derived from a sense of their privileged position in society and the exclusivity of being highly regarded by others in medicine. Playing by the rules and being judged by the rules was an important part of the surgeon's image. This dutiful legacy was all part of the vascular surgeon's deontological set. Adherence to these precepts most likely contributed to good consequences, but it was a teleological perspective that there is a natural or divine order giving them the opportunity to serve humankind, which was a stronger ethical force in every-day surgical practice.

Teleological reasoning is much more in vogue among surgeons than deontological considerations, but if the latter results in greater benefits to the surgeon, it risks potential loss of benefits to the patient. It was in that light of contemporary medicine that the ABMS and ABS continued on their older paths, being duty-bound to their rules. Of course the ABS was aware that if the ABVS became an approved ABMS board, the financial status and public image of the general surgeon doing vascular surgery would be less-ened. This seemed to trump improved care that could be provided by vas-cular surgeons. The conflict between patient care and physician welfare was infrequently discussed in open forums, but it was close to the surface of daily conversation among leading vascular surgeons. The ABS egotism and poor outcomes of general surgeons negated the benefits of following its own rules.

When the primary certificate in vascular surgery was finally approved in 2006, it was considered an important advance. It allowed trainees to complete their specialty training by a number of paths, including the establishment of a 5-year integrated residency in vascular surgery. This path allowed individ-uals to begin their training directly after medical school...such as orthope-dics, otolaryngology, urology, or neurosurgery, all ABMS-approved surgical specialties.

Primary certificate programs were first initiated in 2007 at 3 institutions, Dartmouth, the University of Pittsburgh, and the author's institution, the University of Michigan. It did not void the opportunity to enter a vascular fel-lowship for individuals completing their general surgery residency, but it did designate vascular surgery as a more distinct specialty. Most extraordinarily, in the succeeding years, greater than half of those trainees in the 5-year pro-grams nationwide were women; a figure never achieved when completing a general surgery residency was prerequisite to entering a vascular fellowship. Women never accounted for more than 20% of the general surgery trainees in those days. This stands in contrast to the more than 50% of women in the student body at many medical schools who may now enter vascular training without the burden of a lengthy general surgery residency.

Some advocated a less-specialized approach to surgical care, citing the argument that "generalists" were needed in the remote rural areas. However, in New York, Chicago, Los Angeles, and other populated areas where 95% of our citizens live, the generalist concept does not apply to treating vascular 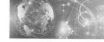 disease. There is simply little justification for a generalist to care for compli-cated vascular disease in most of the nation.

There are those that stubbornly refuse to recognize the value of specialization. They need a little more intellectual honesty and a little more personal responsibility. Trying to do everything should not get a surgeon a medal, and referring a patient to another practitioner is not a sin. They may not remember it, but most physicians made a commitment to this, as they recited the Hippocratic Oath when they became doctors. It is reasonable to conclude that organizations such as the ABS, like individual surgeons, should also recognize the importance of giving up some of its control over their specialty if it would bring greater beneficence to society.

There appeared to be many missteps in the events surrounding the maturation of vascular surgery as a distinct specialty and the efforts to have the ABVS recognized as an independent ABMS board. Among the most egregious involved a vascular surgeon in Boston, Massachusetts, who was an ABS director. He said "There will (be) no way to create continuity of education if everything becomes particulate." He was referring to the fragmentation of general surgery, typified by vascular surgery's attempt to divorce itself from the ABS and general surgery control. However, his statement, if applied to the field of surgery decades ago, would never have seen specialty care evolve in any discipline. Such backward thinking would find general surgeons setting fractured bones one day, performing urologic or thoracic procedures the next day, and operating on an abdominal aortic aneurysm the following day. It is a true example of deontological thinking…following traditional rules that are duty-bound no matter the value or desirability of the outcome. Such rules may have sufficed in the early 1900s, but not a century later.

This particular Bostonian had 2 breeches in ethical behavior that were easily recognized by others. First, as the president of the New England Society for Vascular Surgery, he self-nominated himself to be that Society's representative ABVS director. While maintaining that appointment, he then appeared before the LCSB as a representative of the ABS, testifying against the ABVS proposal. To state that he had a conflict of interest and that he should have resigned his ABVS directorship would be an understatement. His position was dishonest and unethical. That was not his only deviation from ethical behavior. In a different role, as the president of the APDVS, he presented the slate of new officers to be elected, including a surgical colleague of his as the sole nominee to become the Association's future president. But that individual had left his position in Buffalo, New York, and he was no longer a program 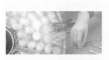 director. When confronted with this fact, he refused to acknowledge that his nominee was ineligible for election or that the reason he supported him was because of the nominee's opposition to the ABVS independence effort. This action was unethical and represented blatant misconduct. Nevertheless, his misbehavior carried the day, going unrecognized by many in the room who were voting. But it was not forgotten.

There were many other intended and unintended lapses in judgment and ethical behavior. At an organizational level, it is noteworthy that the ABS never acknowledged the emergence of endovascular procedures in vascular surgery that would necessitate many more years of training in a traditional general surgery residency. The burden that would have been placed on the already time-heavy training of general surgery residents must have been irrelevant to the ABS, compared with the importance of their maintaining control of vascular surgery.

Certainly, the LCSB as an agent of the ABMS and AMA acted in an unacceptable manner by rejecting the ABVS application with no record whatsoever regarding the precise reason for their denial. It is near-impossible to ignore the apparent self-interest in protecting their own turf and that of existing ABMS boards... at a perceived cost to patient welfare. The lack of recorded minutes of their deliberations and decisions for a body professing 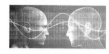 the best interests of the public is dishonest and not how a major medical organization should act. The words "integrity and transparency" have no place in describing the LCSB's action in hearing the 2002 ABVS application.

The unrestrained self-interest of certain leaders of the SVS, found many accepting appointments to positions in the ABS and APDVS, in turn for their overlooking the apparent mandate of the SVS membership to have the ABVS become an ABMS board. Throughout the decade from 1996 to 2006, the vascular surgery communities' strong commitment to an independent ABVS had been expressed in 4 separate surveys overseen by an independent consulting firm, as well as by a majority vote at both the SVS and NA-ISCVS business meetings. To hold a different perspective about independence is understandable, but it escapes rational thinking for one to take diametrically opposite action regarding the Societies' role in defining the future of the discipline, while at the same time serving as an officer of the organization. The ethical behavior of such individuals is subject to question.

In the final analysis, the issue at hand is the role individual physicians have as an instrument of a noble calling in the caring for the sick versus their need to abide by the rules promulgated by organized medicine. These 2 issues, frequently perceived as the profession versus the business of medicine, are often in conflict. That seemed to be the case with the ABS defending the practice of general surgeons doing vascular surgery despite their poorer outcomes compared with vascular surgeons. It took more than a decade for the ABS with its primary certificate to place patient care above the tradition of protecting those holding its certificates. During that time, many patients treated by general surgeons for the ravages of vascular disease were not being well served by the profession. If one assumes medicine has a covenant with society to provide the best care, then organizations representing the practice of clinical medicine should cease acting like trade unions and they should consider better patient care to be more important than physician welfare. Individual surgeons, supporting the primacy of providing the best care for the sick, may at times find themselves at political and financial risk, but doing the right thing for the patient is both ethical and moral in character.

# References

1. Veith F. Presidential address: Charles Darwin and vascular surgery. *J Vasc Surg.* 1997;25:8–18. From the Society for Vascular Surgery.
2. The American Board of Vascular Surgery: rationale for its formation. *J Vasc Surg.* 1997;25:411–413.
3. Stanley JC. Presidential address: The American Board of Vascular Surgery. *J Vasc Surg.* 1998;27:195–202.
4. Burton TM. The surgery your doctor should not perform. *Wall St J.* December 30, 2003.
5. Abelson R. Vascular surgeons bang on the specialists' door. *NY Times.* February 11, 2005.

# 41 Ethics of Introducing Innovative Procedures

Ramon Berguer, MD, PhD

PROLOGUE ▶ On December 3, 1967, Christiaan Barnard transplanted the human heart for the first time. Although this was hailed as a breakthrough by the lay media, within the discipline it was recognized to be a small progression of existing knowledge and skill. Within weeks several more heart transplants had been performed at several centers around the country, indicating a broad readiness for this innovation. Similar stories could be told about many surgical innovations, including operations for obesity, abdominal aortic aneurysm, and hepatic resection for cancer.

It has been pointed out, critically often, that this phenomenon differs dramatically from the prolonged and perhaps too careful testing of a new drug. There are, therefore, those who believe that far greater surveillance is needed of surgical innovation. Contrary to this view is the recognition that surgical innovations develop slowly in small cumulative steps, that heart transplant was preceded by a prolonged period of learning to conduct cardiopulmonary bypass and to anastomose vessels, and that heart transplant represented an inevitable and small step.

There is great force in the analogy of surgical innovation to Darwinian evolution. Near random innovations arise spontaneously, which are subsequently winnowed by a process akin to natural selection. Some survive, whereas others do not. If bleeding at an anastomosis is encountered, a figure-of-eight suture may

**369**

be tried. If the bleeding stops, the surgeon is almost certain to use it again in similar circumstances. If the bleeding does not stop, the maneuver is culled. Natural selection of small incremental innovations occurs daily in the operating room.

Is it valid to "try something?" What of patients' rights and patient autonomy? These considerations demand from the surgeon the utmost of self-knowledge and true mastery of his/her craft. Mastery allows the surgeon to see in the theater 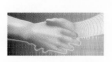 of the mind possible solutions to never-before-encountered problems. Self-knowledge dictates whether an innovation is merely a natural progression or a departure requiring a protocol and peer review. Sometimes the answer is obvious. Often it is nuanced and blurred. The essay that follows should be read together with the paragraphs on innovation in chapter 15 on pediatric surgery and chapter 14 on pediatric cardiac surgery.

Dr Ramon Berguer has been an innovator in vascular surgery. His innovations have been based on a true mastery of that discipline as it has evolved in the past several decades. He has served as a wise mentor, an intrepid operator, and a talented researcher at multiple major institutions.

Dr Ramon Berguer is a professor emeritus of surgery at the University of Michigan Medical School. He is also a professor of biomedical engineering at the University of Michigan.

The fruits of innovation in surgery have been experienced by generations of humans: our lives are longer and more enjoyable because of them. In my own field, I can mention aortic aneurysmectomy, carotid endarterectomy, endografts, arterial grafts, and stents among others. These advances are inscribed into the ethics of surgeons because their aim is to provide the maximum of beneficence to the patients they serve. When these new procedures were tried, the limits for their feasibility and indications were not known and some patients died or became disabled. Only after the innovations were refined did they result in the benefits we know today.

In addition to providing *beneficence* to our patients, our ethical covenant as surgeons requires that we must respect their *autonomy* and *justice*, the 3 fundamental parameters listed in the Belmont Report, the most recent (1974) accepted document concerning human research.

We cannot assume that all innovation amounts to human research. For a new procedure to be called research, it must be structured within a protocol that will permit a scientific analysis of the results. Surgical innovation has a wide spectrum that can be at one end a simple change or variation in technique and at the other an entirely new procedure for which there is no precedent in the surgical practice.

An innovative solution may also occur when a surgeon is trapped in the operating room into an adverse situation for which there is no accepted or described solution.

An innovation, as mentioned earlier, may be a mere technical change (eg, eversion vs standard carotid endarterectomy) or the application of an established procedure in a new location or system (eg, angioplasty of congenital aortic coarctation or laparoscopic aortic bypass). Usually, once the surgical team acquires basic experience with the "new" technique, the latter will be presented to a professional meeting or published as a retrospective study. At this point it behooves the surgeon who proposed it to begin a prospective case series with an established protocol. Only then the project can be considered "human research," and it is at this point that an institutional review board (IRB) or a professional society committee should oversee it. The prospective studies of the innovations cited earlier showed the technique of eversion to be a worthy development, while the angioplasty of coarctations and the laparoscopic bypass were discarded.

Some of our colleagues, mostly in the medical field, have raised objections to the freedom that surgeons have to develop new procedures before being vetted by their IRBs or similar agencies. In their argument, they went as far as stating that federal agencies protect laboratory animals to a greater extent than we do to the patients in whom we operate. Leaving aside the difficulty of determining the boundary in a surgical innovation between a technical variation and new unprecedented innovation, it is worth considering that IRBs or similar agencies exist for the purpose of guaranteeing the ethical norms that must be observed in all biological research studies. They are not there to promote the progress in general welfare that follows innovation. If all the processes involved in guaranteeing the safe outcome of an experiment were applied to a proposed surgical innovation, the latter would never occur. And by drowning innovation those agencies would be denying to the general population the large benefits that derive from it.

Those that criticize the general lack of Food and Drug Administration vetting in new surgical procedures (excluding, of course, those that involve a new device or biomaterial) are in the habit of demanding that any new procedure must be tested through a prospective randomized clinical trial (RCT). When a surgical innovation has already been seen to be beneficial and a prospective observational study has been started, the methodological difficulties of testing it through an RCT cannot be ignored. The poor fit of the methodology of RCT to surgical procedures has been amply discussed; let alone the deontological contradictions that would involve a double-blind study with a sham surgical arm. A prospective case study that follows a previously established research protocol is the best way to assess a surgical innovation. And in fact this has been the way that most life-improving innovations have been incorporated into surgical practice. This includes, among many others, 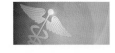 coronary angioplasty, laparoscopic cholecystectomy, and aortic endografting.

To discuss the ethics of innovative procedures, it is helpful to attempt to define what constitutes surgical innovation. This is not an easy task because the spectrum of innovation in surgery runs, as mentioned earlier, from frequently enacted variations in surgical technique to the rare introduction of an unprecedented new procedure based on an idea that has not been validated through standard scientific methods. Unlike with new drugs or devices, there are no Food and Drug Administration regulations to guide the testing and approval of such new surgical procedures. The ethics for the development of these new operations lies on the surgeon and on the institution or professional society of which he/she is a part.

The boundary between gradual improvements of a surgical procedure—which are part of the natural evolution of the surgical skill set—and the radical new innovations is not clear. The former may be a mere change in technique (eg, eversion carotid endarterectomy vs its standard form) or the use of a previously proven method in a new location (eg, the angioplasty of an aortic coarctation or a laparoscopic aortic bypass). Another instance of innovation in the practice of a surgeon occurs when he/she wants to incorporate to his/her practice a new procedure developed elsewhere.

The acceptance of these innovations in surgical practice usually follows the path of the first being presented to a professional society or published as a case series (as a retrospective study). From this point on, a prospective clinical research protocol is instituted that should be vetted by either a societal committee or, in some cases, an IRB.

In the evaluation of all instances of innovative surgery—from the mere changes in technique to the entirely new procedures—it is evident that it has 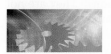 an element that separates it from all other medical and pharmacologic innovations: the "learning curve" of new surgical procedures. New surgical procedures are not fully developed at their birth; their progress toward their final form requires repetition and refinement of elements that will impinge on the final results. The prospective clinical study should be conducted early because we want to learn about its outcomes, particularly the disadvantageous ones, before it becomes incorporated into the practice of surgeons at large.

Consideration of the learning curve—for the surgeon and for the surgical team—is also relevant when entering a new procedure into a clinical trial. This became evident when the results of the North American Symptomatic Carotid Endarterectomy Trial were published. This study compared the outcomes of patients with symptomatic carotid artery disease treated by either surgical endarterectomy or medically with aspirin. In the medical arm of the study, all patients received an identical dose of aspirin. In the surgical arm, they were operated by an array of surgeons who, in this particular study, did not have expertise with the operation: they were mostly general surgeons who did an occasional endarterectomy. This resulted in a significant asymmetry of treatments. The study reported an unacceptable rate of stroke and death of 6%. Now, during this time and across the country, centers experienced in this particular operation were reporting stroke and death figures between 1% and 3%. One may conclude that the North American Symptomatic Carotid Endarterectomy Trial results addressed the question of the indication for endarterectomy for a subset of population served by surgeons with limited expertise.

Surgical innovations (such as aortic aneurysmectomy, carotid endarterectomy, intravascular stents, and grafts) have improved and prolonged the life of entire populations. I mentioned earlier that, early in their development, some of these advances did result in the loss of lives although, once they were finely tuned, they saved or improved thousands of them. While we ask the surgeon who has developed an innovative procedure to seek beforehand the advice of experts proximate to the field or to the pathology that concerns these human experiments, we must acknowledge that entrusting the birth of new procedures to an overzealous IRB may impede future advances. There is an intrinsic element of uncertainty in every new procedure, and some of these uncertainties may only be revealed later when a prospective study is under way. In surgical procedures, as in research, innovation derives from induction and empirical observation; on the contrary the scientific judgment and validation of these advances is obligatorily a deductive process. An IRB or an institutional committee whose mission is to safeguard against risk is to be naturally unreceptive to inductive propositions. This is the eternal tension between guardians and innovators. When Kurt Semm, a gynecologist at the University of Kiel, performed the first laparoscopic appendectomy, his faculty colleagues ordered him to undergo a computed tomography scan of the brain, alleging that only a brain-damaged person would perform laparoscopic surgery. Laparoscopic procedures are today a standard practice in surgery. When Juan Parodi submitted his original work on treating aortic aneurysms with an endograft to the *Journal of Vascular Surgery*, not only the paper was rejected but he was also admonished in writing by its Editor for having performed such an inappropriate operation. Endovascular grafting is today the larger part of a vascular surgeon's practice.

There are 3 situations in which a surgeon is involved in an innovative procedure. The most frequent is when *a new technique developed elsewhere has been brought to a surgeon's attention as a "new" or "better" procedure* and the surgeon wishes to incorporate it into his/her practice. If the technique, as is often the case, involves steps that are not part of his/her established vascular practice, the surgeon should acquire a minimum exposure to it before proposing it to a patient. In the preoperative discussion the surgeon must make clear that although he/she has obtained the requisite education in the new procedure, this is the first time that he/she will be doing this operation. In the operating room the presence of the surgeon who developed the new procedure will serve to reassure the patient that the pertinent safeguards have been put in place. Eventually the ascending part of the learning curve 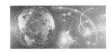 for the surgeon will result in refinements of the procedure and improved outcomes.

A second instance in which a surgeon is confronted with an innovative solution occurs in the operating room when he/she faces *a situation in which the standard methods of treatment cannot resolve the problem.* Years before endografting was available, I encountered a patient who had developed a

15-cm-diameter aneurysm 2 years after being radiated for a retroperitoneal sarcoma. The size of his infrarenal aneurysm suggested that a rupture may occur soon, and I advised him to have an aneurysmectomy. At operation I found the entire retroperitoneal aorta—up to and including its transdiaphragmatic segment—enveloped by a 2-inch-thick, lymph node–like mass that bled on any attempt to dissect through it and defied any attempt to isolate the aorta. I eventually closed the wound and informed the disappointed patient that I had not been able to perform the intended operation. The patient was terrified at the imminence of a rupture that would not be treatable. I told him I would try to figure out a solution.

I thought I could attempt to thrombose the aneurysm and reestablish flow to his pelvis and legs by means of an axillo-bifemoral bypass. I discussed my plan with Dr Alex Walt, then the chair of the Department of Surgery, and with the hospital administration. We met with the patient and explained that this was an untested procedure, but it was the only solution we could offer to avert a rupture that in his case would be fatal. An ad hoc operative consent form was drafted. To perform the procedure, I severed both the common iliac arteries above their bifurcations and occluded them with balloon catheters at their aortic origin (we did not have detachable balloon catheters then). The common iliac arteries with the catheter inside were exteriorized through the abdominal wall. We then constructed the axillo-femoral bypass. Finally we lowered a catheter introduced in the axillary artery into the sac to inject thrombin into it while perfusing saline at a high rate at the level of the renals to avoid proximal propagation of thrombus. The aneurysmal sac thrombosed immediately. The balloon catheters were removed, and the tied off iliac arteries were buried into the abdominal wall. A postoperative arteriogram showed the aneurysm thrombosed up to the level of the renal arteries. The patient was discharged without complications.

I thought this might be a solution for high-risk patients and repeated the operation in another patient. In this patient, the induced thrombosis of the sac stopped 1 inch below the renal arteries. She died 3 months later of a rupture that occurred in the nonthrombosed proximal portion of the sac immediately below the renal arteries. This minimal second observation sufficed to disqualify the innovation. I had performed the same procedure in a third patient with the same resulting incomplete thrombosis. This patient was recalled and underwent a successful standard aneurysmectomy. I never repeated the procedure. Today, similar patients would be offered an endovascular graft.

One should also consider the limitations attending the use of innovation in the case where an *established surgical technique is used in a different* 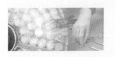 *territory*. I wish I had done so in a case involving a technique as common as an arterial thrombectomy. I had done a distal vertebral bypass on a crane operator who experienced syncope with rotation of the head. In those years, I was obtaining postoperative arteriograms before discharge. In this patient, the postoperative arteriogram showed a thrombus of half-inch length at the distal anastomosis of the bypass at the level of C1. I assumed that I had made a technical error in the construction of the anastomosis and told the patient that I should redo it. The anastomosis was taken down exposing a nearly occluding thrombus that was adherent to the artery and fragmented when I tried to pull it out with the forceps. To remove the thrombus completely, I inserted a fine (#2) thrombectomy catheter for about 3 cm. The anastomosis was redone, and when I reestablished distal flow, the anesthesiologist reported uncontrollable hypertension. The patient never woke up from anesthesia and died after being in coma for several hours. At postmortem there was a large subarach-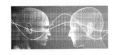noid hemorrhage caused by a minute perforation in the intracranial vertebral artery. I should have been aware that the vertebral artery is so thin at this level that it is translucent and that a technique as banal as a thrombectomy that has been used in all extracranial territories cannot be used in the intracranial territory without great risk. Shortly after this sad event, I read a report from the Mayo Clinic describing the death (from subarachnoid hemorrhage) of 3 out of 5 patients who had undergone catheter manipulation of the intracranial vertebral.

I will discuss my experience with vertebral artery surgery to consider the steps to be taken to ensure the *safeguards required to respect the beneficence and autonomy that must accompany any first human experiments*. It was a neurologist, Raymond Bauer, a professor of neurology at Wayne State University, who encouraged me to reconstruct the vertebral artery. Ray Bauer had hands-on experience in the pathology of the vertebral artery. He had been the national secretary for the first extracranial occlusive disease study in the 1960s and had demonstrated angiographically the mechanics of osteophytic compression and trauma to the vertebral artery. We discussed the potential for brain ischemia secondary to interruption of flow in the vertebral artery, and it appeared to us to be less than what it was for carotid endarterectomy giving the bilaterality of supply in most patients and the often-reported asymptomatic occlusion of the vertebral artery. I was familiar with the anatomy involved and, in what concerns the actual technique, we were routinely placing vein bypasses in arteries smaller than the vertebral artery. And so the first repairs I did were subclavian-vertebral bypasses (after having acquired some experience with this operation, I switched to the simpler and more elegant vertebral to carotid transposition).

We were also looking for ways to correct symptomatic vertebral artery compression along the cervical spine. As it had been the case with proximal vertebral disease, I started by placing a trusted vein graft in the distal vertebral artery to bypass the entire cervical course of the former. Finally, when time came to correct the compression of the vertebral artery by the arch of the atlas (the bow hunter syndrome), I did some prior cadaver dissections to familiarize myself with the suboccipital space and consulted with a neurosurgeon about the management of the subarachnoid plexus of veins and the best tools for the osteotomy. In summary, before introducing a new procedure, it is mandatory to consult with experts in the new territory or system and to consider whether the techniques used can be safely applied in the new location being considered.

I conclude by restating the difficulty of establishing a line between innovations that are a stepwise progression of clinical surgery and innovations that include new methods that have never been tried or tested in humans. For the latter, expert peer consultation and a sincere and thorough conversation with the patient are necessary. The validation of the results of new operations can be done through prospective research protocols.

# 42 Health Care Disparities

Janine E. Janosky, PhD

PROLOGUE ▶ Thomas R. Malthus opined and Charles Darwin came to agree that population tends to increase geometrically and the supply of food and water and other elements of life sustenance tended, at best, to increase linearly. Whether this theoretical construct has validity or not, it is true that there have been grave disparities in the availability of food and water throughout history.

We have emphasized that the surgeon's ethical base honors a principle of proximity that one owes an obligation to one's neighbors or, in the case of a surgeon, to one's patient in the surgeon-patient relationship.

But what of a more broad obligation? Does the average working surgeon have an obligation to the starvation that has throughout history been evident in the world? Many surgeons and their families believe the answer is "yes."

Dr Janine E. Janosky is a professor in the Department of Health and Human Services and the dean of the College of Education, Health, and Human Services at the University of Michigan—Dearborn.

Emulation is an important mechanism for learning in the discipline of surgery. A statement of abstract principle may provide a cognitive framework for a surgeon's altruism, but only an understanding of the life of another can ultimately model the well-lived life. Many surgeons have devoted much or all

**377**

of their professional lives to the alleviation of the great inequalities of health care throughout the world. The following paragraphs are meant to serve as a very small sample of hagiography in this area.

Harvey Doorenbos, MD, devoted 35 years of general surgery practice in Oman and subsequently Africa. He participated in the construction of a hospital in Ethiopia.

Robert Foster, MD, spent 60 years in Zambia and war-torn Angola at significant risk to his own life. He was a practicing surgeon throughout and founder of no less than 3 hospitals.

Harold Adolph, MD, FACS, along with his spouse Bonnie Jo Adolph built a training center for surgeons in Soddo, Ethiopia, a city of 3 million inhabitants.

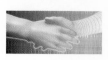

Glenn Geelhoed, MD, was a professor of surgery at The George Washington University. He was not only a practicing surgeon but also an expert in tropical medicine. He led more than one hundred missions to developing countries, accompanied by medical students and residents to whom he exemplified the life of an altruist.

John Tarpley, MD, has spent, in the aggregate, many years in Kenya. He is a full professor at Vanderbilt and a person who best displays the virtues of commitment, courage, and agape. Tarpley retired from Vanderbilt and from the VA Hospital in Nashville on June 30, 2016. He has served as the associate chief of surgery at the VA and program director of the Vanderbilt surgical residency program. He has operated on general surgical patients throughout his career. Tarpley finished his residency at Johns Hopkins in 1978 and went immediately to spend 3 years in Nigeria. He returned to spend a year in Baltimore, then 3 years again in Nigeria and continued this pattern for 15 years. He began his career at Vanderbilt 23 years ago when the pattern ended.

Tarpley trained residents in surgery at the Baptist Medical Center in Ogbomosho, Nigeria, throughout the earlier portion of his career. He has returned to Nigeria annually since he began at Vanderbilt.

Only a few days after he returned he began traveling to Kijabe Hospital in Kenya, once again as a trainer and mentor of surgeons there. He plans to spend his postretirement years in Africa with occasional returns to the United States.

One of the obligations a surgeon owes to the society in which he/she finds himself/herself is to assume some sense of responsibility toward that society as a whole, notwithstanding that the surgeon usually works with individual patients, one at a time. Unequal access to surgical and medical procedures, including testing, occurs in the United States based on socioeconomic status (SES), race, ethnicity, gender, language, culture, sexual identity, citizenship, residence, and disability. There are a complex and interrelated set of individuals, providers, health systems, and societal and environmental facts that contribute to these disparities.[1] The population of the United States is becoming more diverse in that 41% are people of color,[2] with projections that people of color will be the majority of the population by 2045.[3] This means that access must increase or certain segments of the population will have adversely affected health status and outcomes.

"Understanding the demographic and socioeconomic composition of U.S. racial and ethnic groups is important because these characteristics are associated with health risk factors, disease prevalence, and access to care, which in turn drive health care utilization and expenditures."[4] Overall, disparities often disappeared as measures of access to and quality of care achieved high levels of performance across groups, although parallel gains in access and quality led to persistence of most disparities.[5]

There are also well-documented racial/ethnic and SES disparities in health care.[6,7] Health and health care are impacted by the policies, systems, and environments in which people live and function day-to-day. Population health is differentially affected by health behaviors, clinical care, social and economic conditions, and physical environment.[8] Although this model does not include genetic and biologic factors, it estimates that 40% of health is affected by social and economic conditions followed by 30% by health behaviors, 20% by clinical care, and 10% by the physical environment.[8] Disparities in surgical care in the United States are also a combination of complex patient, social, and institutional factors.[9] These disparities include higher rates of chronic conditions, greater comorbidity, and greater risk of premature death. In some conditions such as cancer, some populations may present with more advanced disease.

The United States, one of the wealthiest nations in the world, is far from the healthiest.[10] Although life expectancy and health improved over the past century, these gains have lagged behind other high-income countries.[10] The health disadvantage is present even though the United States spends more per person on health care than any other nation. Among the 17 high-income peer countries, Americans face the second highest risk of dying from a noncommunicable disease and the fourth highest risk of dying from a communicable disease in 2008.[11] American men rank last for life expectancy and women are second to last.[10] The United States is also the fourth highest for deaths from chronic disease.[10] When compared with peer countries, Americans had the highest level of income inequality and poverty, particularly child poverty.

There are significant disparities in the burden of disease and illness experienced by different identity groups. Although these disparities hold true for individual states, such as residents of Michigan, overall and across individual counties, the data become nuanced at the community level. In 2010, for example, Michigan was tied with Arkansas with the 13th highest rate in the nation for adult diabetes with the prevalence of diabetes among African American (5%) and Latino/Hispanic adults (5.4%) aged 18 to 44 years being twice that of their Caucasian counterparts (2.5%). The disparity between Caucasians 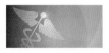 and African Americans is present for older adults but was not clearly determined for the Latino/Hispanic population.[11] According to County Health Rankings and Roadmaps,[12] Macomb, Oakland, and Wayne counties vary in their health outcomes ranking for the State of Michigan. Oakland (23rd of the 82 ranked counties) ranks better than two-thirds of Michigan counties. Macomb (47th) and Wayne (82nd) are worse than half the counties in the health outcomes. With the exception of Wayne County, whose rank for health factors remains the same, Oakland and Macomb have improved rankings in health factors in the most recent few years.

## Disparities in Medical Procedures

Unequal access to medical procedures, including testing, occurs in the United States based on SES, race, ethnicity, sex, language, culture, sexual identity, citizenship, residence, and disability. There are a complex and interrelated set of individuals, providers, health systems, and societal and environmental facts that contribute to these disparities.[13] The population of the United States is becoming more diverse in that 41% are people of color,[14] with projections that people of color will be the majority of the population by 2045.[15] Increased access will certainly lead to the lessening of the adversely affected health status and outcomes.

Many groups face significant disparities in access to and use of care. For example, bisexual individuals have more limited access to care, whereas lesbian and gay individuals have rates comparable to heterosexual adults.[13]

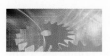
Nonelderly adult Latinos, African Americans, and American Indians, and Alaska Natives are more likely than Caucasians to delay or go without needed care.[2] People of low SES generally experienced less access and poorer quality of medical care.[5] Persistence of most disparities were maintained as all groups gained in access and quality.[5] Although declines in the rates of the uninsured were larger among African American and Latino adults aged 18 to 64 years than among Caucasians, there is still a large gap by race in the percent uninsured.[5] The disparity between African American and Caucasian smokers worsened among adult smokers who had a medical examination in the past year and received advice to quit smoking.[5] The measure of hospice patient caregivers who perceived patient referral to hospice at the right time showed marked differences when comparing American Indian/Alaska Native with Caucasian.[5] Disparities worsened between Latino and non-Latino patients who received hospice care consistent with their end-of-life wishes and who received the correct amount of pain management medicine.[5] Overall quality of care varies by geographic region when coupled with the average differences among African American, Latino, and Asian in comparison with Caucasian.[5] Adolescents aged 16 to 17 years in nonmetropolitan areas were less likely to receive meningococcal conjugate vaccine than metropolitan adolescents.[5]

The percentage of children whose Latino and African American parents reported poor communication with their health provider was higher in comparison with Caucasian parents. It was also higher for poor, low-income, and middle-income families compared with high-income families.[5]

Although from 2005 to 2012 the percentage of hospital patients with heart failure who were given complete written discharge instructions increased overall, for both sexes and for all racial/ethnic groups, the percentage was lower among American Indians and Alaska Natives in comparison with Caucasians.[5] Rates of cancer incidence are lower for Asians/Pacific Islanders and American Indians and Alaska Natives compared with Caucasians.[2] In general, African Americans have higher cancer rates than Caucasians.[2] African Americans have higher death rates because of diabetes, heart disease, and cancer compared with Caucasians.[2] Caucasians have a lower diabetes death rate than Latinos but high heart disease and cancer death rates.[2] For the 3 conditions, Asians have lower death rates.[2] Overall, in an Agency for Health care Research and Qualityreport, disparities often disappeared as measures achieved high levels of performance.[5]

In a comparison of self-identified lesbian-gay-bisexual individuals with adults in New York City, individuals identified as lesbian-gay-bisexual had higher rates of emergency department use than the general public.[14] In addition, in a multilingual population-based survey in New York City, researchers found that women who have sex with women were significantly less likely than other women to have had a Pap test in the past 36 months or a mammogram in the past 24 months.[14] Another study examined access issues for sexual minorities in the use of mental health services and found that self-identified homosexual or bisexual individuals used mental health services more than self-identified heterosexual individuals.[14] A convenience sample of African American lesbians compared with African American heterosexual women found that the former attended counseling or therapy at significantly higher rates than the latter.[14]

Some research also suggests that preventive screening may be less frequent among lesbians and bisexual women than among heterosexual women. The researchers found that self-identified lesbians/bisexual women were less likely to have a pelvic examination in the last 5 years compared with women in the general population as well as those in their 40s were less likely to receive a mammogram.[14] In addition to lower preventive screening rates, lesbian women on average have higher rates of some risk factors for breast cancer. These include greater alcohol use and lower likelihood of childbearing.[13]

Perceived discrimination by health care providers may be a barrier to access to and use of health care services. For example: Although self-reporting that the providers felt comfortable and prepared to work with sexual minority patients, less than 20% of the sample received education in the area.[14] There was a wide variability in attitudes to sexual minority patients in providers of substance abuse treatment that may influence the effectiveness of the 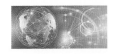 treatment.[14] Those who are transgendered report negative experiences such as hostility or insensitivity in interactions with health care providers.[14]

Both youth and adults who identify as a sexual and/or gender minority experience higher rates of mental illness, substance abuse, violence, and discrimination compared with the general population.[13] Approximately 40% of homeless youth are identified as lesbian-gay-bisexual-transgender, and the leading reasons for homelessness among this group are due to family rejection.[13] Parental rejection increases the likelihood that lesbian-gay-bisexual-transgender youth will suffer from depression, attempt suicide, use illegal drugs, and/or engage in risky sexual behaviors.[13]

## Disparities in Surgical Procedures

There are well-documented racial/ethnic and SES disparities in health care.[6,7] Health and health care are affected by the policies, systems, and environments in which people live and function day-to-day. Population health is differentially affected by health behaviors, clinical care, social and economic conditions, and physical environment.[8] Although this model does not include genetic and biologic factors, it estimates that 40% of health is affected by social and economic conditions followed by 30% by health behaviors, 20% by clinical care, and 10% by the physical environment.[8]

Disparities in surgical care in the United States are also a combination of complex patient, social, and institutional factors.[9] These disparities include higher rates of chronic conditions, greater comorbidity, and greater risk of premature death. In some conditions such as cancer, some populations may present with more advanced disease. For example, African Americans, Native Americans, Hawaiians, Indians, Pakistanis, Mexicans, South and Central Americans, and Puerto Ricans are 1.4 to 3.6 times more likely to present with advanced (stage IV) breast cancer than non-Latino Caucasians.[15]

In addition to the timing of clinical presentation, another explanatory variable for outcome differences may be access to specialists or clinician-level factors.[7] Research findings reveal that clinicians caring for African American patients generally deliver lower-quality health care than when caring for Caucasian patients. African American patients may receive their care from a subgroup of physicians whose qualifications or resources may differ from those of the physicians who treat Caucasian patients.[15] Findings that included clinicians caring for African American patients were less likely to report access to 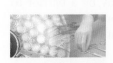 high-quality subspecialists, high-quality diagnostic imaging, high-quality ancillary services, and nonemergency hospital admission.[15] In a study of 8 major cardiovascular and cancer procedures and with adjustment for illness severity, African American patients' outcomes were associated with an increased risk of death following surgery for 7 of the 8 procedures. Once controlled for by the hospital where the patient was treated, the results owing to race were reduced.[16]

Physician-patient communication may be adversely affected by discordant health care for racial/ethnic minorities in comparison with Caucasian patients,[7] which can affect ascertainment of informed consent, collection of social history, and postoperative care instructions adherence.

One study investigated racial disparities in the use of commonly performed medical procedures in US hospitals.[6] Relative risks of age-adjusted rate of procedures used by Caucasians, African Americans, Latinos, Asians or Pacific Islanders, and Native Americans were calculated. Caucasians were compared with all other races based on use and insurance types. Racial disparities were found in the use of cardiac catheterization and coronary arteriog-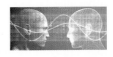raphy, with Caucasian patients significantly more likely to receive the procedure. These differences were maintained by insurance status.[6] Insurance status differences were found between races in upper gastrointestinal endoscopy as well.

Caucasians were twice as likely as Native Americans, more likely than Latinos, and less likely than African Americans to receive fetal monitoring. Caucasians were more likely than all other races to have a cesarean section. Regardless of patients' insurance status, Caucasians were significantly less likely to receive blood transfusions compared with other races. African Americans used this procedure at a higher rate than others. The findings were attributed to sickle-cell anemia, which is mostly diagnosed in African Americans.[6] The findings suggest that "in order to identify the root causes of racial disparities to receive medical procedures, issues such as patients' education and financial status, language barrier, socio-cultural factors involving physician decision making, physicians' attitude towards races, co-morbid diseases, after procedure complications, mistrust to healthcare systems, and patient-physician interaction need to be carefully examined."[6]

As much as 11% to 30% of the global burden of disease requires surgical care and/or anesthesia management.[17] Most recent estimates from the Centers for Disease Control and Prevention are that approximately 51 million inpatient and 53 million outpatient surgical cases are performed in the United States every year.[18] Disparate surgical care may result in poorer functional outcomes, mortality, prolonged rehabilitation and recover, and lower quality of life. For example, the patient SES is a predictor of mortality during surgery, in that mortality is greatest among patients in the lowest SES.[19] The effect of SES of a patient on mortality is not reduced by other explanatory hospital-level or patient-level factors. Access, availability, and affordability to the health care services are disproportionately affected by SES and racial/ethnic minority status.[18] Patients with low SES are less likely to receive appropriate surgical services when compared with more affluent patients.[7] Trauma patients without health insurance have a 50% increase in adjusted odds of death.[20]

Sex, also, affects surgical outcomes. Coronary artery bypass grafting, mitral valve procedures, and other surgical outcomes are disparate for women in comparison with men.[7] Numerous factors are associated with differences in surgical outcomes for men and women. These factors range from sex-determined differences in anatomy, physiology, and the immune response.[21]

Surgeons are, whether by conscious choice or by happenstance, thought to be leaders in their communities and in the world. The principle of distributive justice is one of the fundamental obligations of our discipline. Many surgeons have, at some point in their careers, become actively engaged in work that would promote a more just distribution of the health care advantage enjoyed by many in the developed Western world. Most in our discipline believe that to be at least cognizant of and to perhaps participate in the amelioration of health care disparities is our obligation.

# References

1. The Henry J. Kaiser Family Foundation. Disparities in health and health care: five key questions and answers. Available from: http://kff.org/disparities-policy/issue-brief/disparities-in-health-and-health-care-five-key-questions-and-answers/. Accessed 01 September 2016.
2. The Henry J. Kaiser Family Foundation. *Key Facts on Health Care by Race and Ethnicity*. Kaiser Family Foundation. Available from: http://files.kff.org/attachment/Chartpack-Key-Facts-on-Health-and-Health-Care-by-Race-and-Ethnicity. Accessed 02 September 2016.
3. United States Census Bureau. Table 11. Percent Distribution of the Projected Population by Hispanic Origin and Race for the United States: 2015 to 2060. Available from: http://www.census.gov/population/projections/data/national/2014/summarytables.html. Accessed 02 September 2016.
4. National Center for Health Satistics. Health, United States, 2015: In Brief. Hyattsville, Maryland: Centers for Disease Control and Prevention, U.S. Department of Health and Human Services; 2016.
5. Agency for Healthcare Research and Quality. 2014 National healthcare quality and disparities report. Available from: http://www.ahrq.gov/sites/default/files/wysiwyg/research/findings/nhqrdr/nhqdr14/2014nhqdr.pdf. Accessed 02 September 2016.
6. Haque SS, Faysel MA, Khan HMR. Racial differences in the use of most commonly performed medical procedures in the United States. *J Health Dis Res Pract*. 2010;4(1):14–25.
7. Haider AH, Dankwa-Mullan I, Maragh-Bass AC, et al. Setting a national agenda for surgical disparities research: recommendations from the national institutes of health and american college of surgeons summit. *JAMA Surg*. 2016;151(6):554–563.
8. County Health Rankings and Roadmaps. Our approach. Available from: http://www.countyhealthrankings.org/our-approach.
9. American College of Surgeons. Statement on health care disparities. Available from: https://www.facs.org/about-acs/statements/67-health-care-disparities. Accessed 31 August 2016.
10. Institute of Medicine. *U.S. Health in International Perspective: Shorter Lives, Poorer Health (Report Brief)*. Available from: http://iom.edu/~/media/Files/Report%20Files/2013/US-Health-International-Perspective/USHealth_Intl_PerspectiveRB.pdf.

11. Michigan Department of Community Health. Diabetes in Michigan update. Available from: http://www.michigan.gov/documents/mdch/Diabetes_in_Michigan_Update_2013_416620_7.pdf. Accessed 19 October 2015.
12. County Health Rankings and Roadmaps. 2015 Michigan rankings. Available from: http://www.countyhealthrankings.org/app/michigan/2015/overview. Accessed 19 October 2015.
13. The Henry J. Kaiser Family Foundation. *Health and Access to Care and Coverage for Lesbian, Gay, Bisexual, and Transgender Individuals in the U.S.* Available from: http://files.kff.org/attachment/Health-and-Access-to-Care-and-Coverage-for-LGBT-Individuals-in-the-US. Accessed 02 September 2016.
14. Institute of Medicine. *The Health of Lesbian, Gay, Bisexual, and Transgender People: Building a Foundation for Better Understanding.* The National Academies Press. Available from: http://www.nap.edu/download/13128. Accessed 02 September 2016.
15. Bach PB, Pham HH, Schrag D, Tate RC, Hargraves JL. Primary care physicians who treat blacks and whites. *N Engl J Med.* 2004;351(6):575–584.
16. Lucas FL, Stukel TA, Morris AM, Siewers AE, Birkmeyer JD. Race and surgical mortality in the United States. *Ann Surg.* 2006;243(2):281–286.
17. Meara JG, Leather AJM, Hagander L, et al. Global Surgery 2030: evidence and solutions for achieving health, welfare, and economic development. *Int J Obstet Anesth.* 2016;25:75–78.
18. National Institute on Minority Health and Health Disparities. NIH launches research program to reduce health disparities in surgical outcomes. Available from: https://www.nih.gov/news-events/news-releases/nih-launches-research-program-reduce-health-disparities-surgical-outcomes. Accessed 31 August 2016.
19. Bennett KM, Scarborough JE, Pappas TN, Kepler TB. Patient socioeconomic status is an independent predictor of operative mortality. *Ann Surg.* 2010;252(3):552–558.
20. Haider AH, Chang DC, Efron DT, et al. Race and insurance status as risk factors for trauma mortality. *Arch Surg.* 2008;143(10):945–949.
21. Guth AA, Hiotis K, Rockman C. Influence of gender on surgical outcomes: does gender really matter? *J Am Coll Surg.* 2005;200(3):440–455.

# 43 Gender Inclusion and Equity in Surgery

Dee E. Fenner, MD
Timothy R.B. Johnson, MD, AM, FACOG

PROLOGUE ▶ The student of the history of surgery is often surprised and occasionally dismayed at the clearly evident presupposition that surgeons are male. Early writers repeatedly state that the goal of their program is to "produce men" of great competence. Historically, at least our discipline was largely closed to women.

If war may ever be judged to have a positive impact, the rise of women in every aspect of American life may to some extent have been quickened by World War II. In recent decades, women have assumed power and leadership in every institution of the Western world. Predictably, the discipline of surgery has been slow to embrace this trend, notwithstanding the now long list of great female contributors to the discipline. This chauvinism is now changing rapidly; one well-known integrated vascular surgery training program has a preponderance of female trainees.

Obstetric and gynecologic surgery has been a leader in the recognition of the value that women bring to our discipline. Dr Dee E. Fenner and Dr Timothy R.B. Johnson have been both champions and chroniclers of this movement.

Dr Dee E. Fenner is a professor and chair of the Department of Obstetrics and Gynecology and a professor of Urology at Michigan Medicine

Dr Timothy R.B. Johnson is a professor and former chair of Obstetrics and Gynecology and a professor of Women's Studies at the University of Michigan

As women assume an equitable share of places in American medical schools, it is not surprising that women are increasingly pursuing professional training and careers in surgical specialties. It is equally unexceptional that they face barriers of acceptance by a brash, often oppositional fraternity with questions about technical and professional competency, cost-effectiveness, commitment to practice, and patient acceptance. Professional ethics and fairness require the evidence-based embrace of women surgeons as full participants in contemporary practice. Using a framework commonly applied to clinical ethics, nonmaleficence and beneficence should be assured, as should patient autonomy and preference, and finally issues of social justice.[1]

## Quality, Safety, and Surgical Skills

Evidence shows that women physicians demonstrate quality and safety metrics comparable to men and achieve the technical and surgical dexterity required of successful surgeons. A random sample of Medicare fee-for-service beneficiaries older than 65 years hospitalized with medical conditions from January 2011 to December 2014 with male and female attending physicians in the same hospital was compared. The outcome measure was 30-day readmission rate. The study showed that elderly patients treated by female internists have a lower mortality and readmissions compared with those cared for by male internists.[2]

Several studies of surgical skills acquisition using training models have shown no differences between men and women. Van Hove and colleagues[3] tested 35 first-year surgical residents using the McGill Inanimate System for Training and Evaluation of Laparoscopic Skills (MISTELS) before and after a 4-week skills training program. The correlation between trainee characteristics, including age, sex, designated surgical specialty, and laparoscopic skill level, was assessed. Nineteen (41%) were female. At intake, there was no significant correlation to age, sex, or designated field. There was a significant negative correlation between trainee age and both degree of improvement during training and final score ($P = .02$ and $.05$). Gender did not correlate with performance on initial or posttraining MISTELS testing; however, women demonstrated better skill retention with a higher mean score (34.3 vs 29.9) on the posttest ($P = .02$).

In a study evaluating obstetrics and gynecology and general surgery residents using the validated Fundamentals of Laparoscopic Surgery, the authors aimed to determine whether female surgical residents underestimate their surgical abilities relative to males on a standardized test of laparoscopic skills. Twenty-six general surgery residents (13 males and 13 females) from

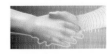

Stanford University and 25 female obstetrics and gynecology residents from Stanford and University Hospitals/Case Medical Center were included. Actual and predicted score as well as delta values (predicted score minus actual score) were compared between residents. Multivariate linear regression was used to determine variables associated with predicted, actual, and delta scores. There was no difference in actual score based on residency or gender. The results showed that predicted scores, however, were significantly lower in female versus male general surgery residents (25.8 ± 13.3 vs 56.0 ± 16.0; $P < .01$) and in female obstetrics and gynecology residents versus male general surgery residents (mean difference 20.9, 95% CI 11.6–34.8; $P < 0.01$). Male residents more accurately predicted their scores, whereas female residents significantly underestimated their scores. They concluded that gender differences in estimating surgical ability exist that do not reflect actual differences in performance. This finding needs to be considered when structuring mentorship in surgical training programs that reinforce women surgical trainees that their gender does not predict or have a negative impact on their surgical skills.[4]

Women have been shown also to have the physical and mental toughness long thought required to be successful surgeons, and they have the ability to undertake taxing and extended procedures with the requisite "toughness." A survey was sent to all the graduates of a general surgery residency that had

matriculated from 1985 to 2006. There were 75 respondents (75% response rate) of which 16 were women and 58 were men. Twice as many men as women pursued fellowship training (46% vs 27%, $P = .2$). Similar factors motivated the career choices: appeal of their field, clinical opportunities in that field, and having an influential residency mentor. However, significantly more women listed lifestyle as an important factor in choosing their future career pathway (69% vs 43%, $P = .03$). Of the most recent graduates (1996-2006), there was no difference in completion of fellowships based on gender. But lifestyle continues to be more important to women. Surgical residency programs might improve the recruitment of women by addressing the perception of the lifestyle associated with choosing a surgical career.[5] Women are more likely than men to leave a training program because of family reasons or to follow a spouse.[6]

## Challenges of Surgical Training and Practice

Medical students, surgical residents, fellows, and fully trained surgeons affiliated with at least one of the 4 major surgical societies were asked to complete a level-specific survey located on the American College of Surgeons Web site. There were 4308 respondents (76% men). Men and women selected similar reasons for choosing a surgical career and residency program and criteria critical to a successful residency program, with women placing greater emphasis on clerkship experience and faculty diversity. There were no statistically significant differences between the men's and women's perceptions of their own training. Although, when asked to evaluate whether certain aspects of training were comparable for male and female residents, women were statistically less likely to agree that their experiences were comparable with those of their male colleagues. Male and female surgical residents, fellows, and trained surgeons identified almost identical training needs and priorities, yet women perceived disparate treatment.

Both male and female respondents cited family and childbearing concerns related to training in general surgery. Earlier studies confirm this common interest in maternity and paternity policies.[7,8] Data also showed that female residents, trained female surgeons, and male fellows consider on-site childcare to be an important component of a successful training program, although male residents and female fellows are considerably more likely than their opposite gender colleagues to look for training programs that are considered "family friendly." Implementation of systems to support bearing and raising children will make programs more appealing to all applicants.

Although the questions were not phrased to imply that one gender received preferential treatment over the other, women residents and trained surgeons were considerably more likely to agree with a statement that read "female residents are treated in an inferior manner compared with male residents." Clearly this is a major problem for surgeons in practice and training. Dissimilar treatment could prevent female surgeons from achieving their ultimate potential, dissuade female medical students from pursuing a career in the field, affect morale, or contribute to attrition and poor productivity.

Also concerning was the minority of respondents who agreed that, in their residency programs, residents might be verbally abused or humiliated in front of colleagues or subjected to sexually inappropriate comments and behavior. Despite this perceived maltreatment, more than half of the male and female respondents agreed that they would definitely do surgery again and encourage medical students to consider careers in surgery. Perhaps female residents, fellows, and trained surgeons have grown to accept a different standard of treatment or simply put up with it in exchange for training in their field of interest. Although most respondents appeared content with their choice to enter into a surgical career, a notable minority disagreed that they would make the same career choice or encourage others to do so. The authors suggested that changing some aspects of surgery training programs might help attract the best candidates and minimize attrition. Disparities in treatment of male and female residents need to be better clarified and addressed, and any and all resident mistreatment must cease. Future studies should be designed to identify particular scenarios in which female surgery 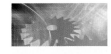 trainees feel alienated, so that education interventions could be directed at those involved in particular negative behaviors.[9]

The persistent, well-described disparity between the salary and earning of female and male surgeons, with women earning less, must be addressed at all levels.[10–12] This gender disparity mirrors a similar disparity in most US job classifications and professions.

Evidence has shown that women surgeons are well accepted by patients and usually their communication score and empathy exceed those of their male counterparts. Johnson et al reported on a self-administered survey designed for and distributed to patients ($N$ = 264) in 13 obstetrics and gynecology waiting rooms in Connecticut. The survey was used to determine whether there were any patient preferences with regard to the gender of physicians providing obstetric and gynecologic care within this population. Of the women surveyed 5.9% preferred men to be their obstetrician-gynecologists, 27.6% preferred women, and 66.6% indicated that they had no preference regarding the sex of their obstetrician-gynecologists.[13]

Much has been written about gender differences in obstetrician-gynecologists, the projected supply of men and women in this specialty practice field, and the potential implications of a shift in gender distribution among providers. Although the practice of obstetrics and gynecology still has more male than female providers, the number of women in this field has been growing steadily for many years. If current trends continue, it is estimated that women will soon outnumber men in the field of obstetrics and gynecology, with a paucity of men in training programs. If most patients prefer to seek care from women, then the current trend should be encouraged; if it is not true, however, there may be a "shortage" of men in obstetrics and gynecology.[13]

## Burnout, Maternity, and Two-Career Families

One critique raised against the training of women is that they do not work the long hours and extended years of male colleagues making the "cost-effectiveness of women" a question.

A special issue of importance, when considering the increasingly important role of gender in the profession, is the role of maternity and dual-career families. Of course, maternity issues, including maternity leave, breastfeeding, and so forth, must be treated fairly. The increasing number of women in dual-career professions requires consideration for both parties.

A questionnaire was mailed to all women and men surgeons who were board certified in 1988, 1992, 1996, 2000, or 2004. Of the 3507 surgeons, 895 (25.5%) responded. Of those, 178 (20.3%) were women and 698 (79.7%) were men. Most men and women would choose their profession again. Male sur-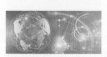geons (odds ratio [OR] 2.5) and all surgeons of younger age (OR 1.3) were less likely to favor part-time work opportunities for surgeons. Most were married, 75% of women and 92% of men. On multivariate regression, women (OR 5.0) and surgeons of younger generation (OR 1.9) were less likely to have children. Women were twice as likely as men to have their first child after entering practice. The spouse was the offspring's primary caregiver for

27% of women and 80% of men ($P < .001$). More female surgeons than males thought maternity leave was important (67% vs 31%, $P < .001$). Overall, women are happy with their professional choices but favor alternative work schedules, maternity leave, and childcare as serious considerations to maximize recruitment and retention of women surgeons.[14]

Members of the American College of Surgeons were surveyed to evaluate the differences in burnout and career satisfaction between men and women surgeons. Of approximately 24 922 surgeons sampled, 1043 women and 6815 men returned the surveys (31.5% response rate). Women surgeons were younger, less likely to be married, less likely to be divorced, and less likely to 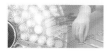 have children (all $P < .001$). No differences between women and men in hours worked or number of nights on call per week were observed. Women surgeons were more likely to believe that child-rearing had slowed their career advancement (57.3% vs 20.2%; $P < .001$), to have experienced a conflict with their spouse's/partner's career (52.6% vs 41.2%; $P < .001$), and to have experienced a work-home conflict in the past 3 weeks (62.2% vs 48.5%; $P < .001$). More women than men surgeons had burnout (43.3% vs 39.0%; $P = .01$) and depressive symptoms (33.0% vs 29.5%; $P = .02$). Factors independently associated with burnout on multivariate analysis were generally similar for men and women and included recent experience of a work-home conflict, resolving the most recent work-home conflict in favor of work, and hours worked per week. Work-home conflicts appear to be a major contributor to surgeon burnout and are more common among women surgeons. Although the factors contributing to burnout were remarkably similar among women and men surgeons, the women were more likely to experience work-home conflicts than were their male colleagues.[15]

Physician recipients of a KO8 or K23 from 2006 to 2009 were surveyed. There were 1049 respondents for a 74% response rate. Women were more likely than men to have a full-time employed spouse or domestic partner (86.5% [95% CI, 82.7%-89.2%] vs 44.9% [95% CI, 40.8%-49.8%]). Among married or partnered respondents, after controlling for work hours, spousal employment, and other factors, women spent 8.5 more hours per week on domestic activities.[16]

Dual-physician relationships are more common among women surgeons (42% to 50%) compared with male surgeons (15% to 30%). For women in the dual-physician relationship, they are more likely to have depressive symptoms and low mental quality of life compared with surgeons whose domestic partner stays home. Surgeons whose domestic partner stays home appear to be more satisfied with their careers, regardless of gender ($P < .0001$). Surgeons in dual-physician relationships more often experience a career conflict. Health care organizations should strive to help dual-physician partners by facilitating their careers with flexible scheduling, daycare in the workplace, and adjusted timelines for promotion and tenure and by planning for dual spousal recruits.[17]

In dual-career couples, there has been an increase for one of the partners to work a reduced schedule. Fifty-one full-time physicians and 47 reduced-hour physicians, all female, were interviewed. Reduced-hour physicians were more likely primary care, spent more time at home, and were less involved in research. There was no difference between the 2 groups in perception of work interfering with family life. All physicians who worked their preferred number of hours—full time or reduced—reported better job-role quality, lower burnout, better marital-role quality, and higher life satisfaction. So women physicians who work their preferred number of hours achieved the best balance of work and family outcomes.[18]

## Conclusion

Gender bias cannot be an acceptable form of professional behavior or a reason for exclusion of women from training and practice. Hong and Page[19] introduce a general framework for modeling functionally diverse problem-solving agents. In this framework, problem-solving agents possess representations of problems and algorithms that they use to locate solutions. They use this framework to establish a result relevant to group composition and found that when selecting a problem-solving team from a diverse population of intelligent agents, a team of randomly selected agents outperforms a team that comprises the best-performing agents. This result relies on the intuition that as the initial pool of problem solvers becomes large, the best-performing agents necessarily become similar in the space of problem solvers. Their relatively greater ability is more than offset by their lack of problem-solving diversity. "Mathematically, diversity trumps ability."[19-21] Women surgeons are occupying a larger space next to their male colleagues. Equity, consistency, and other human rights and civil rights principles, as well as federal job requirements, state and institutional regulations, and internal human resource rules, must be respected. Reimbursement must be consistently and repeatedly attended to as a matter of fairness. Inclusion must be sought at every level of the professional pipeline, and ethical principles should always be considered to remain controlling the professional imperatives.

## References

1. Jonsen AR, Siegler M, Winslade WJ. *Clinical Ethics: A Practical Approach to Ethical Decisions in Clinical Medicine.* 8th ed. McGraw Hill Education; 2015.
2. Tsugawa Y, Jena AB, Figueroa JF, Orav EJ, Blumenthal DM, Jha AK. Comparison of hospital mortality and readmission rates for Medicare patients treated by male vs female physicians. *JAMA Inter Med.* 2017;177:206–213. doi: 10.1001/jamainternmed.2016.787.
3. Van Hove C, Perry KA, Spight DH, et al. Predictors of technical skill acquisition among resident trainees in a laparoscopic skills education program. *World J Surg.* 2008;32:1917–1921.

4. Flyckt RI, White EE, Goodman LR, Mohr C, Dutta S, Zanotti KM. The use of laparoscopic simulation to explore gender differences in resident surgical confidence. *Obstet Gynecol Int.* 2017; Article ID 1945801, 1–7.

5. McCord JH, McDonald R, Leverson G, et al. Motivation to pursue surgical subspecialty training: is there a gender difference? *J Am Coll Surg.* 2007;205:698–703.

6. Bergen PC, Turnage RH, Carrico CJ. Gender-related attrition in a general surgery training program. *J Surg Res.* 1998;77:59–62.

7. Baxter N, Cohen R, McLeod R. The impact of gender on the choice of surgery as a career. *Am J Surg.* 1996;172:373–376.

8. Mayer KL, Ho HS, Goodnight JE. Childbearing and child care in surgery. *Arch Surg.* 2001;136:649–655.

9. Saalwachter AR, Freischlag JA, Sawyer RG, Sanfey HA. The training needs and priorities of male and female surgeons and their trainees. *J Am Coll Surg.* 2005;201:199–205.

10. Desai T, Ali S, Fang X, Thompson W, Jawa P, Vachharajani T. Equal work for unequal pay: the gender reimbursement gap for healthcare providers in the United States. *Postgrad Med J.* 2016;92:571–575.

11. Ly DP, Seabury SA, Jena AB. Differences in incomes of physicians in the United States by race and sex: observational study. *BMJ.* 2016;353:i2923. doi: 10.1136/bmj. i2923.

12. Weeks WB, Wallace A. The influence of race and gender on family physicians' annual incomes. *J Am Board Fam Med.* 2006;19:548–556.

13. Johnson AM, Schnatz PF, Kelsey AM, Ohannessian CM. Do women prefer care from female or male obstetrician-gynecologists? A study of patient gender preference. *J Am Osteopath Assoc.* 2005;105:369–379.

14. Troppmann KM, Palis BE, Goodnight JE, Ho HS, Troppmann C. Women surgeons in the new millennium. *Arch Surg.* July 2009;144:635–642.

15. Dyrbye LN, Shanafelt TD, Balch CM, Satele D, Sloan J, Freischlag J. Relationship between work-home conflicts and burnout among American surgeons: a comparison by sex. *Arch Surg.* 2011;146:211–217.

16. Jolly S, Griffith KA, DeCastro R, Stewart A, Ubel P, Jagsi R. Gender differences in time spent on parenting and domestic responsibilities by high achieving young physician researchers. *Ann Intern Med.* 2014;160:344–353.

17. Dyrbye LN, Shanafelt TD, Balch CM, Satele D, Freischlag J. Physicians married or partnered to physicians: a comparative study in the American College of Surgeons. *J Am Coll Surg.* 2010;211:663–671.

18. Carr PL, Gareis KC, Barnett RC. Characteristics and outcomes for women physicians who work reduced hours. *J Womens Health.* 2003;12:399–405.

19. Hong L, Page SE. Groups of diverse problem solvers can outperform groups of high-ability problem solvers. *Proc Natl Acad Sci.* 2004;101:16385–16389.

20. Page SE. *The Difference: How the Power of Diversity Creates Better Groups, Firms, Schools, and Societies.* Princeton, NJ: Princeton University Press; 2007.

21. Makary MA, Sexton JB, Freischlag JA, et al. Operating room teamwork among physicians and nurses: teamwork in the eye of the beholder. *J Am Coll Surg.* 2006;202:746–752.

# 44 Autonomy in Excess

Lloyd A. Jacobs, MD

PROLOGUE ▶ The notion of an individual's autonomy has deep roots in English common law. It derives originally from the prohibition of "unlawful touching" and is to a significant degree embodied in the amendments to our constitution. The notion has, therefore, wide implications beyond its applications to health care. Ultimately, a person, of whatever gender or persuasion, has nearly absolute authority over his/her body. Behaviors and utterances, unless clearly unlawful, have much of the same sanctity.

Surgeons, by the very definition of their work, intrude on this sanctity. What is important is that we do our work with the full, clear, and usually expressed directive of the patient. One's autonomy in this regard is nearly absolute.

The surgeon has an obligation to promote the autonomy of his/her patients. Recent parlance has begun to replace the term "autonomy" with the phrase "respect for persons." Adoption of this usage emphasizes that autonomy is the only one aspect of what it is to be a human being; interdependence and connection with others are an equally compelling need of human flourishing. Still, throughout this book we will continue to use the term "autonomy" because it is this aspect of human need that stands opposite the traditional authoritarian posture of our discipline.

The patient may exercise his/her autonomy in a way that the surgeon believes is detrimental to the patient's own health. One example of such behavior is a failure to comply with a regimen of wound care or the inappropriate use of medications. Such behaviors may not only affect the patient but also be unlawful as when opioids are sold on the street. This phenomenon is particularly relevant to the surgeon as pain management is an integral and important aspect of surgical care.[1]

A second example of far-reaching consequences resulting from an individual patient's noncompliance is the development of antibiotic resistance. Failure to complete the prescribed course of antibiotics is thought to contribute to this problem. A patient's demands for antibiotics, even when inappropriate, may overcome the surgeon's scruples and also contribute to the problem.

Occasionally, patients will express to the surgeon attitudes, which in any current culture are unacceptable. It is not uncommon for patients to impugn a race or religion or sexual orientation in comments clearly unrelated to the illness under discussion. Worse, patients may refuse to be examined or operated on by a person of some particular category. Once again there are no easy answers. Full planned chart documentation should be shared with the patient. Ultimately the surgeon may be justified in terminating the relationship. No matter how painful, the surgeon must not abandon the patient.

In these examples the surgeon's role is largely educational. Ultimately an impasse may be encountered. As so often said in this book, unresolvable tensions may come to exist between the patient's autonomy and his/her own or society's welfare.

Autonomy is also often seen as a context for end-of-life decisions and in discussions of informed consent for an operation or procedure. However, a situation even more difficult may face the surgeon when the patient refuses care. Paradoxically, this occurrence seems to be more frequent in this age of transparency. Concomitants of that transparency, which may conduce to patient refusal, are a lessening of the surgeon's authority and a fuller understanding by patients of procedural complications. However, in most instances, a patient's refusal of a procedure is not due to a careful calculated assessment of risk. More often the refusal may rest on reasons that seem to most of us to be irrational.

Patients may refuse needed surgical intervention for a wide variety of reasons, and the surgeon has an obligation to try to understand those reasons. It is important to remember that rational arguments in opposition to irrational thinking are unlikely of success. Somehow, the surgeon must earn the trust of the patient; this may best be accomplished by showing a reciprocal respect for the patient's objections.

There are 3 reasons generally that cause patients to refuse a needed operation or procedure. These are neither distinct nor mutually exclusive. The patient may have misinformation about the risks and benefits of a procedure. A patient may be frozen by fear. And, occasionally the patient refuses on 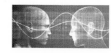 recognition of a power gradient in rote defiance of authority. Although these are not distinct, they require distinct responses from the surgeon.

More than 90% of households in the United States have immediate Internet access, and a high percentage of patients indicate that they have searched the Internet for information about their health before their consultation with a surgeon. The search heading may be a diagnosis given by a primary care provider or a guess based on the patient's perceptions of his/her symptoms. Used this way the Internet is a powerful promoter of patient autonomy and in general has promoted good within the meaning of the word implied throughout this book. However, it is a truism that the Internet may also be the source of a great deal of misinformation. Such misinformation may consist of an inaccurate description of the natural history of a disease or unwarranted focus on complications of a procedure and occasionally may consist of clear charlatanry. Indeed, it is sometimes unclear why the patient consulted with the surgeon at all; his/her mind appears to have been fixed before the consultation. The surgeon should not be misled by this appearance. A patient's refusal of needed surgical care is often a cry for help.

When patient refusal results from misinformation, the surgeon has an obligation to provide accurate information. This may not be easy because an accurate description of many procedures is technically complex and beyond easy communication. Moreover, a myriad of emphases in description is possible for any operation. The surgeon must choose. A "just trust me attitude" or a "take it or leave it" ultimatum is to be avoided. It is often best to advise the patient to consult with family members, trusted advisors, or others within the constellation of his/her own network rather than trying to force the issue to a conclusion. Leave the issue open; do not, by act or utterance, signal closure.

A second reason for patient refusal is fear. This fear is rarely quelled with information; it is not fear of complications or pain or a changed lifestyle. It is more accurately, perhaps, called dread: dread of death, dread of dismemberment, or dread of the loss of life's meaning, which is tantamount to annihilation. Such dread "doth make cowards of us all."[2]

Pressing the patient to realize and act on his/her autonomy and freedom to choose will avail nearly nothing in this circumstance. In fact the fear and dread they experience are nearly synonymous with the alienation end of the autonomy spectrum. Here is where the only patient support is succor, and a modicum of maternalism or paternalism is the only tool. "We will care for you; you may depend on us," is the only message likely to avail. Consultation with specialists in mental health or pastoral care may be of great assistance.

Intoxication with alcohol or other substances as a cause for patients to 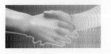 refuse needed procedures is most frequently encountered in trauma and emergency surgery settings. It should be noted again that none of these causes of refusal are pure; intoxicants may increase fear or even render alternative care more appealing. Here the conundrum may be truly Gordian.

The urgency of the circumstances may be such that there is inadequate time for intoxicants to be metabolized. There is inadequate time to seek a judge's order. There is inadequate time to find surrogates or to establish their authority. And if legitimate surrogates are present, they may be hesitant to speak contrarily to the patients' irrational utterances. This is an almost classic example of a situation wherein whatever you do will be wrong. Seek consultation, not only for corroboration of information but also in the hope that a show of consensus may prevail. Consultations therefore need not be from another surgeon; an emergency department physician or whoever is available will be helpful.

Courts have ruled that a notion called "implied consent" has validity when a patient is comatose. In that instance, most hospitals have procedures for the documentation of patient unconsciousness and dire need of operation under the rubric of implied consent. Surgeons should familiarize themselves with these policies before they are needed.

It sometimes occurs that a patient refusing intervention becomes unconscious during discussion of the need for intervention. This may initially appear to simplify the situation; many experienced surgeons have witnessed situations in which further discussion seemed futile, and the surgical team hoped for or waited for unconsciousness. This is not a good solution. The surgeon is still left with his/her obligation to being the patient's agent and to do or behave as the patient would have wanted. Moreover, waiting for unconsciousness to ensue is somehow contrary to the principle of beneficence however salutary the outcome may be.

There are no easy answers here. Ultimately, a patient in possession of his/her faculties is perfectly within his/her rights to refuse intervention; such refusal must be honored. A patient not in possession of his/her faculties by virtue of intoxication or even dread is more difficult to treat. But here also, at great psychologic cost to all involved, patient autonomy must ultimately prevail.

## References

1. Baker DW. History of the Joint Commission's Pain Standards. *JAMA*. 2017;317(11):117.
2. Shakespeare W. To Be or Not To Be. Soliloquy from Hamlet; 1603.

# 45 The Ethical Obligations and Opportunities to Participate in Peer Review

Richard E. Burney, MD

PROLOGUE ▶ Although the surgeon's obligation to his/her individual patient is clearly a deontological one and nearly obsolete, the surgeon's relationship to society at large is complex and confusing. Much of this book, therefore, focuses on societal obligations and the tension felt by the surgeon to stand between the obligation to his/her individual patient and the utilitarian ethic of "the greatest good for the greatest number." Moreover, this tension may remain unconscious, and its ill effects may be experienced only indirectly.

Surgeons exist and work within a societal matrix. Consequences of alleged substandard performance have been extant for centuries: The Code of Hammurabi in ancient Mesopotamia specified a lex talionis, eye for an eye, set of consequences. The societal matrix and its obligation are ancient, pervasive, and sometimes odious. Still it is always a surgeon's obligation to reckon with them.

Dr Richard E. Burney has been both a champion for the society's prerogative and a champion for justice and due process for surgeons. His long history and wise balance have made him a nationally recognized expert in the world of peer review. Some of his narratives are shocking; all are instructive. Every surgical trainee should read this chapter carefully.

Dr Richard E. Burney is a professor emeritus of surgery at the University of Michigan Medical School and continues to actively practice general surgery.

## Introduction

Among the ethical obligations of all physicians is the duty to participate in peer review. The purpose of this chapter is to describe the scope, themes, and variations of that obligation. These range from self-review, consisting of self-assessment and individual quality improvement efforts, to engagement at a variety of higher levels of participation, beginning at the local group or department level and extending to the hospital, region, state, and national levels. The common theme across this range of activities, regardless of the level at which one might be working, is a fiduciary duty, which in the medical context means the responsibility of putting your patient's interests above your own. This duty comprises the ethical requirements of honesty, altruism, and beneficence, in combination with knowledge, lack of bias or conflict, objectivity, transparency, and the ability to engage in open-minded inquiry. This obligation is described in the policies of major medical organizations.

> Statement of the American Board of Internal Medicine on Medical Professionalism in the New Millennium: *As members of the profession, physicians are expected to participate in the processes of self-regulation, including remediation and discipline of members who have failed to meet professional standards. The profession should also define and organize the educational and standard-setting process for current and future members. Physicians have both individual and collective obligations to participate in these processes. These obligations include engaging in internal assessment and accepting external scrutiny of all aspects of their professional performance.*[1]
> Principles of Medical Ethics of the American Medical Association (AMA): *A physician shall uphold the standards of professionalism, be honest in all professional interactions, and strive to report physicians deficient in character or competence, or engaging in fraud or deception, to appropriate entities.*[2]

As will become evident, there are many different types of obligations, each with its own set of challenges. Peer review can cover a range from self-discipline to reporting substandard conduct on the part of your peers without any conflicts of interest, to reviewing submitted articles for publication, to ensuring that members of your profession act properly 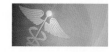 through service on various internal and external oversight boards and committees.

I hasten to add that it is not possible to examine the surgeon's role in peer review without concurrently examining the ethical values and behaviors of the leadership in the various institutions and systems that support peer review, which can either enable it or undermine it. I will therefore touch on this important aspect of peer review as well.

## Origins of Peer Review

One can logically argue that no one is more qualified to make judgments about physician performance than other physicians, and although this seems obvious today, it is actually a relatively recent achievement. A century or more ago, as the era of modern science–based medical practice began to emerge, physicians could for the first time differentiate between medical practice based on empiric and scientific observation and testing and that based on folk remedies and quackery. To remedy this and to protect the public, some physicians began to band together to form associations and institutions that could render judgments on the qualifications and performance of unqualified persons advertising themselves to the public as physicians.

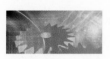 Thus, the AMA was founded in 1847 by "regular" physicians (ie, those with Doctor of Medicine [MD] degrees), who found themselves competing with the graduates of dubious schools—eclectic, herbalist, homeopathic, and so forth—who expounded alternative medical theories and sought a way to become formally recognized for the first time as a true profession, with the privilege of self-governance. At that time, in the late 19th century, the legal status of a "profession" was recognized only for lawyers and military officers. The first official state boards of medicine were established at least in part to accord to medicine the same privileges as a legally recognized profession. (However, remember that the AMA also fought against midwives to establish themselves as the only legitimate providers, thus cutting poor rural women off from support, and opposed abortion to make themselves the governing body from health care for women. There are economic motives to establishing a monopoly, not just peer review.) The new state boards, for the first time, could require physicians to be licensed if they wished to practice. In other words, physicians were for the first time enabled to render judgments regarding the education and qualifications of those seeking to enter medical practice. The constitutionality of the regulation of medical practice through state boards of medicine was promptly challenged, but the legitimacy of the power of state medical boards was upheld by the US Supreme Court in the landmark 1889 decision, Dent v. West Virginia.

Then, as now, there was concern regarding the inherent conflict of interest that existed in professional self-regulation. George Bernard Shaw in his preface to "The Doctor's Dilemma" argued that a doctor paid fees for services could not be trusted to regulate his/her own professional behavior. This is actually an argument for external peer review and poses the questions how and by whom? Should this be done exclusively within the profession? Was the legal protection that "regular" physicians sought to perform their duties on a medical board mainly for the purpose of protecting their own turf and excluding non-MDs (in the 19th century, that meant physicians from alternative schools and diploma mills; today, it might mean alternative care providers such as advanced practice nurses) from engaging in medical practice? Or was the purpose truly to protect the public from charlatans? Could peer review within the profession, giving it a form of monopoly power, be done in a way that avoided economic self-interest? Or was some degree of self-interest inevitable and inherent in any peer judgment? Although most believe that peer review can be structured and performed in such a way as to avoid contamination by self-interest, and that the higher-level goal of protecting the public outweighs such concerns, there will always be those who argue otherwise. And for peer reviewers, it will always represent an ethical challenge.

## Immunity for Peer Reviewers

Physicians are called on to make judgments on other physicians at many levels. The examination of one's qualifications by peers usually starts with the application to join a specialty society or be admitted to a hospital medical staff. These are among the most basic levels at which the profession assures the quality in the care that patients receive because such acceptance is an acknowledgment that a physician has met an accepted standard for education and training. The physicians participating in these decisions are presumed to have the reputation and best interests of the institution or society in mind but may also be influenced, or appear to be influenced, by bias or prejudice. Thus, those making the decisions must ensure that they have no conflicts of interest, apparent or real. The decision to admit a professional to a hospital staff or specialty society also carries with it a more difficult job, which is the need to oversee subsequent performance and impose discipline if performance or behavior is substandard or puts patients at risk.

Criticism of peer review is most evident at the hospital level when admission to a medical staff and delineation of privileges are at stake and when one or another dominant specialty group seeks to keep out possible competitors under the guise of preserving quality. Peer review processes within hospitals have been challenged on the one hand for being ineffective and on the other for being biased or unfairly punitive, which has put peer reviewers at risk of being sued as a result of their decisions. Should physicians engaged in 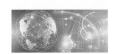 these peer review activities have legal protection? The need to protect physicians on peer review committees from legal harassment has been recognized as critically important for quality oversight. Immunity protection for good faith peer review activities was enacted at the federal level as part of the

Health Care and Quality Improvement Act of 1986. As a result of this law, physicians engaging in peer review of quality of care can do so without the fear of incurring personal liability. Their ethical responsibilities remain unchanged.

## Hospital Staff Review

The effectiveness of peer review activities for both overseeing admission to a medical staff and imposing disciplinary actions depends in large part on the size, organization, and structure of the institution, as well as the nature of the infraction or complaint. This is particularly true in small hospitals where a physician is likely to have few peers or where external, usually financial, pressures on the hospital create an environment that affects judgment. Let me give an example in which there were both individual and system failures.

A young surgeon with a growing family, having completed his surgical training at a large community teaching hospital and not wishing to uproot his family, takes a job in the same region at a nearby small community hospital that has advertised for a general surgeon. The one surgeon at that hospital is older, and although he has acknowledged the need for another surgeon, he has no interest in helping someone new. The hospital, which is paying the young surgeon's salary to help him get started in practice, strongly encourages the new surgeon to take on all the cases he can, including some for which he has had little, if any, exposure during his training. Having no senior guidance from his sole colleague and fearing displeasure of the administration, he tries to do these cases. Some of his patients have serious complications, which lead to a large malpractice settlement and termination of his privileges at the hospital and a report to the state Board of Medicine.

During the investigation by the Board, a number of ethical and other issues pertaining to this surgeon came to light, but concerns about the behavior of the other surgeon and the hospital administration were raised as well. In this situation, what were the obligations of the various parties? The surgeon in question had an obligation to provide good care for his patients, which included not taking on cases for which he was ill-prepared. The other surgeon at the hospital had the obligation to offer assistance and advice to a younger colleague. The hospital had an obligation to the patient population it served 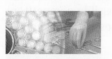 to provide the best care it could. All three parties had an obligation to serve the public honestly and skillfully. The Board of Medicine's chief obligation is to protect the public, but at the same time, the Board was fully aware that this young surgeon's career hung in the balance. It has both legal and ethical obligations that may be in conflict.

In the end, the young surgeon in this story recognized his errors and behaved responsibly, even if the hospital and the other surgeon did not. The surgeon had sufficient self-awareness to seek counseling and to recognize that he had made serious errors in judgment. He was interviewed for a new position in a multihospital group in another state, and during his interviews, he was completely honest about his mistakes and the problems he had encountered. An arrangement was worked out that allowed him to start work there with a limited scope of practice, with mentoring and close monitoring. The licensing board in the other state, given all the facts, limited his license accordingly by placing him on probation with the requirement that his new employer give regular reports regarding his performance. He successfully rehabilitated his career.

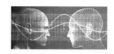

## When Should Peer Review Start?

At what point in our professional careers should we become subject to peer review? Should it be deferred until application for a medical staff position or membership in a national specialty organization? The answer is no. The most important times may be during medical school and postgraduate training. The competition for medical student admission, which more and more has come to be based primarily on presumably objective measures such as test scores and grades, is so intense that it has led to the presumption that all students are qualified and capable; they would have to be to get where they are. Moreover, one cannot easily pass judgment on a medical student's knowledge while the student is presumably still learning. The giving of grades has given way to giving feedback intended to help students succeed. Testing has been outsourced to the United States Medical Licensing Examination. Failure has become the fault of the school, not of the student. Character is hard to judge and ethics, hard to inculcate. Nevertheless, I have encountered a small number of students who one could reasonably predict, based on their medical school performance, would fail in their careers because of personal failings.

"Peer review" at this stage must consist of more than looking at grades and test scores. The failure is less often one of intelligence or knowledge; more often it is one of motivation, absence of altruism, and deficits in personal behavior, manifested by cheating, laziness, dishonesty, or substance abuse. Other personality disorders might include a lack of empathy, an inability to get along with ancillary personnel, a lack of caring, and inappropriate decision making. Some cases were particularly troubling: I was once asked to help make recommendations for how to deal with a third-year medical student, a faculty member's son, who had been found to be stealing drugs from the anesthesia carts. Another legacy student was found to have cheated on a test. The first was dismissed from school; the second was asked to take a year off. In both instances, the physician parents faced with these difficult situations involving their children did not contest the recommendations but put the integrity of the profession above their personal disappointment.

If a student has been disciplined in some way during medical school but has successfully completed his/her studies and graduated in good standing, should that be considered a black mark on his/her career? 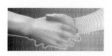 As a member of the Board of Medicine, I was involved in adjudicating a case in which a physician who, in the course of applying for a license in another state to enter a fellowship there, answered "no" to the question, have you ever been subjected to disciplinary action, assuming that the question referred to disciplinary action by a hospital or state licensing authority. He was penalized by that state licensing board because his medical school transcript showed that in his third year he had been dismissed from one of his clinical rotations, which he later made up. He graduated in good standing, currently held a state license, and had no reason to consider this a disciplinary action for another state's licensing purposes. For this, a heavy fine was imposed. Rather than spending the additional money to contest this decision, he paid the fine, unaware that by so doing he would become subject to additional penalties imposed by any other states in which he was or wished to be licensed because of failure to report the other state penalty. The case came to me because of this failure to report. After ascertaining the facts and interviewing the physician in person, I could find no reason for the first state to have imposed a disciplinary action, which in my view had been based almost entirely on a legal technicality of word interpretation. It was certainly not the cause for imposing additional penalties. In my view, the other state medical board seemed to be acting in its own self-interest by imposing an unwarranted fine on this physician. He ultimately chose to go elsewhere for fellowship.

## Peer Review During Postgraduate Training

Peer review of physicians during postgraduate training has some of the same characteristics as peer review of medical students: Is there a fundamental deficiency in character or performance that should disqualify someone from continued training in that specialty? It is rare for a surgical resident to be dismissed from a training program, and such disciplinary actions can be, and frequently are, challenged by accusations of discrimination and bias. The peer review role in such situations is to assure both procedural and substantive due process that there has been adequate notice of deficiencies with opportunity for corrective action and remediation, the availability of adequate mentoring and monitoring, and fairness of the hearing process. If the failure is one of knowledge and skill, or uncertainty as to whether the resident is in the right specialty, the best solution is to help the resident transition to a new field. I have seen successful transitions from surgery into anesthesiology, emergency medicine, psychiatry, or industry made by self-aware young residents who found themselves after 1 or 2 or 3 years in the wrong field. On the other hand, if the failure is one of honesty, integrity, psychiatric issues, or substance abuse, the challenge is much greater. I know of one senior surgical resident whom I reported for failure to take proper, attentive care of his patients. He was fired from the program. I ran into him 10 years later and was surprised when he thanked me for having helped him to recognize and deal with his substance abuse problem, something neither I nor anyone else had known about at that time. He was now in successful practice in another field.

That story had a happy ending, but these situations do not always work out that way. What I sometimes saw during my service on the Board of Medicine was the file of a physician who as a resident exhibited substance abuse or personal behavior problems and instead of being fired, was allowed to resign or to finish the year and drop out of the program. The physician, with no black marks on his record, would find another training position that, again, lasted only a year. Although failing to successfully complete any postgraduate training program, but having in the process accumulated enough years of postgraduate training with no reported disciplinary actions on his record, he became eligible for an unrestricted license and in this case become a potential menace.

The ethical obligation of the postgraduate program director is to monitor not just the technical performance but also the behavioral characteristics of the trainees in the program. That obligation should not be ignored in the case of a trainee who drops out by failing to terminate the trainee. The reluctance to put something negative on a physician's record, to avoid hassle, to sweep it under the carpet, and let him/her become someone else's problem represents a failure of peer review. It is important to recognize that imposing a disciplinary action and putting it on the record does not prevent a physician from going on to have a successful career. Quite to the contrary, it forces the physician to confront the fact that he/she has a problem, while at the same time giving notice to others, eg, training programs, hospitals, licensing boards, that this physician has had problems and needs special supervision.

The failure to do this can negatively affect both the trainee and the program director when the latter is called on to exercise peer judgment at the end of residency training and when the program director must sign off on young surgeons completing their training and attest to the fact that they are both competent and of good moral character. One chairman, new to an academic department, found he had a chief resident whose behavior raised questions in his mind. On the other hand, the resident was almost at the end of a long period of training, the new chairman had only limited exposure to him, and there were no black marks on his evaluations. No one else had raised alarms. In the end, he signed off on the trainee. 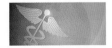 He regretted his decision 2 years later when the young surgeon's subsequent performance was so substandard that he was dismissed from his position. This failure reflected poorly on the program, which was seen as no longer trustworthy in its recommendations.

In practice, character traits are the chief determinants of competence.

## Department-Level Review

At the department level, it is incumbent on the department leaders to exercise peer review whenever a new surgeon is brought on to the staff. This has been done in a variety of ways, the most time-honored of which is the personal phone call to someone reliable who is or should be familiar with the person in question. (Which is why my future father-in-law, a surgeon, placed such a call to my department chair when he learned that I might wish to marry his daughter.) The quality of this anecdotal evidence can be variable. I know of at least one instance in which a highly respected institution gave its blessing to a candidate my institution was recruiting, who by all appearances and on paper was stellar, but about whose behavior the institution harbored serious reservations, so much so that later it admitted it was pleased to see him go. After a couple of years his egocentric, narcissistic tendencies led to his dismissal from the institution that had recruited him.

Assessments of personal behavior are often subjective. Who is to say there is no inherent or unrecognized bias in one's personal assessment of someone else? Moreover, if poor surgical results have occurred, there is always an explanation for the apparent lapses or errors in care or judgment. When someone is

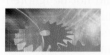

persuasively confident about what he/she is doing, it can overcome a degree of doubt in the mind of the evaluator, or perhaps engender skepticism. How does the surgical leader gather objective data, for example, evidence of poor quality care or financial mismanagement that can unequivocally support a decision to fire someone, particularly someone prominent in his/her field?

An internal conflict is faced by every surgeon asked to judge a colleague, in particular a colleague who is a friend or acquaintance, when something bad has happened, because one cannot help putting oneself in the other's shoes and thinking, "there but for the grace of God, go I": the same thing could have happened to me. This empathic tendency tempers the kind of judgments that one might make, tending to shift one toward forgiveness, but an argument can be made that this is a false benevolence. There is a difference between personal forgiveness and professional forgiveness. I may forgive the person but at the same time condemn his/her actions.

A valued colleague in a large surgical department seemed to get himself into trouble when doing certain types of complex cases. This was not recognized, however, until the chair of the department had to reoperate on one of the patients to correct an obvious error in both judgment and technique. The chair, who had recruited the surgeon in question, was faced with some troubling questions. He now knew of "one bad case." He chose to inquire further, and other anecdotes of poor judgment or technique surfaced. There were only a few egregious cases; was this a situation in which "there but for the grace of God" obtained? The surgeon he had recruited had a glowing national reputation; it would be embarrassing to all parties if he were to be disciplined or fired. Why had not these deficiencies surfaced during the recruitment process? Was the surgeon in question aware of his limitations? Was the surgeon taking on complex cases beyond his capability? If so, why? What were the ethical responsibilities of the surgeon and of the chairman? The hospital legal office got wind of the problem and, fearing possible malpractice actions, put pressure on the chief of the medical staff to force the issue.

During a subsequent conversation with the surgeon, the chair began to see that the surgeon did not recognize he might be taking on cases he should not and that a combination of ego, hubris, and pride prevented him from both altering his practice and accepting criticism. The surgeon, confronted with this opinion, felt the chair was biased and was judging him unfairly based on the one case with which he had been personally involved. How then should the chair proceed in a fair and ethical way?

His first step was to assemble a panel of peer reviewers who were unaware of the alleged problem and ask them to review 25 or more randomly selected cases for quality: judgment, decision making, surgical planning, operative performance, complications, and postoperative care, without indicating in advance what the concerns were. The review was structured in a way that focused on the patient's point of view and minimized as much as possible the exercise of hindsight. The panel was not asked to offer opinions with regard to what should be done should deficiencies be found. They found deficiencies in judgment and technique with regard to certain types of cases.

The end result was a negotiation in which the surgeon, confronted with the peer review results, was forced to recognize that his sphere of competence was narrower than he wished it to be, and he accepted "voluntary" limitations in operating privileges. The medical staff office instituted a monitoring program. The surgeon did the kinds of cases he could do well. There were no further problems.

This example argues for some form of ongoing monitoring to be sure professionals are not practicing outside their area of expertise. This is particularly true when new or innovative techniques are introduced. Hospitals and care organizations must establish appropriate credentialing procedures to assure adequate training and experience, as well as monitoring outcomes, which can only be done by peers.

## Peer Review at the Institutional Level

Peer review at the institutional level or higher always involves the interaction or collaboration of physicians and lawyers in joint medical and legal review. There is no question that the workings of the legally trained mind are different from those of the medically trained mind. The lawyer is trained 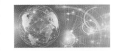 to advocate for one point of view, and the legal process generally leads to a decision for one side over another with little room for compromise. The legal process can have a harsh, black-and-white, Manichean quality, one in which gray areas are eschewed. Physicians, on the other hand, work daily in gray areas and are constantly reminded that not all situations are black and white; and although they can advocate for their patients at times, they have no enforcement power over them. This divergence in thinking can make for challenging confrontations, whether the setting is a hospital peer review committee, a medical board disciplinary hearing, or a malpractice proceeding. The ethical physician's role in any of these settings is to see to it that the standard of medical care prevails or at least has a fair hearing. It is not necessary to advocate for one point of view or another, for the patient or the hospital, for the plaintiff or the defendant.

The intersection of medicine and law has always been contentious and an often misunderstood ground on which to tread. The law has rightly established the principle that persons who have been harmed are entitled to compensation. However, the associated legal proceedings to determine whether compensation is warranted are by their very nature adversarial, and adversarial interactions are something that physicians are not comfortable with and work hard to avoid. Patient care is, after all, based on establishing therapeutic trust and cooperation. Nevertheless, errors and harms occur in the course of medical practice and when they do, it is up to peers to acknowledge them. Uncomfortable as this may be, it, too, is a role for peer review.

I have served on a hospital medical liability review committee (MLRC) for more than 30 years and observed how, at least where I work, this activity has evolved over time. Currently, under the leadership of Richard Boothman, it is a thoughtful process that puts the patient and physician first. Mr Boothman, an attorney who spent the first half of his career defending physicians and hospitals in malpractice cases, had the insight to recognize that the adversarial process was seriously flawed and frequently served neither patients nor physicians well. After moving from his private legal firm to the University of Michigan Health System, he developed what has been described as the "Michigan Model" for dealing with malpractice allegations and improving patient safety (http://www.uofmhealth.org/michigan-model-medical-malpractice-and-patient-safety-umhs). Whereas in the distant past the liability review committee might have focused on whether it could defend against an allegation of malpractice, committee members now focus as peer reviewers on the quality of care that the patient received. Was the care provided reasonable or was it substandard? If it was substandard, how and why, and what can the institution do to improve the quality of care going forward? This kind of internal self-criticism may not only be difficult but also recognize 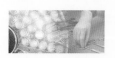 that the goal is improvement and prevention of harm. It is OK to admit you made a mistake, but with it comes the obligation to work diligently to do better. If harm has occurred, the patient may be entitled to compensation in some form. (It is up to a different committee to determine if compensation is warranted.) For faculty members, the ability to try to think objectively as much from the patient's point of view as the physician's and to criticize the work of colleagues without losing respect for them or their work is required. We are fortunate to work in a safe environment in which it is acceptable, indeed expected, for one to offer and accept criticism in this way and in so doing improve the quality of care.

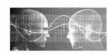

## Peer Review of Research Program Integrity

The University of Michigan is a "research university," and as such the integrity of the research done here is paramount to the university's reputation. Allegations or complaints related to research integrity are therefore handled at the highest university level through the office of the Vice President for Research, even if they involve medical care issues or concerns within one of the schools.

I was called on a few years ago to serve on an ad hoc advisory committee that was asked to conduct a peer assessment of possible violations of research integrity by a newly appointed medical faculty member who had brought with him a large amount of grant money and potentially important connections to industry related to the development of new technology. The testing of this technology required human subjects. It was clear from the evidence we gathered that although no patient harm had occurred, this faculty member's research team had violated critical aspects of informed consent in conducting the work. At the same time, the faculty member was young, had brought unique qualifications to the university, and had shown great promise on the basis of his prior work. This is the kind of situation in which there are competing interests. The Vice President for Research, to whom the committee reported, made quite clear in the instructions to the committee that the integrity of the university's research work and the protection of the patients were the paramount considerations. The medical school had an interest in preserving the promising career of the newly appointed faculty member. The medical school institutional review board, charged with the protection of human subjects in research, needed to be assured that any violation of the human subjects protocol was dealt with appropriately, lest all of its government research funding be jeopardized. Needless to say, the multiple competency interests made this situation particularly difficult. The surgeon involved in the peer review process must exercise patience, justice, and a modicum of mercy in such situations. There are no easy solutions.

## Billing Compliance

At one time, I served on what was called the "compliance committee." This committee was charged with overseeing the billing practices of the faculty to ensure that all of the Medicare and other insurer standards were being adhered to, and specifically that adequate faculty supervision was occurring and documented and that systematic overbilling, which whether intentional or not could be considered fraud, was not occurring. This required on the one hand swallowing hard and accepting arcane, nit-picking rules being imposed 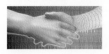 on us from the outside. However, it also required making judgments about the behavior of peers and about the administrators and supervisors in various departments, who were under pressure to maximize revenue. Here again, one must examine and criticize the behavior of esteemed colleagues without creating destructive disharmony. The committee encountered some starting outliers. It is hard to know if the behavior was willful or simply arose from ignorance, but some clinical departments, which were unable to justify their billing practices on the basis of the existing documentation, had to return substantial revenues that could not be justified. The compliance committee could not take all the credit for this, but when the Government Accounting Office spent a year at our hospital as part of the infamous Physicians at Teaching Hospitals (PATH) audits that began in 1998, it found little if any evidence of improper billing.

## Self-assessment

Physicians are increasingly being called on to do their own personal peer review, that is, to monitor and report on their own practices with regard to criteria laid down by specialty boards, insurers, and government payers, such as the Centers for Medicare and Medicaid Services. For surgeons, this comes in several forms. One of these is the requirement for maintenance of certification by the American Board of Surgery, which now requires 90 hours of relevant continuing medical education (CME) every 3 years as well as a self-assessment of the understanding of what one has learned. Another is the Physician Quality Reporting System, which Centers for Medicare and Medicaid Services will use to adjust payments up or down depending on compliance with national quality improvement goals. This is soon to be replaced by a new acronym, MIPS (merit-based incentive payment system), which is a component of the Quality Payment Program to take effect in 2017. This structured reporting and self-assessment minimizes, but does not eliminate, conflicts of interest. Its effectiveness depends on the honesty and completeness of the reporting.

Another opportunity for peer assessment in Michigan is through a set of quality collaboratives, sponsored by Michigan Blue Cross Blue Shield, the Michigan Quality Reporting System, in which surgeons can collect and compare outcomes for high-volume, potentially high-risk procedures, such as bariatric surgery and major joint replacement. The American College of Surgeons (ACS) sponsors an analogous quality initiative designed to assist surgeons in self-assessment, the National Surgical Quality Improvement Program, which is designed to help meet Physician Quality Reporting System goals.

Self-assessment of hospital performance is also now required by the Joint Commission as part of its efforts to assist hospitals in evaluating the performance of members of the medical staff. The requirements for accreditation now call for Ongoing Professional Practice Evaluations (OPPEs) based on objective performance criteria to be determined by the hospital medical staff and administration. The result of this is that every quarter, for example, I am asked to evaluate the physician assistant who works with me, while at the same time, I am evaluated by one of my superiors and receive a quarterly report on my performance with regard to quality-related events such as catheter-associated urinary tract infections and postoperative surgical site infection rates.

## Joint Commission Mandated Review

As a result of Joint Commission mandates, a variety of opportunities for peer review exist at various institutional levels, usually as a member of a medical staff committee or departmental committee. Medical staff regulations as stipulated by the Joint Commission call for oversight of admission to the medical staff and credentialing as well as delineation of privileges. (Credentialing verifies one's qualifications and training for medical staff membership; privileging delineates what one is allowed to do once admitted to the staff.) One essential element of this process is "documentation of current evidence, including peer and/or faculty recommendations, of the individual's ability to perform the privileges requested."[3]

Teaching hospitals continue to have regular morbidity and mortality conferences at which peer participation is expected. This may not be possible in smaller, nonteaching settings. The same is true in single specialty or multi-specialty groups. Whether one has the opportunity to participate or be evaluated by peers will also depend on group dynamics. Important peer activities include mentoring and assisting colleagues.

Another form of oversight of surgical practices in the hospital, now abandoned, was surveillance by a "tissue committee." This was a hospital staff committee that reviewed surgical specimen reports and clinical charts looking for how often surgeons, without apparent good reason, removed normal tissues. In this way the committee tried to identify discrepancies or failures in patient evaluation or errors in diagnosis and looked for patterns of substandard care. Thanks to computer-based, searchable medical records, this has now been replaced by newer, more focused, data-based measures of quality, such as monitoring rates of surgical site and catheter-associated urinary tract infections. With the advent of the electronic health record, it is also now possible to monitor metrics, such as total operative time, amount of blood used, returns to the operating room (OR) and readmissions to the hospital 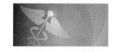 within a set time frame, and surgical site infection rates, to determine if someone is an outlier in need of focused review.

In the 1970s and 1980s, at the same time when Medicare instituted prospective payment for hospital admission, hospitals were required by the Joint Commission to have quality assurance (QA) and utilization review (UR) committees of the medical staff. The QA committee did retrospective reviews comparing care, as reflected in the chart, with various criteria and standards. For example, were the proper antibiotics given for a patient with pneumonia? UR was conducted to ensure that patients did not linger in the hospital longer than needed, using "severity of illness/intensity of care" criteria.

These programs were intended to remove or minimize the role that subjectivity, with its inherent potential biases, might play in decisions about medical care quality and use, thus unburdening reviewers from accusations on unethical practices. Unfortunately, physician reviewers quickly recognized that the review criteria were inadequate to the task and lost respect for the programs. In the end, neither was very effective in achieving the desired goals of ensuring high quality and efficient medical care, although some insurance companies and government payers continue to use them in some form.

## Medical Staff Quality Committee

In my institution, there is a unique peer review committee that deals not directly with quality of care but rather with the personal behavior and 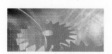 integrity of both house officers and physicians on the medical staff. While quality-of-care issues are evaluated by the Patient Safety office, the medical staff quality committee (MSQC) handles concerns related to professionalism. And while the MLRC deals only with allegations after the fact, the MSQC tries to identify behaviors that may lead to poor quality care and to prevent problems that might turn into errors and patient harm. As part of its work, the MSQC also oversees OPPE performance in the various departments of the medical center to meet Joint Commission requirements.

Members of this committee must be able to distinguish between medical quality issues that may have systemic roots and those that arise or are likely to arise because of personal failings. The MLRC does not impose penalties on medical staff members; the MSQC can and does do so. In this way it plays a role quite similar to that of the state Board of Medicine, which I will talk about later. Is a physician's behavior becoming erratic? Are his/her prescribing practices out of line? Have concerns been raised about a physician's judgment? Is there evidence of sexual harassment or inappropriate behavior? Is someone falsifying records? Using drugs? If any of these things are happening, what is the potential for rehabilitation? If the physician in question is a prominent member of the medical staff, is prominent in the community, or sees a large number of patients, how will it be handled if the person must be suspended or privileges revoked? It is far better for all concerned, and certainly more timely, if these kinds of issues are dealt with fairly and firmly at the institutional level and the results are reported to the state Board of Medicine than the other way around.

With regard to individual practice evaluation, the old, subjective assessments have been replaced by newer requirements, the OPPE and the Focused Professional Practice Evaluation, instituted in 2007, which call for much more frequent examination of practice performance than the usual biennial or triennial recredentialing process and are intended to assist in credentialing decisions.

As a member of the MSQC, I have tried to answer these questions and assist departments or clinical services to figure out how to do this. It is much harder than it sounds, in part because surgeons are not accustomed to using data for improvement; they are more accustomed to using data for criticism and fear becoming the target. Nevertheless, it is critically important that surgeons become familiar with this kind of professional oversight and participate in the committees that are responsible for seeing it done. Pressure from the outside, in this example being accountable to physicians outside the inner circle of surgical colleagues, is more likely not only to cause discomfort but also to identify the need for change.

I have been asked on more than one occasion to be a participant in a Focused Professional Practice Evaluation and fill out a 360° evaluation of a colleague, medical or surgical, who was acknowledged to be a good doctor but whose behavior was potentially disruptive. The behavior in question might be characterized by intolerance, by being "hard" on nurses or subordinates, not controlling anger, and being hypercritical. One concern in such a review is that the physician in question might have underlying, remediable, medical, social, or behavioral problems that need to be addressed. Or it might be that the person was simply not aware that the behavior was disruptive; or was aware of it but thought it was acceptable. Whatever the case, peer review in an environment of peer support is what is needed and most likely to create a win-win for both physician and hospital.

## No Surgeon Is an Island: Team Interactions and Evaluations

No surgeon is an island; we are all dependent on the teams of people we work with in the office, in the OR, and on the patient care floor. How one interacts with team members has gained new attention in recent years and has been shown to correlate with quality of patient care. Surgeons encountering OPPE requirements for the first time find themselves having to learn about the 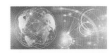 evaluation of aspects of physician performance, such as behavior in the OR and interactions with nursing staff that have never been closely scrutinized in the past. Moreover, they may find themselves and their colleagues being evaluated on these newer measures by nonsurgeons who are skeptical about the insular environment in surgery and believe that surgeons are inclined to go easy on one another rather than be appropriately critical. The following are the questions surgical leaders are being asked: How do you know how good a job you are doing? How do you know how good a job the others in your department are doing? What observations are you making? How are you gathering data on performance? From whom are you gathering them? How objective and reliable are they?

Two highly skilled colleagues of mine, with whom I had operated and worked with side by side, began after a few years on the faculty to be more irritable and argumentative or demanding with subordinates, and OR nurses began to voice complaints. This led to the leadership asking the surgeon to participate in an in-depth voluntary analysis of behavior—a forced self-assessment—using a PULSE 360 evaluation, which obtains and records perceptual feedback for health care workers from everyone around you. PULSE stands for Physicians and Professionals Universal Leadership-Teamwork Skills Education (www.pulseprogram.com). It is a Web-based survey, filled out anonymously, that is perceived to be more objective than one that might be devised locally. The intent is to identify behavioral issues before they become destructive. Its use is not without its critics, however, depending on how it is used and why. In the present example, one surgeon found it helpful, leading to more self-awareness, and demonstrated improved performance; the other did not and chose to retire.

## Government-Sponsored External Peer Review: Professional Standards Review Organizations

In 1972, in an effort to control the spiraling costs of Medicare, Congress passed amendments to Title XI of the Social Security Act establishing Professional Standards Review Organizations (PSROs). These were local physician-directed agencies whose purpose was to apply UR and QA methods using individual professional judgment to Medicare admissions in an effort to reduce cost and align care with accepted professional standards. They could also initiate medical care evaluation studies. PSROs were never well accepted by the physician community, but a small group of physicians who believed that quality of care was enormously variable continued work to preserve the role of peer review in quality oversight.

In 1976, C. Gardner Child, III, the recently retired Chairman of the
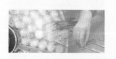
Department of Surgery at the University of Michigan, who had a long-standing interest, unusual for surgeons, in broad issues of health care quality and manpower, took me to one of the first organizing meetings of the Michigan Area VII PSRO, which had jurisdiction over a 5-county area that included Ann Arbor. This was the beginning of a long career in the field of quality oversight

and peer review outside the usually recognized boundaries. The PSROs had access to Medicare and Medicaid records on which some basic statistical analysis could be done, looking at types of admissions, diagnoses, procedures, and lengths of stay. Although the data were rudimentary, they were also revealing and showed hugely disproportionate numbers of procedures 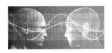 such as tonsillectomy and upper gastrointestinal endoscopy in some small community hospitals. They also uncovered many admissions that could not be justified on the basis of diagnosis and treatment. The program took me into the record rooms of 15 regional hospitals, none of which were like any I had been in before. Chart review, albeit based mainly on individual professional judgment, confirmed many of the findings of overuse and substandard care suggested by the statistical analysis.

This voluntary, unreimbursed work placed the physicians who were doing the review, like myself, in direct conflict with those whose practices were being questioned by government outsiders. Complaints regarding professional judgment, personal autonomy, competitive bias, and the motives of the reviewers and the review organization were immediately raised. I can remember one uncomfortable meeting with members of a small hospital's medical staff explaining our findings and pointing out that unless changes were made, penalties could be imposed up to and including preprocedure review and denial of Medicare reimbursement. I in particular, coming from an academic setting, could be accused of bias, making judgments on artificial and unrealistic standards of care. On the other hand, when one-third of all tonsillectomies in the 5-county area were being done in one 50-bed hospital, it was pretty obvious that something was awry.

What is the obligation of the reviewer like me in this situation? On the one hand, he is working for a government-supported agency, conducting a contract obligation. He has an obligation to preserve the integrity of that organization and its employees. He is looking at medical care that is being conducted in institutions that may be thought of as competing with his own. He is also an academic surgeon on salary and not at all like the individual private practitioners whose practices he is evaluating. Are his judgments therefore unavoidably tainted by inherent bias?

There was a bigger picture as well. This program was initiated at a time when small community hospitals were struggling. If they closed, possibly as a result of our review results, the community might be denied a valued resource. On the other hand, one could also ask if that community was really benefitting from the substandard care this institution was delivering. Could we, through our findings, help the hospital to rehabilitate itself? In the end, more than a third of the small hospitals in Michigan closed their doors or were assimilated into larger hospital systems over the next decade. This happened not because of any actions of the PSRO, but someone familiar with our findings could have predicted it.

## External Review: Professional Standards Review Organization to Professional Review Organization to Quality Improvement Organizations

In 1984, 10 or more PSROs in Michigan were consolidated into 1 Professional Review Organization (PRO) at the same time that prospective payment on 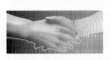 the basis of diagnosis related groups was instituted by Medicare. I served as one of the founding members and the president of the board of the Michigan PRO for more than 20 years. At the outset, I presided over a board consisting almost entirely of physicians. The biggest ethical challenge was to get the board members to understand that their role was not to protect physicians from government oversight—although one role was to ensure that any oversight was fair—but rather to ensure that patients under the Medicare and Medicaid programs were receiving necessary and appropriate care, ie, care that taxes should be paying for. The addition of public, nonphysician members to the board assisted greatly in this regard.

The reorganization of the Medicare peer review program and the dramatic changes brought about by prospective payment for hospital admissions raised a completely new set of issues both for hospitals trying to adjust to new payment realities and physicians directing and working in government-funded quality oversight. Admissions to the hospital now had to be justified on the basis of preestablished criteria for Medicare to pay for them. New efficiency in medical care delivery had to be achieved by hospitals. Care previously delivered inside the hospital moved to the outpatient realm. Patients were no longer routinely admitted on the day before elective operations, and hospital admission for routine postoperative care for some operations would no longer be reimbursed. The specter of hospitals discharging patients "sicker and quicker" was raised. Whose side were the physicians doing external oversight on?

I remember vividly meeting with surgeons in the community in 1986 when the rule was imposed that patients undergoing elective inguinal hernia repair would no longer qualify for hospital admission. Only a few years earlier, these patients could be hospitalized for up to 5 days. Who was I to carry the message that these patients could only be admitted to the hospital if they were very sick or had a complication requiring hospital treatment. What was the evidence that this policy would not lead to many unanticipated negative consequences?

The chief problem with the PRO program in its first decade of existence was that it was still using the retrospective, ineffective tools that had been introduced at the time of the PSRO program and could only penalize doctors and hospitals, not help them improve. This finally changed in 2006 as a result of a report from the Institute of Medicine calling for the transformation of "PROs" into Quality Improvement Organizations.[4] Physicians working in quality oversight under the newer mandate are not burdened with the ethical concerns raised in the past. They can help their colleagues and the public at the same time.

## Government-Sponsored Peer Review: State Medical Boards

As discussed earlier, the licensing of physicians by states across the country began after the Civil War in the mid- to late 19th century, in conjunction with the passage of state laws establishing occupational licensing of all professionals, whether architects or engineers or doctors, to protect the public from fraudulent practices and quacks. This history and the decisions by the US Supreme Court establishing the legitimacy under the US Constitution of states to do this with regard to the medical profession are recounted in detail in 2 books. One book is by Johnson and Chaudhry titled *Medical Licensing and Discipline in America: A History of the Federation of State Medical Boards.*[5] The second source is titled *Licensed to Practice* by Mohr[6]; both books are well worth reading.

The chief roles of state boards of medicine are to establish standards for the education and training of physicians who wish to practice medicine and to ensure that, after being licensed, they meet acceptable standards of practice. The actual structures, organization, powers, and practices of state boards vary from state to state. Some have more independence and financial support than others. Although at one time state boards conducted their own testing of applicants, this role has now been delegated to the Federation of State Medical Boards (FSMB), which along with the National Board of Medical Examiners develops and administers the United States Medical Licensing Examinations, which all medical students take. They produce a separate examination for foreign medical graduates. State boards continue to set the rules for when the test must be taken and how many failures are allowed before the candidate becomes ineligible for a license.

A state license is required for a physician to provide care for a patient physically located in that state; that is, it is the location of the patient not the location of the physician that determines in which state licensing is necessary. States ordinarily give at least 2 types of medical license: general (unlimited) for most physicians in practice and educational limited for residents in training, although other types of limited licenses may be available in some states. Requirements for training may also vary. At present no state requires more than 3 years of postgraduate training to apply for a license and no state requires that a physician successfully complete an accredited residency program before obtaining a license to practice.

Having delegated the education and training aspects of licensing, state medical boards devote most of their time and energy to investigating questions of competence and moral character and deciding on disciplinary actions. Medical boards have neither the resources nor the mandate to monitor individual medical practices or deal with variations in quality of care that may exist in their states. They can respond only after the fact to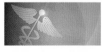

complaints. The following are the chief questions that they have to answer, when given a complaint: Is this physician competent or impaired? Does he/she represent a threat to the general public? Each medical board has a process, which has been established by state health code and rulemaking, for providing peer review of the complaints that come before it and for meting out penalties and disciplinary actions, which may take the form of fines and required CME, limitations on scope of practice, suspension, or revocation of one's license.

In all states most members of state medical boards are physicians. Several large states have separate medical and osteopathic medical boards. The number and level of participation of nonphysicians on state medical boards vary widely. Most state medical boards have only a small number of nonphysicians or public members. Michigan has the most public members, 8 of 19, 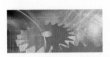 and requires that a public member chair its disciplinary subcommittee. The important role of public members on state medical boards has been described in detail in a recent book by R. Horowitz titled *In the Public Interest: Medical Licensing and the Disciplinary Process.*[7]

Complaints brought to the state medical board fall into several distinct categories. These are as follows:

1.  Suspicion of substance abuse involving alcohol or drugs: Physicians who admit to or are found to have confirmed problems with substance abuse are, in the best-case scenario, entered into treatment and rehabilitation programs and monitoring.
2.  Inappropriate prescribing practices involving opioids and other schedule II drugs: These are identified through statewide prescription monitoring programs, through complaints from the public, from the Drug Enforcement Agency, and from federal and state prosecutors.
3.  Billing fraud: Physicians prosecuted and imprisoned for Medicare fraud, usually related to fraudulent billing but also systematic overbilling, will come before the state board to have their licenses suspended.
4.  Physicians reported for boundary issues, such as inappropriate touching of patients during examinations, and failure to use chaperones when indicated.
5.  Physicians reported for having sex with patients or engaging in inappropriate sexual liaisons, for example, exchanging sex for prescription drugs.
6.  Physical or mental incompetence: This can be a much more difficult determination to make. Incompetent physicians are the last ones to recognize their incompetence, and others are reluctant to make judgments despite it being their duty to do so. Physically impaired physicians, for example, after suffering a stroke, are expected to report their disability but most often do not. They are sometimes identified later by failure to complete their CME requirements.

7. Malpractice: Often large malpractice settlements must be reported to the state medical board, but alleged malpractice can also be reported by patients and families. Medical errors or patient harm leading to legal settlements is not always indicative of the incompetence requiring state board action. State boards are quite limited in their ability to protect the public from slips, lapses, and stupid mistakes leading to harm for which patients should rightfully be compensated. Those decisions are best dealt with by the legal system. The state medical board cannot compensate patients for their injuries; the legal system can.

8. Medical incompetence: Physicians, however, are often uncomfortable in reporting suspected incompetence. Patient reports of medical incompetence or malpractice are often problematic because one "bad" case is almost never sufficient to warrant an action against a practitioner's license. Such concerns are best dealt with at the local level. The standard of practice as interpreted at the level of the state board may be less strict than it might be in a hospital peer review committee or in a court of law. The potential penalty, loss of license, is much greater and less beneficial to the public at large than are the remedies that might be available through other, more local agencies. Moreover, the state board's ability to enforce remediation is much weaker than that of the hospital.

9. Failure to accumulate the requisite hours of CME: Renewal of license in all states requires somewhere between 50 and 150 hours of AMA Category I CME in a 3-year period. Unless this failure is found to be the result of a serious underlying problem, the penalty is normally a fine and mandate to make up the deficient hours.

One of the most difficult challenges I have faced in all my years of doing peer review was learning how to work while under constraints imposed on the state Board of Medicine by legislators for mainly political reasons and how to get along with the political appointees placed in charge of overseeing the work of the Board. Physicians and public members of state boards may have widely divergent views on moral and ethical issues that come before the Board. The attorney or attorneys providing legal advice to state board may bring yet a third point of view. At times, legal counsel acts to restrain board members or assure that proposed disciplinary actions are legally allowable under state laws. At other times, lawyers and administrative personnel feel impelled, sometimes under political pressure, to follow the letter of the law rather than common sense and can push for technically allowable penalties in situations that physicians believe do not warrant them. Some regulations make no sense at all. Many of these were the result of so-called out-of-state actions in which a physician is sanctioned in one state for a minor infraction 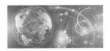 and the penalty is reported to another state in which the physician holds a license. In Michigan, there is legislation that stipulates that the state board *must* act in some way on all out-of-state actions regardless of whether the board in Michigan would have acted on the alleged infraction in the first place or even if the infraction is minor, such as having failed to report the out-of-state action within 30 days.

What is one's ethical obligation to serve on such a board when you disagree with much of the way in which it is forced to operate? The primary ethical obligation is to serve and protect the public, even if it means putting up with the limitations of the position, while trying to alter those limitations if possible.

## Dealing With the Impaired Physician

The impaired physician is one who is mentally or physically unable to practice medicine or surgery competently. The term "impaired" is used principally to refer to problems associated with substance abuse, but physicians can also become impaired from a variety of causes, including mental illness and behavioral aberration, cognitive and/or physical decline, and acute or chronic medical illness. During my tenure on the Board of Medicine, I saw them all.

The topic is well covered in the literature and the AMA, the FSMB, and other national organizations on their Web sites have published policy papers on how to recognize it and what to do about it. The first and foremost duty is to report impairment if one observes it. States and large employers have physician health programs (PHPs) to assist physicians in treatment, recovery, and monitoring, but only if the physician admits to having a problem. All agree that physicians have a duty to report suspected impairment in a colleague, arguing that one should not wait until a patient is harmed or the physician has been arrested for repeated driving under the influence or prescribing irregularities. From the peer review perspective the 2 most important aspects are when and how to report suspected substance abuse and how to deal with it.

One physician I dealt with was reported to the Board of Medicine because of irregularities in opioid dispensing and was found to have hidden in his office and home thousands of pills. He had been under great emotional stress because his wife was slowly succumbing to metastatic breast cancer over a 4-year period. He had resorted to taking opioids to deal with the mental pain and was taking, at the time his problem was discovered, a staggering amount of hydrocodone on a daily basis. He readily admitted his problems and entered into a health recovery program. At the same time, the Board imposed a number of limitations on his license, stripping him of his ability to prescribe controlled substances and requiring peer monitoring and reporting on his practice for a 2-year period after he emerged from detox and was released from the PHP.

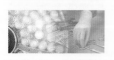 Although the ideal situation is one in which the physician recognizes the problem and self-reports, more often than not this is not what happens. One physician, who was identified as a result of repeated citations for driving under the influence, rejected the evaluation of the PHP and claimed that she had found a counselor to assist her in her recovery. Her "recovery" turned out

to be a perpetuation of the same problem, with the assistance of a colleague whose behavior was equally unethical. In another case, family members also played an enabling role.

Physicians who seem to be most at risk are anesthe- 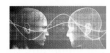 siologists, emergency physicians, and psychiatrists, but the problem is certainly not limited to these specialties. An addictionologist who ran a clinic treating patients for substance abuse was reported by his nursing staff for erratic behavior and found to be self-medicating.

## The Aging Surgeon

Dealing with physicians, particularly surgeons, whose mental and physical capabilities may be waning as they age presents a difficult challenge. The physician is going to be the last one to recognize declining abilities. I remember a conversation I had on this topic with C. Gardner Child, III, a nationally renowned surgeon, before his retirement from the University of Michigan 40 years ago. He said that he would stop operating at age 70 years to avoid having to face the dilemma of declining ability. He was true to his word. Today, however, age 70 years is not necessarily thought of as old, and laws and court rulings against "ageism" have restricted the ability of employers to impose arbitrary age restrictions on employment. There is no restriction on professional practice, including medical practice, with regard to age, and research on physician age and quality of care has not found age, per se, to be an important variable.[8] The problem, however, of declining ability is no less real. In recognition of this, the ACS has outlined a set or recommendations in its Statement on the Aging Surgeon (https://www.facs.org/about-acs/statements/80-aging-surgeon) in which it states that "gradual decline in overall health, physical dexterity, and cognition generally occurs after the age of 65." The ACS recommends baseline and regular comprehensive health evaluations for older surgeons. The statement reiterates the duty of physicians to report concerns about declining ability in colleagues.

One way to avoid dealing with the whole issue of declining ability is to create in advance and enforce contractual agreements that require surgeons to retire earlier than they might wish. One way to do this is by writing into either the medical staff bylaws or the department of surgery regulations the requirement that surgeons who, because of their age, wish to no longer take emergency night call can remain on staff for only a limited period, such as 2 years, before their privileges expire.

In my time on the Board of Medicine, I encountered 2 other types of problems related to declining abilities. One was the physician who developed serious medical illness, and the other was the physician who wished to reenter the profession after an extended period of absence or move into a different specialty. The most egregious example of the latter was the retired physician who reemerged as an expert in medical marijuana and dispensed large numbers of certifications for its presumed medicinal use. Another physician had a disabling stroke, which took him out of practice for more than 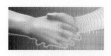 6 months. He failed to report this change in his condition to the Board as required under his "general duty" obligation and saw no reason why he should have to submit to a comprehensive examination regarding his recovery. Compounding these ethical lapses were the abetting actions of colleagues who attested to his abilities without actually having done any objective examinations. The behavior of both the physician and his colleagues represents failures of professionalism.

The question arising from this case that confronted the Board was that it is difficult to define what kind of illness might constitute a disability sufficient to prohibit one from practicing medicine and what duration of absence from practice should be considered sufficient to impose testing and/or retraining requirements, a limited license, and/or monitoring of practice (that is expensive and would have to be paid for by the physician).

## Medical Practice Reentry and Transitions

With regard to reentry into practice after a period of absence, the FSMB has looked into this question stimulated by the number of retired physicians whose retirement income was drastically reduced by the economic crisis of 2008 and who might wish to reenter practice because of financial hardship. Its report on reentry to practice outlined the issues and challenges facing both physicians and regulators (https://www.fsmb.org/Media/Default/PDF/FSMB/Advocacy/pub-sp-cmt-reentry.pdf). There are many reasons, however, for reentry, and the physicians who wish to do this are not always old.[9] Among women, reentry into practice was desired after time taken off for child-rearing, for example. A physician who chaired a health maintenance organization credentialing committee on which I served set the best example in this regard in my experience. He had held an administrative position for a number of years. When he decided to return to practice, he was self-aware enough to know that having done enough CME to maintain his license was not sufficient to ensure he could practice safely to a high standard. He planned to spend 6 to 12 months in a program of voluntary reeducation, essentially becoming a resident once again. One can only applaud this degree of professionalism.

The same principles should apply to physicians who try to make the transition from one specialty to another, but this is not always the case. Before the development of training programs in emergency medicine in the 1980s, almost any physician could moonlight in the emergency department, and many surgeons, internists, and general practitioners made the transition to work in the emergency department full time. Today, during my service on the Board of Medicine, I saw transitions of a different kind. Physicians failing in their practice who were filling newly discovered lacunae in the health care system would find jobs doing home care visits, operating pain clinics, and peddling medical marijuana certifications. One such physician, who came before the Board, was basically filling an empty space in her life by visiting old people in their homes and billing Medicare. A retired anesthesiologist in his late 80s traveled the state selling medical marijuana certificates at shows and rallies.

## Incompetence

Professional incompetence, as distinct from mental incompetence, such as Alzheimer disease, comes in many forms. Because the finding of incompetence always involves professional opinion, it is always in the eye of the beholder to some extent. Moreover, it must be distinguished from simple error or unintended complication. In general, it is much easier to prove impairment than incompetence. And often the question must find a locus of responsibility before it can be answered. Let me offer an example.

An older, prominent surgeon in his mid-70s came to the attention of the Board of Medicine because of a complaint from a patient who had undergone a lap-band procedure for body mass index more than 50. Having not lost weight after almost 2 years, he grew frustrated with the first surgeon's care and sought a second opinion. The second surgeon recommended a sleeve gastrectomy. At the time of the second operation, however, the surgeon discovered to his surprise that the previously placed lap band was not around the stomach at all, but rather was around a collection of fat in the gastrohepatic ligament.

The case suggested incompetence on 2 counts. First, the patient was too obese to have been a candidate for a lap-band procedure to be effective. Second, the surgeon then manipulated it for more than a year, stringing the patient along even though he was not losing weight, without looking into why. The patient finally went to another surgeon, who reoperated, discovered the error, and did a more appropriate bariatric procedure.

This case raised a number of questions, among them: Should this be considered an accepted complication of the procedure? Or was the surgeon to perform this procedure in view of the egregiousness of the intraoperative error? Why had he done a lap-band procedure on a patient with a body mass index more than 50 when the current literature argued that this is an ineffective procedure for such a patient? Why when the procedure had so clearly failed had the surgeon not recognized this failure over a 2-year period and not done any follow-up imaging to determine whether something was awry? What was the scope and nature of his surgical practice, given his age? 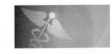 How many of these operations was he doing and what were his results? Did he participate in the regional bariatric surgical collaborative that had been active for several years and allowed surgeons to compare outcomes and improve their practices? What kind of supervision was being carried out by the hospital in which he worked? From what I could tell he was not doing enough operations to maintain his surgical privileges, yet his privileges were not limited or revoked.

When I interviewed him, I was more than a little concerned about these questions. Not only did he do the wrong operation but also he did it incompetently and steadfastly maintained otherwise. The surgeon did not admit a lack of competence but made a video publicizing the error as a "complication" of the procedure. My conclusion after interviewing this surgeon was that he exhibited a number of personal and ethical failures, starting with hubris, and extending to dishonesty with himself and others, especially his patients. His ego prevented objective self-assessment, and the institution in which he practiced had chosen to ignore the fact that his practice was in effect a scam.

Unfortunately, the Board of Medicine could act only on the 1 complaint before it and did not have the legal authority or resources to conduct a more thorough investigation or even talk to the hospital where he practiced. His attorney quickly cut off the line of questions when I tried to probe into the nature of the surgeon's actual practice.

The Board of Medicine, at least in Michigan, has the authority only to recommend penalties, such as fines and mandatory CME, or certain limitations on a physician's license, such as probation or suspension for a limited period, 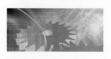 but to suspend someone's license, it has to prove that the physician is a threat to the public. In a case like that of the surgeon mentioned earlier, the authority to investigate further and determine whether he should have his privileges altered lies with the hospital, which is the primary locus of responsibility for such actions. Without more information, there was very little the Board could do beyond a slap on the wrist.

I was once asked by the attorney of a large hospital to review the performance of a surgeon who had been on staff for several years and seemed to have a high rate of deaths and complications. The hospital was considering taking action to revoke this surgeon's privileges but needed an independent review from someone who had no knowledge of the surgeon and no conflict of interest, which any internal reviewer might have had. After reviewing a large number of randomly selected charts—not just the ones the hospital was concerned about—it became clear that this surgeon was operating inappropriately on elderly nursing home patients, many of whom never recovered. This surgeon had come from a top-tier academic training program. It was not possible to determine without more investigation how his values had become so distorted as to engage in the practices that I saw and that his hospital, to its credit, had investigated. I recommended that his privileges be terminated, an action that would automatically be reported to the Board of Medicine. Could he be rehabilitated? Was his residency director notified? I do not know.

Action by the Board of Medicine in a case such as this would depend on judgments as to whether the surgeon was competent, ie, conformed to minimal standards or acceptable and prevailing practices and whether he/ she was of good moral character, which would include engaging in ethical practices.

Some hospitals, it seems, prefer not to know what their surgeons are doing, even when the surgeon is exemplary. Another case in which I participated involved a surgical oncologist with a busy referral practice in a large private hospital. A complaint was filed against him with the Board of Medicine by a patient who had suffered a complication after surgery. The complication in question was a known risk of the complex procedure, and after interviewing the surgeon I had little doubt about his competence. I asked him if he knew how often this complication occurred in his practice, because if he could come up with some actual numbers, I could make a better case that no action was needed on the part of the Board. He said he would try. He asked the hospital to pull the charts for his last 100 similar cases, but when he explained the request originated with the Board of Medicine, the hospital legal office blocked the request. The surgeon in this case was acting ethically. The hospital in my view was acting both irresponsibly and unethically.

## Boundary Issues

Not all unethical professional practices are immoral, but all immoral behavior is unethical. Most unethical practices that come before the Board of Medicine involve morality and relate to what are called the boundary issues, including appropriate sexual conduct. Examples include trading opioid or anxiolytic prescriptions for sex; entering into sexual affairs with patients; inappropriate touching, molestation, or fondling of patients during examinations; and doing breast and gynecologic examinations without a qualified chaperone present. Some cases are egregious and clear, but others may reflect differing perceptions of what appropriate boundaries are. Resting a hand on a patient's thigh may be intended by the doctor as a means of reassurance but interpreted by the patient, especially if no qualified chaperone is present, as a sexual advance.

## Spiraling Down

I witnessed several stories reported to the Board of Medicine of surgeons whose careers started in a promising way and then deteriorated, spiraling downward from a respected position as a specialist on a hospital staff to an unemployed surgeon taking sporadic locum tenens jobs to make a living. They were not surgeons with drug problems or alcoholism. In some cases, well and highly trained surgeons, once they started making mistakes, failed to  take responsibility and find a remedy, while the system in which they worked also failed to seek a remedy. Having lost one position, they face increasing isolation, lose peer support, and, of necessity, become itinerant surgeons. A plastic surgeon began to exhibit inappropriate and unethical behavior by cutting corners related to proper sterilization in an effort to avoid bankruptcy. Another physician simply ignored all the basic rules for sterilizing instruments he used in his office. Each case has its own unique sad story, but all raise the question, from an ethical standpoint, how did this happen? How many failings, personal, professional, and systemic, contributed to this decline over the course of years?

One of the dilemmas facing surgeons, and physicians in general, is that if they cannot practice medicine, there is not much else they can do. They are not employable outside the field of medicine. The tragedy of unethical behavior is that it arises out of personal failings that may not become evident until after completion of training. This is a strong argument for terminating the surgical training of physicians who exhibit unethical or unsocial behavior during residency.

## Caring for a Colleague

As a surgeon, one of the highest complements one can receive is to be considered a "surgeon's surgeon," which is to say one who is asked to care for one of his/her colleagues. There are 2 sides to each such choice. On the one hand, is the surgeon who needs care really in the best position to know whom to ask? Is the decision made on the basis of friendship or on the basis of objective knowledge? On the other hand, do you as a surgeon feel comfortable taking care of your colleague or a colleague's family member? Would you feel loss of privacy while being cared for in your own hospital? Because of discomfort that might arise in such a situation, some surgeons prefer to go to another institution for care, which could be interpreted as implying the care in their own institution is substandard.

One case I was involved with in my time on the Board of Medicine involved a physician who asked a colleague to treat him for gallbladder disease. The surgeon, who practiced primarily vascular surgery, felt obligated to agree to the request for a variety of social and cultural reasons and thought he could do this safely even though he would not ordinarily accept such a referral. The outcome was catastrophic for both. The patient suffered a bile duct injury and serious complications after attempted repair; the physician was devastated by the harm he had caused on his friend who was permanently disabled.

## The Perfect Storm

I know of another analogous situation in which the outcome was less than satis-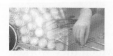factory and represented a failure of peer review in the case of an older surgeon who did not want to limit his practice despite warnings and was enabled by the hospital to get into further trouble. The warnings came from his malpractice carrier, which had begun to notice a series of complaints and canceled his policy. Because this surgeon had for years performed over 900 major cases a year, the hospital was concerned about what would happen to their bottom line if he had to stop operating. The surgeon had made no plans for slowing down or taking on a partner as he passed age 70 years and continued to operate a solo practice with the help of a nurse/surgical assistant. His caseload was such that 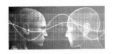 he could not follow patients closely or deal with complications in a timely way. He did not have good working relationships with other surgeons, hence no peer support. Nevertheless, the hospital agreed to cover his malpractice and allowed him to continue operating without any restrictions and with an incentive in his contract that encouraged him to do as many cases as possible.

The personal and institutional failures here are obvious and led to a series of serious complications that led to justifiable legal actions against both the surgeon and the hospital. I was called on to review the situation. What I found could only be characterized as the perfect storm: Self-interest on the part of both the surgeon and hospital led to incentivizing an older surgeon whose capabilities had begun to wane, to continue a high-volume practice involving cases in all branches of general surgery that no younger surgeon could begin to sustain today.

This last example brings up the role of the physician's participation in the legal system. As mentioned earlier, malpractice litigation does not always serve either the patient or the medical care providers well. Does this mean that surgeons have an ethical obligation to offer expert testimony or not? I do not believe there is an obligation to do so, but given that patients are harmed in the course of medical care and are entitled to compensation, without the availability of fair and honest expert analysis and opinion, no party is well served. If at all possible, expert opinion to be ethical should not be adversarial; that is, it should not be intended deliberately to help either plaintiff or defendant; that is the job of the attorneys. Rather, the proper role is to present an analysis of the facts with regard to standard of care or what was reasonable under the circumstances. When asked to review a case, whether internal or external, my first rule is do not do it for the money or agree to review something you are not an expert in. The second rule is to do it in such a way as to avoid hindsight bias, which means starting at the beginning without knowing what happened in the end or what the complaint actually is. The third rule is to tell the person requesting the opinion what you think, not what they might hope to hear. If your analysis elicits the response, "so you can't help me," so be it. This topic is covered in more detail in a separate chapter.

## The Future of Peer Review

Peer review in its many forms will continue to be a responsibility of all physicians, as much if not more tomorrow than it is today. Its forms and mandates will continue to change. Peer review today is being transformed by collaborative quality initiatives sponsored by both private and public insurers, by the promise and also the failings of the electronic health record, by the analysis of "big data," and by new forms of mandated external review, of which OPPEs and self-assessment are just the beginning. Physicians involved in the new forms of peer review, analyzing large administrative data sets and participating in large collaborative projects, will face the same pressures as the peer reviewers of the past, to improve quality and reduce cost, and the same challenges, to do this in an ethical manner, with honesty and altruism in combination with knowledge, objectivity, and the ability to engage in open-minded inquiry.

# References

1. ABIM Foundation/ACP Foundation/European Federation of Internal Medicine; 2005.
2. Brotherton S, Kao A, Crigger BJ. Professing the values of medicine. *JAMA*. 2016;316(10):1041.
3. Pellegrini C. Credentialing and privileging: five tips for ASCs. *Bull Am Coll Surg*. 2016;101(2):40.
4. Institute of Medicine. *Medicare's Quality Improvement Organization Program: Maximizing Potential*. Washington, DC: National Academies Press; 2006.
5. Johnson DA, Chaudhry HJ. *Medical Licensing and Discipline in America: A History of the Federation of State Medical Boards*. Lanham: Lexington Books; 2012.
6. Mohr JC. *Licensed to Practice*. Baltimore: Johns Hopkins University Press; 2013.
7. Horowitz R. *In the Public Interest: Medical Licensing and the Disciplinary Process*. New Brunswick, NJ: Rutgers University Press; 2013.
8. Kupfer J. The graying of US physicians. *JAMA*. 2016;315:341–342.
9. Grace E, Korinek E, Weitzel L, Wentz D. Physicians reentering clinical practice. *J Med Regul*. 2011;97:16–23.

# 46 Burnout, Substance Abuse, and Suicide: A Surgical Perspective

Chandrakanth Are, MD, MBA,
FRCS, FACS
Alexander J. Caniglia, BS
Ashish Sharma, MD
Jeffrey P. Gold, MD

PROLOGUE ▶ When Dr John Flynn, who we left meeting with his program director and his chairman, finally got home that night, his daughter was already asleep. His wife, however, had a surprise planned for after their TV dinners. She had rented a cassette version of Arthur Miller's *Death of a Salesman.*

Flynn had great difficulty following the thread of the play. As in a dream, he attempted to synthesize the story of Willy Loman, the traveling salesman. The narrative became confused with Flynn's own life, and for a time Willy Loman was attempting, unsuccessfully, to get a Swan-Ganz catheter to wedge in a pulmonary artery branch. Flynn was moved at Loman's unraveling and wept when Willy, at Frank's Chop House, blurted out that he had been fired from his job. However, Dr Flynn was asleep again at the denouement and Loman's suicide.

Dr Jeffrey P. Gold, a skilled and successful cardiac surgeon, now Chancellor at the University of Nebraska Medical Center, has assembled a stellar multidisciplinary team to analyze one of the most critical issues within our profession. The medieval had a word for it: acedia or accedie. Its usage emphasizes what may be the most important etiologic factor for the modern syndrome of burnout. Acedia speaks of despair and loss of meaning or joy in life. Acedia may be identical to Kierkegaard's *Sickness Unto Death.*

**429**

Substance abuse and suicide, Gold and his colleagues argue, are extremi-
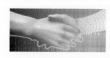 ties on the spectrum of burnout: similar but more severe.
In the spirit of careful understanding being a prerequisite
for correction, Gold and colleagues present a wealth of
data concerning the syndrome and freely admit that there
may be no easy solutions.

Dr Chandrakanth Are is in the Department of Surgery, Division of Surgical
Oncology, at the University of Nebraska Medical Center.

Mr Alexander J. Caniglia is in the College of Medicine at the University of
Nebraska.

Dr Ashish Sharma is in the Department of Psychiatry at the University of
Nebraska Medical Center.

Dr Jeffrey P. Gold is the chancellor and chief executive officer at the
University of Nebraska Medical Center.

There are several causes that contribute to the ongoing rise in physician
burnout, substance abuse, and suicide (BSAS). It seems that the frequency
and intensity of these causative factors is on the rise. Although the canvas of
this chapter is painted intentionally with a surgical brush, what is outlined
probably applies not only to the surgeons but in variable degrees also to the
entire profession regardless of the specialty. BSAS may be perceived as different shades of the same color to some physicians, whereas for others, they
may be perceived as derived from an entirely different palate of different col-
ors. This chapter will attempt to clarify for the readers that these 3 terms
are distinct and are related to each other, with the manifestations dependent
on the specific setting. It is important to be cognizant of this, as there is significant overlap across the knowledge base and outcomes spanning these 3
important manifestations of dysphoria.

It is painful to witness these trends, considering that most enter the surgical
profession with a real powerful desire and passion to heal the sick. Most medical students who choose surgery have compelling reasons to do so as noted by
the passion displayed along their educational pathway and as described in their
personal statements. For some, the desire stems from an inspiring mentorship
experience or a personal tragedy, and for others it may stem from a life-chang-
ing event involving a surgical procedure or some other event related to the field
of surgery. They choose to heal the sick by holding themselves to the highest
ethical standards demanded by any profession in the world.

These lofty standards date back to the Hippocratic Oath and continue to
be emphasized even in the present day as embodied by the Fellowship pledge
of the American College of Surgeons (ACS). The Fellowship pledge of the
ACS states the following:

*I pledge to pursue the practice of surgery with honesty and to place*
*the welfare and the rights of my patient above all else. I promise to*

*deal with each patient as I would wish to be dealt with if I was in the patient's position, and I will respect the patient's autonomy and individuality.*

*I further pledge to affirm and support the social contract of the surgical profession with my community and society.*

*I will take no part in any arrangement or improper financial dealings that induce referral, treatment, or withholding of treatment for reasons other than the patient's welfare.*

*Upon my honor, I declare that I will advance my knowledge and skills, will respect my colleagues, and will seek their counsel when in doubt about my own abilities. In turn, I will willingly help my colleagues when requested.*

*I recognize the interdependency of all health care professionals and will treat each with respect and consideration.*

*Finally, by my Fellowship in the American College of Surgeons, I solemnly pledge to abide by the Code of Professional Conduct and to cooperate in advancing the art and science of surgery.*

Most young women and men who come into the discipline of surgery enter with idealism and an iron-clad ethical intent. Unfortunately, as they go through their surgical training and into practice, they may witness one or more aspects that may alter their perception of the field of surgery. Most are fortunate enough to rely on an intrinsic fortitude and continue to maintain an ethical framework of practice. The accumulation of these influences, both positive and negative, in the context of long hours and high stress over the length of a surgical career can be devastating and contribute to BSAS.

The 4 basic principles of professional ethics consist of the following:

1. The principle of autonomy
2. The principle of beneficence
3. The principle of nonmaleficence
4. The principle of justice

The first ethical principle of autonomy states that we have an obligation to respect the autonomy of other persons, who in the case of surgeons are their patients. The word autonomy stems from Latin and stands for "self-rule." The ability to make decisions without adverse influence or coercion respects 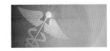 the individual's human dignity. We see many examples on a daily basis, where surgeons are influencing patients to consent for procedures that are appropriately indicated, yet can be associated with significant risk and sometimes with unknown outcomes. Balancing the risk and outcomes and respecting a patient's autonomy forma foundation of daily surgical practice.

The second ethical principle of beneficence states that we have an obligation to "do good" in all our actions. Doing good does not always consist of an act of commission; the rule could also require obedience to obeying the rules of appropriate omissions. We as surgeons are bound to be forceful in justifying a procedure when indicated. We should be equally forceful in preventing an operation when it is not indicated.

The third ethical principle of nonmaleficence consists of doing no harm. A foundation of our discipline depends on the principle of "primum non nocere"—do no harm. Surgeons are witnesses to many practices that when done for the wrong indications or at the wrong time may indeed do harm to patients.

The fourth ethical principle of justice consists of treating all patients equally, fairly, and impartially. Although this may be difficult in the present day because of the difficult or noncompliant patient, it nonetheless behooves us to uphold this principle of justice as much as we can. Similar to the principles of autonomy, beneficence, and nonmaleficence, the potential problems with the ethical principle of justice are not limited to patients and transcend into the professional and societal relationships as well.

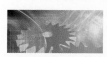 These 4 principles of ethics permeate every aspect of our day-to-day surgical practice. Adherence to these 4 major ethical principles by all surgeons in all domains of practice and all levels of leadership can nourish happy and healthy surgical careers. Likewise, failure to adhere to these core principles can lead to devastating consequences, not only to the surgeon but also to his/her patients and the core of the "social contract" of the profession of surgery.

In this review, we will address the professional wellness-related areas that may derive from any of the 4 core principles of surgical ethics, which in turn can have a direct or indirect relationship to BSAS.

The first section of this chapter will address the definitions and quantify the BSAS in surgeons. The second section will outline several of the recognized causes contributing to BSAS collectively, to account for the potential overlap between these manifestations. The third section will attempt to provide detailed strategies for prevention and management of these key areas.

## Definition of Burnout

It is clear that although physician burnout receives much attention currently, we do not have a clear, coherent, and agreed-upon definition of burnout in this setting.[1-3] Other conditions such as depression are well-defined diagnostic entities within our medical and layperson's lexicon, whereas until recently there was no standardized and validated definition of burnout. Some of the oldest references to the term appear in the Old Testament, Exodus 18:17-18.[3] Recent references relate to William Shakespeare alluding to burnout around the time of the 16th century. The German-born American psychologist Herbert Freudenberger is credited with coining the term burnout as we know it presently.[1,2,4] He used the term to describe the consequences of severe stress and high ideals affecting people in "helping" professions such as doctors and nurses.

We have come a long way from the etymological and definitional ambiguity of the term burnout. Burnout is currently defined in many ways such as exhaustion of physical or emotional strength or motivation usually as a result of prolonged stress or frustration; or loss of motivation, growing sense of emotional depletion, and cynicism; or consisting of the 3 main components that include emotional exhaustion, alienation from job-related activities, and reduced performance. Burnout is now a clinically recognized entity similar to any other diagnoses such as depression or cancer with a specific ICD-10-CM code (Z73.0) that can be used for purposes of reimbursement.[5] Although many symptoms may overlap with depression, it is nonetheless recognized as a separate diagnostic entity. It is also becoming clear that burnout causes structural and organic damage that affects the neural circuits, which eventually lead to a vicious cycle of neurologic dysfunction.[6] Golkar[6] compared the findings on resting-state functional MRI between 40 subjects formally diagnosed with burnout symptoms and 70 controls. They noted key differences in the size of the amygdala between the 2 groups, which are believed to be critical in emotional reactions.

Burnout is now a more clearly understood entity with a model that outlines its phases of progression[7] and is also measurable by several scales of which the most used is the scale developed by Maslach and Jackson in 1981[8] (see Table 46.1), Maslach Burnout Inventory. This inventory is considered by many as the standard tool for measuring burnout. In addition, it is acknowledged that burnout has diffused out from the original "helping" professions to affect any or all professions.

## Burden of Burnout in Surgeons

The burden of burnout can be gleaned from various sources. Campbell[9] conducted a survey of the graduates ($n = 1706$) of various University of Michigan surgical residencies and members of the Midwest Surgical Association to measure the rate of burnout. With a response rate of 44%, they documented a burnout rate of 32%. Shanafelt[10] conducted an anonymous cross-sectional survey of the members of the ACS. Of the 24 922 surgeons sampled, 7905 returned the surveys giving a response rate of 32%. In this large national study, the noted rate of burnout was alarmingly high at 40% and was documented as the single greatest predictor of surgeon's satisfaction with career and specialty choice. In a more recent study, Pulcrano noted that the burnout rate 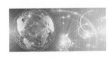 was variable among various surgical specialties, with general surgery ranging from 12% to 31.8%.[11] Data on the rate of burnout specific for individual surgical specialties have been published. In surgical oncology, for example, the rate of burnout has been documented to be in the range of 28%[12] to 36%.[13] Kuerer[12]

TABLE 46.1 ▶ MASLACH BURNOUT INVENTORY

|  | Every Day | A Few Times a Week | Once a Week | A Few Times a Month | Once a Month or Less | A Few Times a Year | Never |
|---|---|---|---|---|---|---|---|
| I deal very effectively with the problems of my patients | | | | | | | |
| I feel I treat some patients as if they were impersonal objects | | | | | | | |
| I feel emotionally drained from my work | | | | | | | |
| I feel fatigued when I get up in the morning and have to face another day on the job | | | | | | | |
| I have become more callous toward people since I took this job | | | | | | | |
| I feel I am positively influencing other people's lives through my work | | | | | | | |
| Working with people all day is really a strain for me | | | | | | | |
| I do not really care what happens to some patients | | | | | | | |
| I feel exhilarated after working closely with my patients | | | | | | | |

conducted a survey of the members of the Society of Surgical Oncology in 2006. Of the 1519 members, 549 responded, which gave a response rate of 36%. Seventy-two percent of the respondents were in academic surgery and worked more than 60 h/wk. Although 79% of the respondents noted that they would choose surgical oncology again, nearly a third of the respondents (28%) were categorized as having burnout. Balch[13] performed a subset analysis of the data obtained from the study[10] that included members of the ACS. Of the

7905 respondents, 407 were surgical oncologists. Surgical oncologists were noted to be younger, more likely to be females, and were noted to have a burnout rate of 36%.

The rate of burnout in surgery is better appreciated when placed in perspective by comparison with other specialties. The Medscape Lifestyle Report[14] published annually provides a comprehensive review of various trends in the physician community. The Medscape Lifestyle Report of 2016 emphasizes that it covers 2 important aspects of a physician's life that could affect patient care: burnout and bias. This report includes 25 special- 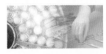 ties and has a large sample size of 15 800. In addition to providing data for all the 25 specialties, the report highlights the data for each of the 25 individual specialties. The overall trends for all the specialties documented a rise in the rate as well as the severity of the burnout.

In the same Medscape Lifestyle Report 2016, surgery ranked high in the second quintile (seventh out of 25 specialties) with a high burnout rate of 51%. When rated for severity (from 1 to 7, 1 = least and 7 = worst), surgery ranked in the third quintile with a rate of 4.3%. Although women (58%) were noted to consistently have a higher rate of burnout, nearly half of the men (49%) also document burnout. Interestingly, the rate of burnout seems to have plateaued in women from 43% (2013) to 59% (2015) to 58% (2016). In contrast, the rate of burnout has increased for men from 39% (2013) to 47% (2015) to 49% (2016). When rated for happiness outside of work, surgeons ranked in the middle at 61%, whereas for happiness at work, surgeons ranked in the second quintile (seventh out of 25) at 32%. Female surgeons reported less happiness both at work (23% vs 35%) and outside of work (57% vs 62%) when compared with men.

---

# Definition of Substance Abuse

The World Health Organization defines substance abuse as the harmful or haz-ardous use of psychoactive substances, including alcohol and illicit drugs.[15] The National Institute of Drug Abuse (NIDA) defines addiction as a chronic, relapsing brain disease that is characterized by compulsive drug seeking and use, despite harmful consequences.[16,17] The NIDA considers addiction a brain disease with structural changes that can be long-lasting and associated with harmful and often self-destructive behaviors.

The NIDA[16] is a section under the National Institutes of Health, and its mission is to advance science on the causes and consequences of drug use and addiction and to apply that knowledge to improve individual and public health. The NIDA accomplishes this through (1) strategically supporting and conducting basic and clinical research on addiction, its consequences, and the underlying neurobiologic, behavioral, and social mechanisms that are involved and (2) ensuring that the findings of research are disseminated adequately to improve the prevention and treatment of substance use disorders and enhance public awareness of addiction as a brain disorder.

Although addiction is not considered a specific diagnosis in the fifth edition of the *Diagnostic and Statistical Manual of Mental Disorders (DSM-5)*, NIDA continues to use "addiction" to describe compulsive drug-seeking 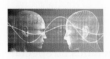 behavior despite negative consequences. The new DSM-5 refers to this as substance use disorder, which is defined as mild, moderate, and severe to indicate the level that is determined by the number of diagnostic criteria met by an individual. The new DSM describes substance use disorder as a problematic pattern of use of an intoxicating substance leading to clinically significant impairment or distress, as manifested by the presence of at least 2 of the following criteria within a 12-month period:

1. The substance is often taken in larger amounts or over a longer period than was intended.
2. There is a persistent desire or unsuccessful effort to cut down or control the use of the substance.
3. A great deal of time is spent in activities necessary to obtain the substance, use the substance, or recover from its effects.
4. Craving, or a strong desire or urge to use the substance.
5. Recurrent use of the substance resulting in a failure to fulfill major role obligations at work, school, or home.
6. Continued use of the substance despite having persistent or recurrent social or interpersonal problems caused or exacerbated by the effects of its use.
7. Important social, occupational, or recreational activities are given up because of the use of the substance.
8. Recurrent use of the substance in situations in which it is physically hazardous.
9. Use of the substance is continued, despite the knowledge of having a persistent or recurrent physical or psychologic problem that is likely to have been caused or exacerbated by the substance.
10. Tolerance, as defined by either of the following:
    a. A need for markedly increased amounts of the substance to achieve intoxication or desired effect.
    b. A markedly diminished effect with continued use of the same amount of the substance.
11. Withdrawal, as manifested by either of the following:
    a. The characteristic withdrawal syndrome for the substance (as specified in the DSM-5 for each substance).
    b. The substance (or a closely related substance) is taken to relieve or avoid withdrawal symptoms.

The media report[17] released by NIDA in October 2016 noted that abuse of and addiction to alcohol, nicotine, and illicit and prescription drugs cost Americans more than $700 billion a year in increased health care costs, crime, and lost productivity. It also notes that illicit and prescription drugs and alcohol contribute to more than 90 000 deaths every year in America.

The relapse rate for addiction ranges between 40% and 60%, which is higher than the rate for some other chronic illnesses such as diabetes (30%-50%). The NIDA also provides a list of the most commonly used addictive drugs, which are summarized in Table 46.2. Although these data may be derived from NIDA-funded annual survey of 8th, 10th, and 12th grade students, it provides a list of commonly used addictive drugs.

The data pertaining to the type of substance abused by physicians were reported by McLellan.[18] They conducted a longitudinal, cohort study over a 5-year period (1995-2001) of all physicians with a substance abuse problem who were admitted to any of the included 16 physician health programs. Laboratory and medical records of the 904 physicians were analyzed.

TABLE 46.2  ▶ MOST COMMONLY USED ADDICTIVE DRUGS

| Most Commonly Used Additive Drugs | Description |
| --- | --- |
| Marijuana (Cannabis) | |
| K2/Spice | Herbal mixtures that produce experiences similar to marijuana |
| Prescription and over-the-counter medications | Opioids |
| | Stimulants |
| | Depressants |
| Alcohol | |
| Amphetamines/methamphetamines | |
| Anabolic steroids | |
| Bath salts | Emerging family of drugs containing synthetic chemicals |
| Cocaine | |
| Hallucinogens | MDMA (Ecstasy, Molly) |
| | LSD |
| | PCP |
| | Psilocybin |
| Heroin | |
| Inhalants | |
| Ketamine/Rohypnol and GHB | |
| Nicotine | |

GHB, gamma-hydroxybutyrate; LSD, lysergic acid diethylamide; MDMA, 3,4-methylenedioxymethamphetamine; PCP, phencyclidine.

The participants were predominantly men (87%) with an average age of 44 years. The commonly abused substances included alcohol (50.3%), opiates (35.9%), stimulants (7.9%), or other substances (5.9%). Fifty percent reported the use of more than one substance, and the rate of intravenous abuse was 13.9%.

## Burden of Substance Abuse in Surgeons

The field of surgery is no stranger to substance abuse considering that the father of American or modern surgery Dr William Stewart Halsted himself was addicted to substances that were not then illicit. William Stewart Halsted (1852-1922) was born in New York to a wealthy businessman. He completed his college at Yale (1870-1874) and entered medical school at the College of Physicians and Surgeons in New York in 1874.[19] After finishing medical school and working for a few years, he accepted the invitation of his long-time friend William Welch and moved to Baltimore. He was appointed the first Surgeon-in-Chief and Professor of Surgery at the Johns Hopkins Hospital.

Halsted is credited with monumental contributions to the field of surgery and medicine as a whole. These include pioneering the residency training system, inventing latex gloves, and developing and advancing concepts in the 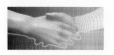 care of breast cancer, hernia repair, aneurysms, intestinal surgery, gallbladder disorders, and fracture management. He emphasized the concepts of safe and meticulous surgery and wide resection including lymphadenectomy for the management of cancer. His other significant contribution was in the field of local anesthesia.

Having realized the local anesthetic benefits of cocaine, he started experimenting on himself along with a few friends.[20] These experiments included injection of cocaine around nerves and observation of its desired anesthetic effects. As a result of multiple experiments, he became addicted to cocaine, which caused him to seek rehabilitation facilities. Morphine was then used to treat his cocaine addiction, and he ultimately became addicted to both.

Oreskovich[21] conducted a cross-sectional voluntary survey of the members of the ACS in 2010. Of the 25 073 surgeons sampled, 7197 completed the survey giving a response rate of 28.7%. The rate of alcohol abuse or dependence was equivalent to 15.4%, with females (25.6%) reporting a higher rate than males (13.9%). The factors independently associated with a higher incidence of alcohol abuse or dependence included female gender, group practice, no children, hours worked per week, nights on call per week, type of practice setting, presence of burnout, positive screen for depression, major error in the past 3 months, and youthful age. In another study by Oreskovich,[22] the highest prevalence of alcohol abuse or dependence was found among dermatologists and orthopedic surgeons and lowest among general practitioners and neurologists.

# Definition of Suicide

The Centers for Disease Control and Prevention categorizes and defines self-directed violence as follows:[23]

> *Suicide: Death caused by self-directed injurious behavior with an intent to die as a result of the behavior.*
>
> *Suicide attempt: A nonfatal, self-directed, potentially injurious behavior with an intent to die as a result of the behavior, which might result in injury.*
>
> *Suicidal ideation: Thinking about, considering, or planning suicide.*

The Centers for Disease Control and Prevention[24] states that suicide is the 10th leading cause of death, with 41 149 suicides in the United States in 2013. Suicide is the seventh leading cause of death in males and the 14th leading cause of death in females. Suicide results in an estimated loss of $51 billion due to medical costs and loss of work. Males are more likely to commit suicide and account for 77.9% of all suicides, although females are noted to have a higher incidence of suicide attempts. Firearms account for the most commonly used (56.9%) method to commit suicide in males followed by poisoning in females (34.8%). Nonfatal, self-inflicted injuries are much higher with an incidence of 494 169 (2013) and are noted to contribute to a loss of $10.4 billion due to medical costs and loss of work.

# Burden of Suicide in Surgeons

Data relating to burden of suicide in physicians overall are published by the American Foundation for Suicide Prevention.[25] It notes several alarming trends about suicide in physicians such as the following:

1. Approximately 300 to 400 physicians commit suicide every year in the United States.
2. In the general population, males have a higher rate of suicide than females, whereas female physicians have rates comparable with male physicians.
3. Female physicians have a suicide rate that is 250% to 400% higher than the general female population in other professions.
4. Contributing to the higher rate of suicide is the higher completion to attempt ratio in physicians, likely due to greater knowledge of lethality of drugs and easier access to the same drugs.

Shanafelt documented the rate of suicidal ideation in surgeons by conducting a survey of the membership of the ACS. Of the 7905 respondents, 501 (6.3%) surgeons reported suicidal ideation during the previous 12 months. They noted that in individuals older than 45 years, the rate of suicidal ideation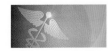

in surgeons was 1.5 to 3 times higher than in the general population. The independent factors associated with suicidal ideation included positive screen for depression, burnout, perceived major medical error in the past 3 months, and having a youngest child aged between 19 and 22 years.

## Causes of Burnout, Substance Abuse, and Suicide

This section will attempt to provide an overview of the causes contributing to BSAS in physicians/surgeons. It needs to be highlighted that the list of causes is not exhaustive and may just represent the tip of an iceberg. Most of the literature cited arises from mainstream media and less from the published medical literature. The outlined causes are not in any particular order of importance, and, more importantly, this section is not intended to confirm causality or offer solutions. A list of causes contributing to burnout as documented in the Medscape Lifestyle Report[14] is outlined in Table 46.3.

TABLE 46.3 ▶ LIST OF CAUSES CONTRIBUTING TO BURNOUT: MEDSCAPE LIFESTYLE REPORT 2016

| Cause | Rate (1-7)<br>1 = Does Not Contribute To Burnout At All<br>7 = Significantly Contributes |
|---|---|
| Too many bureaucratic tasks | 4.84 |
| Spending too many hours at work | 4.14 |
| Increasing computerization of practice | 4.02 |
| Income not high enough | 3.78 |
| Feeling like just a cog in a wheel | 3.71 |
| Maintenance of certification requirements | 3.66 |
| Impact of the Affordable Care Act | 3.43 |
| Too many difficult patients | 3.42 |
| Too many patient appointments in a day | 3.40 |
| Inability to provide patients with the quality care that they need | 3.29 |
| Lack of professional fulfillment | 3.14 |
| Difficult colleagues or staff | 2.97 |
| Inability to keep up with current research and recommendations | 2.92 |
| Compassion fatigue (overexposure to death, violence, and/or other loss in patients) | 2.88 |
| Difficult employer | 2.83 |

Table modified from Peckham C. Medscape Lifestyle Report 2016: Bias and Burnout. *Medscape*. January 13, 2016. Available at: https://www.medscape.com/slideshow/lifestyle-2016-overview-6007335. Accessed March 6, 2018.

## Burden of the Professional Liability System

The medical practice system in the United States is perceived by some, indeed many, to be hostile to physicians and more expensive than in other countries.[26,27] Although indemnity payments and administrative payments account for less than 1% of the health spending, the actual costs are higher (2%-3%) because of the defensive medicine it promotes.[28] The expense associated with the practice of defensive medicine is much higher and highlighted below. The role of professional liability in dictating practice patterns has grown over the last 4 decades. The number of claims and the size of awards per claim increased till the 1980s following which we have seen some stabilization both in the frequency and the amounts awarded. Nonetheless, medical malpractice allegations and the overall professional liability system continue to play a large role in dictating practice patterns directly or indirectly.

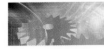

A common notion in the United States is that "every patient is a potential lawsuit." This notion perpetuates the fear of medical malpractice allegations and provides the solid foundation of practicing defensive medicine.[29-32] Ordering more tests than needed or performing more procedures that are not routinely indicated would be categorized as positive defensive medicine. Not performing procedures that could be beneficial but avoiding them because of the high risk profile would constitute negative defensive medicine. In a report (survey of physicians) released by Gallup and Jackson Healthcare,[31,32] it is noted that 9 out of 10 (nearly 92%) of US physicians report practicing defensive medicine. Although physician compensation accounts for only 8% of the health care expenditure in the United States, defensive medicine is felt to account for 26% to 34%, which translates to nearly $650 to 850 billion. In another study, Rothberg[30] estimated the costs of defensive medicine on 3 hospital medicine services in a health system by having physicians assess the defensiveness of their own orders. The authors noted that fully 28% of the 4200 plus orders were reported by physicians as being at least partially defensive.

The fear of professional liability litigation and the perceived need for practicing defensive medicine create a very stressful environment for physicians on a daily basis. The fear may influence physicians and surgeons to pursue treatment pathways or protocols that are not entirely based on science or evidence. These treatment practices can conflict with the ethical principles of the surgeons and can contribute to stress and burnout. This may affect surgeons more acutely because they are called to operate on patients in dire situations. For example, we can consider this patient who was previously diagnosed with stage IV pancreatic cancer with documented carcinomatosis. She is receiving palliative chemotherapy and no discussions were held about her code status. She presents to the emergency room with an acute abdomen, with investigations revealing free air suggestive of a perforated viscus. We as surgeons are called to determine whether she can be considered a surgical candidate. We are meeting the patient for the first time in her prolonged illness and have not had the opportunity to build a relationship or to facilitate 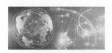 end-of-life discussions. In this situation, it still falls on the surgeon to address the free air even though the outcome will be determined by the pancreatic cancer. Because no one has held end-of-life discussions with her, it certainly would be difficult if not impossible to initiate these discussions with the patient and family who we are meeting for the first time. With respect to the sentiments of the patient and family, we initiate discussions within the short time frame permissible about all the treatment options ranging from comfort care to operative intervention. Although we know that operative intervention to address the perforated viscus is not going to alter the final outcome, the pervasive fear of malpractice prevents us from emphasizing the futility of operative intervention. Finally, the patient is operated upon and as expected, very little was achieved because of the extent of disease. The abdomen was washed out and closed with drains. The patient succumbs to the disease during the same hospital admission. Instead of having the possibility of spending the last few days of her life with family at home with dignity, the patient spent her last days in the hospital. We, as surgeons, could have been more forceful in our role providing advice on the most humanistic and compassionate treatment approach. Such situations are unquestionably stressful to all involved.

There is no specialty that is immune to the disastrous effects of medical professional liability concerns, although some specialties are more prone. A 2015 survey by Medscape noted that obstetrics/gynecology had the highest rate of being sued at 85%.[33] Surgery also had a very high rate at 83%. It was noted that by age 54 years, nearly 64% of the physicians were sued at least once, which increased to 80% at age 60 years. The survey also noted that being sued takes a heavy emotional and physical toll on the physicians. Many physicians who were sued spoke about their feelings, which include feeling helpless while being lied about by colleagues/patients/lawyers, implication of incompetence, self-doubt, being judged by nonpeers (jurors ignorant about medicine), exposure and humiliation, loneliness and isolation, and negative effect on marriage and family. Some state that they no longer trust any patients, which affects their practice and could lead to long-term anxiety, depression, and long-term suffering in general. The omnipresent fear and the significantly negative emotional and mental consequences of being sued play an undeniable role in the rising incidence of BSAS in physicians and surgeons.

## Physician and Surgeon Injury and Abuse

The physician workplace abuse is not an uncommon problem as noted by the Bureau of Labor Statistics.[34] The report published by the Bureau of Labor Statistics in 2010 covers the period from 2003 to 2007 and highlights the problem of workplace abuse.[34] The health care and social assistance industry employed an estimated 15.1 million people in 2007 and is the second largest industry sector in the nation. Women make up nearly 80% of all the private wage and salaried workers in health care and social assistance, whereas they make up only 45.3% of all other industries combined. In 2007, there were 670 600 injuries and illnesses in the health care and social assistance industry with an injury and illness rate of 5.6 per 100 full-time workers, which is higher than the average of 4.2 for the private industry. Hospitals are a major component of the health care and social assistance industry and reported nearly 270 000 nonfatal injuries and illnesses in 2007. Hospitals topped the list with the highest number with 100 000 reported injuries. Although hospitals constituted for only 29.5% of all health care and social assistance employment, they accounted for 40.1% of all injuries and illnesses in the sector. Injuries ranged from nonfatal exertion-related injuries to fatal injuries resulting from assaults on health care workers. The Bureau of Labor Statistics reported that most of the assaults were committed by patients or residents of the health care facility. The most common group victimized included nursing aides, nurses, and orderlies.

Although it might appear that most of workplace abuse does not involve physicians, the burden of violence against physicians/surgeons is not trivial and should not be ignored.[35,36] The elegant report published by Phillips[36] in *The New England Journal of Medicine* in 2016 provides a picture of workplace violence against physicians. Phillips[36] notes that health care workplace violence is an underreported, ubiquitous, and persistent problem that has been tolerated and largely ignored. This combined with the difficulty in performing research in this field due to lack of structured research models gravely underestimates the burden of the problem. Although most of the health care workplace violence may be verbal, other categories include assault, battery, domestic violence, stalking, and sexual harassment. Verbal abuse is more common and is harder to quantify and report but can be just as harmful as the other types of abuse.

Workplace violence can be categorized into 4 types depending on the offender's relationship with the victim and workplace. Type I workplace violence, for instance, would be someone like a bank robber. This is a person with no known relationship or connection to the workplace or employees but is committing the acts for alternate reasons. Each grouping of workplace violence then increases in level of personal relationship and/or connection to the workplace from there. Type II involves an offender who is a client, customer, or patient of the workplace facility or employee. The third group involves an offender who is a current or former employee who then commits the violent acts. Lastly, Type IV entails someone who has a personal relationship with an employee, yet, no relationship or connection with the place of work. An example of this group is a jealous boyfriend who goes to his girlfriend's place of work to then harm her. The common type of abuse in the health care workplace falls into Category II. In fact, the highest number of Type II assaults in the United States is directed against health care workers. In a survey conducted in 2014 on hospital crime, it was noted that the Type II violence accounted for 75% of aggravated assaults and 93% of all assaults against employees.[37]

Physicians seem to be frequent targets of Type II workplace violence. It is noted that violence against physicians occurred at a rate of 10.1 per 1000 workers, comprising 1.1% of all workplace violence. Some of these acts of violence toward surgeons have led to tragic consequences. In 2010, an orthopedic surgeon was shot by a patient's son, which resulted in serious injury.[38] Dr David Cohen, an orthopedic surgeon, was delivering bad news to Warren Davis about his mother. At that time, Warren Davis became upset, brandished a semiautomatic weapon, and fired on Dr Cohen. He was operated on and expected to make a full recovery. Warren Davis subsequently shot his mother fatally and also committed suicide by a gunshot wound to the head.

In another recent event in 2015, a Boston cardiac surgeon was murdered by the son of one of his patients.[39] Dr Michael Davidson, a cardiac surgeon, was 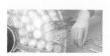 married with 3 children and was shot by Stephen Pasceri, a father of 4 children. Dr Davidson eventually succumbed to his injuries. The 55-year-old accountant walked into the Shapiro Cardiovascular Center at Brigham and Women's Hospital on January 20, 2015 and insisted on seeing Dr Michael Davidson, although he did not have an appointment.

Stephen Pasceri's mother was a patient of Dr Davidson, who had succumbed to her illnesses at an outside hospital. Pasceri felt that it was due to the drug amiodarone and wanted to confront Dr Davidson about it. Dr Davidson was known for his thorough approach and also for spending a lot of time talking to his patients. When seeing Pasceri, he interrupted his clinic and let him in to talk about his mother. As the discussion went on for several minutes, Dr Davidson had asked the physician's assistant to leave the room. Although he could have rushed the discussion to get home to his 3 children and wife pregnant with their fourth child, Dr Davidson explained patiently to Pasceri the benefits of amiodarone. Suddenly gunshots were heard and Dr Davidson came rushing out of the room screaming: "He's shooting, he's shooting," and collapsed at the end of the corridor. After surgery that lasted nearly 8 hours he succumbed to his injuries. A note left by Pasceri on his flash drive stated that a malpractice suit would not constitute adequate justice and that he had to murder Dr Davidson. Such violence is not just restricted to practicing surgeons. Workplace violence is also a problem for our surgical residents. Barlow[40] conducted a survey of surgical staff nationwide to elicit information about workplace violence and obtained responses from 475 respondents from 57 residency programs. They noted that of the 280 residents that witnessed one or more physical attacks, nearly 179 reported being attacked. Female residents were more likely to call hospital security for help in navigating hostile situations. Junior residents were more likely to be assaulted, and these incidents occurred more frequently in public rather than in private hospitals. The main perpetrators of assault on surgical residents consisted of patients followed distantly by family members and staff.

The trend in violence against physicians and surgeons in the United States is frequent and increasing. Assaults that are not fatal, such as verbal and emotional abuse, also add to the burnout and substance abuse rates in the United States. Some patients and families are extremely demanding and perceive that the physician or surgeon should only be a dispenser of care that they seek and not rely on the surgeon's own decision or judgment. Failure to do so could trigger malpractice allegations, losing patients to another practice, lodging complaints with the hospital administration, and, more importantly, providing unfavorable reviews on social media Web sites that rate physicians. In an era when patients are often referred to as customers and the customer is supposed to be the king, physicians do not always feel that they are adequately supported in their interactions with patients and their families. Physicians and other health care workers are frequently asked to "grin and bear it" regardless of the severity or unreasonable nature of demands from patients even if they are not rooted in evidence. This lack of an equitable social contract between the physicians and their patients will continue to add to the physical and emotional toll on physicians and contribute to the rising burden of BSAS.

In addition to fatal injuries, workplace-related injuries are common in surgeons. They can include sharp injuries, latex allergies, musculoskeletal injuries, blood-borne pathogens, laser plumes, anesthetic gases, and so forth. Of these, static/abnormal postures leading to musculoskeletal injuries in surgeons are very common.[41–45] Davis et al[42] conducted a survey of the membership of the Tennessee Chapter of the ACS. Electronic RedCAP surveys were distributed via e-mail to all members in the state. A total of 260 responses (out of 793) were received giving to a response rate of 33%. Nearly 40% of surgeons had sustained injuries in the workplace. Although 50% of surgeons received medical care for their occupational injury, only 20% reported those injuries to their institution. As a result of the injury, 22% missed work and 35% performed fewer operations.

Rambabu et al[43] conducted a cross-sectional survey to determine the prevalence of musculoskeletal injuries in physicians. They noted that surgeons had a high prevalence of 37% surpassed only by dentists (61%). In another study of surgical specialists, Soueid et al[44] noted that plastic surgeons had the highest rate of musculoskeletal injuries with general surgeons, otolaryngologists, and neurosurgeons following. This was further validated by Capone et al[45] in a study estimating the prevalence of musculoskeletal injuries in plastic surgeons. Of the 500 surveys distributed, 339 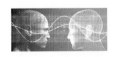 responded with an impressive response rate of 67.8%. Musculoskeletal symptoms were noted in nearly 81.5% of surveyed surgeons. The more common injuries were muscle strain, vision changes, cervical pain, lumbar pain, and shoulder arthritis/bursitis.

It is very clear that surgeons suffer a high rate of occupation-related injuries of which musculoskeletal injuries predominate. In addition to the high rate of occupational injuries, underreporting of the injuries compounds the problem. It is likely that only some surgeons will seek treatment for these injuries and that some may become addicted to pain relievers or other addictive substances. The underreporting of the injury and its treatment with potential addiction and abuse can be another cause of burnout or suicide.

## Bullying, Harassment, and Discrimination

The issues of bullying, harassment, and discrimination in the medical specialties are ancient. Although the awareness may have increased, what has not changed is that how it is underreported and unaddressed. The lack of dedicated high-quality research to even quantify the burden inhibits addressing these issues. However, there are some studies/opinions[46–50] that have addressed the issues of bullying, discrimination, and the presence of unethical practices that permit the 2 to flourish. The Expert Advisory Group (EAG)[46] was commissioned by the Royal Australasian College of Surgeons and tasked with assessing the burden of discrimination, bullying, and sexual harassment. The EAG invited surgeons in practice and in training to participate in the research project and had a good response. The findings and feedback were obtained from 5 major pieces of work: prevalence survey, qualitative research, organizational survey, submissions to the issues paper, and online discussions. Nearly 47% (3516 of 7405) of the invited constituents participated in the research. Of these 49.5% were more than 10 years post examination, 29.5% were less than 10 years post examination, 16.5% were in training, and 4.2% were international medical graduates. Of the 352 hospitals invited, 117 responded to the organizational survey translating to a response rate of 33%. Several surgeons provided personal examples and participated in online discussions as well. All surveys were conducted between April and July 2015.

Based on the findings the EAG noted:

> *"It was shocked by what it heard."*

The research found that nearly 49% of practicing surgeons, trainees, and international medical graduates reported being subjected to discrimination, 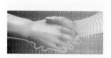 bullying, and sexual harassment. Nearly 71% of hospitals reported discrimination, bullying, or sexual harassment. The problems existed across all surgical specialties and "senior surgeons and surgical consultants" are reported as the primary source of the problems. The report also noted that:

> *"Bullying was noted to be endemic in surgery, common in training and the surgical workplace and central to the culture of surgery. There was general consensus that the worst cases were deliberately orchestrated and perpetrated by a small number of people who abused their institutional positions of power.*

*There is significant gender inequity in surgery, which influences and is influenced by the dominant surgical culture in which inappropriate behavior is rarely "called out." There are reported instances of sexual harassment, and sexism more broadly is commonplace in surgery."*

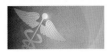

The EAG concluded that:

*"Bullying, sexual harassment are pervasive and pose a serious problem to the practice of surgery in Australia and New Zealand. The effects are significant and damaging. Discrimination, bullying and sexual harassment affect not only individuals who are subjected to these behaviors, but also the health care teams who witness or are part of them, and patients whose safety is risked as a result of them. The research shows that there are some surgeons who do not believe these problems exist."*

The perils of bullying, discrimination, and sexual harassment are not only restricted to practice but also affect surgeons in training.[50,51] The General Medical Council in the United Kingdom conducted a survey of doctors in training in 2013 to assess the prevalence of bullying.[50] Over 13% ($n$ = 6620) of the respondents reported being victims of bullying and harassment in their training position. Female physicians and those who obtained their medical degree outside the United Kingdom were more likely to make a comment on bullying or undermining. Nearly 19.5% ($n$ = 9723) of trainees had witnessed someone else being bullied in their post. Finally, nearly 13 276 physicians (26.5%) had experienced undermining behavior from their senior colleagues. In another study conducted by the Royal College of Surgeons in Edinburgh,[51] it was noted that surgical trainees are 3 times more likely to experience bullying than in other specialties. For most specialties, it was noted that 1 in 5 (20%) have been victims of bullying and just over 2 out of 5 (44%) have witnessed it. Whereas for surgery, the figures are much higher: 3 out of 5 have experienced bullying and nearly 9 out of 10 have observed this damaging behavior in the workplace.

Although most of these data emanate from outside of the United States, Dr Patricia J. Numann, one of our past presidents of the ACS, states, in an elegant editorial,[52] that the data from the study from Australia may be representative of any country including the United States. The inability to confront the perpetrators and the unethical practices they foster is a matter of serious concern. The EAG report from Australia notes that people are frequently afraid to raise an issue or make complaints, fearing risk to their training, career, or livelihood. Until this situation of fear and retribution can be effectively addressed, bullying will continue in the workplace and cause considerable and cumulative stress that can lead to BSAS.

## Electronic Health Record, Electronic Medical Record, and Computerized Physician Order Entry

The introduction of electronic health record (EHR) as part of the Patient Protection and Affordable Care Act has had a significant impact on the work-flow and satisfaction for many physicians. Although the 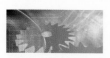 potential benefits can be significant, the EHR has contributed some negative consequences to physician satisfaction, which may ultimately lead to burnout. The 2013 Physician Satisfaction Study sponsored by the RAND Corporation and the American Medical Association[53] explored the factors affecting physician professional satisfaction and their implications for patient care, health systems, and health policy. Although physicians felt that electronic medical record (EMR) was beneficial (better access to patient data, improved tracking, and better communication), there were many more reasons for physician dissatisfaction with EMR. These reasons included time-consuming data entry, EMR and EHR algorithms that do not match clinical patterns, interference with face-to-face patient care, insufficient exchange of information, information overload, mismatch between meaningful use and clinical practice, financial consequences, taking away physicians to perform "low-skilled work," and standardized templates compromising quality and usefulness of documentation.

A more recent time and motion study by Sinisky[54] and sponsored by the American Medical Association highlighted the negative consequences of EHR and clerical work. This study analyzed the allocation of physician time in ambulatory practice and included 4 specialties: family medicine, internal medicine, cardiology, and orthopedics. Fifty-seven physicians were observed for 430 hours and, in addition, 21 physicians also completed after-hour diaries. The authors noted that during the office day, physicians spent 27% of their total time on direct clinical face time with patients and 49.2% of their time on EHR and desk work. While in the patient room, physicians spent 52.9% of clinical face time with patients and 37% of time on EHR and related desk work. Overall, for every hour that a physician spent face-to-face with the patient, he/she spent 2 hours on EHR and desk work. In addition, on average physicians spent an additional 1 to 2 hours of personal nighttime on additional computer and clerical work.

The link between EHR and specifically physician stress and burnout has been studied. Shanafelt[55,56] conducted a survey of physicians across all specialties across the United States between August and October 2014. The study obtained information about the physician usage of EHR/computerized physician order entry (CPOE) and correlated that trend in the usage of electronic patient portals to burnout. With a response count of 6375, they noted that 5389 (84.5%) physicians reported the use of EHR. Of the 5892 physicians, 4858 (82.5%) reported the use of CPOE. The authors noted that physicians who used EHR and CPOE had a lower rate of satisfaction appropriately because of the time spent on electronic clerical tasks. Although EHR was not associated with burnout, an independent association was noted between the usage of CPOE and burnout among physicians (OR = 1.29; 95% CI, 1.12-1.48, $P$ < .001). In addition, 44% of physicians were dissatisfied and 63% noted that EHR contributed to inefficiencies in their work environment.

Data relating to the role of EMR contributing to physician stress and burnout are available for some individual specialties. Babbot[57] assessed the relationships between the number of EMR functions, primary care work conditions, and physician satisfaction, stress, and burnout. Their MEMO (Minimizing Error, Maximizing Outcome) study from 2001 to 2005 included 379 primary care physicians and 92 managers from 92 clinics located in New York City and upper Midwest. The clinics were divided into low, moderate, and high EMR clusters based on the electronic workload. They noted that physicians in the moderate ($P$ = .03) and high ($P$ = .01) had lower satisfaction than those in the low cluster. In addition, physicians in the high EMR cluster were noted to have much higher rates of burnout. Although these findings are from the primary care environment, it is plausible that they are equally applicable to surgeons. The study by Sinisky,[54] which included nonsurgical and surgical specialties, noted similar negative consequences of EHR across specialties.

In addition to the administrative work related to direct patient care emanating from EHR/EMR, other administrative demands are also increasing. Some of these relate to maintaining compliance and the significant changes associated with it. For example, compliance with the new International Classification of Diseases (ICD) system is expected to add to the physician stress on a daily basis. The World Health Organization's ICD is a system of diagnostic codes established for uniform defining and reporting of disease so as to develop a common global language of communication.[58] Since the 1980s the United States has used this coding system for the purposes of billing and reimbursement. The recent version of ICD-9 was replaced by ICD-10, which took effect on October 1, 2015. The ICD-10 system is purported to have significant benefits over its predecessor. Some of these include (1) greater number of codes to cover more diseases, (2) more specificity to define laterality (left or right) when needed, and (3) more detail such as the ability to differentiate a burn injury between the arm and forearm instead of labeling it as arm alone. Although the benefits may be real, there are negative consequences of ICD-10 that have added to the administrative burden for physicians. ICD-10 boasts of nearly 70 000 codes compared with only 13 000 for ICD-9. The sheer magnitude of this large volume of new disease-based codes that physicians have to become familiar with is a major administrative burden. Although increasing the details of coding in ICD-10 may be helpful for better billing and 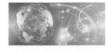 reimbursement, it is not without its adverse consequences. It is certainly beneficial to know which part of the pancreas is affected by the malignant neoplasm (ICD-10) when compared with ICD-9 that simply codes of pancreatic

TABLE 46.4 ▶ SOME CODES FROM ICD-10 SYSTEM

| ICD-10 Code | What It Codes for |
|---|---|
| V95.43XS | Spacecraft collision with injuries |
| V97.33XD | Sucked into jet engine, subsequent encounter |
| R46.1 | Bizarre personal appearance |
| W61.62XD | Struck by duck, subsequent encounter |
| Z 63.1 | Problems in relationship with in-laws |
| W61.33XA | Pecked by a chicken |
| Y92.253 | Hurt at the opera |
| V91.07XA | Burn due to water skis on fire |

cancer. On the other hand, having 3 codes for injury sustained by "walking into lamppost" certainly calls for questions about the true benefits of the bloated ICD-10. W22.02XA codes for injury sustained by initial encounter of walking into lamppost. W22.02XD codes for injury sustained by walking into a lamppost again. W22.02XS stands for sequela originating from injury resulting from walking into a lamppost. Some of the other codes in the ICD-10 system that can add to the administrative burden of physicians are highlighted in Table 46.4.

Physicians cannot avoid the new ICD-10 system, as it is integrally related to coding/billing, which determines reimbursement. Unless the new system is made more user-friendly or we find an easier system for reimbursement, it will continue to add to the stress levels for physicians and other health care professionals.

Another cause of stress at the workplace for physicians is the implementation of the Physician Payments Sunshine Act as a part of the Affordable Care Act. The Sunshine Act is implemented by the Centers for Medicare and Medicaid Services through its Open Payments Program. Open Payments is a federal program that collects information about the payments drug and device companies make to physicians and teaching hospitals for activities such as travel, research, gifts, speaking fees, and meals. It also includes ownership interests that physicians or their immediate family members have in these companies. These data are then made available to the public each year on this Web site. The process involves 3 steps that need to be done every year: complete an e-verification process by logging into Centers for Medicare and Medicaid Services, register in open payments, and review and dispute any data by December 31. The theoretical purpose of the Sunshine Act is to weed out unethical liaisons between industry and the physicians. However, in practice, this creates an enormous amount of work for most of the ethically committed physicians. It adds a significant amount of work and stress to the majority to weed out the minority of physicians with unethical liaisons. The burden of correcting the wrong information lies on the individual physician, which has been noted to be very time-consuming. In addition, the microscopic level of detail required is burdensome as well. Accepting any food worth more than $10 to 25 needs to be reported and will show up on the Web site for the public to review. Similarly, accepting even trivial items such as stationery or pens is now forbidden.

The Maintenance of Certification (MOC) was heralded as a method to keep physicians current with specialty-specific evidence-based practices. The older model consisted of recertification every 8 to 10 years depending on the specialty. The newer MOC model adds another layer of certification that needs to be met every 2 to 3 years depending on the specialty. Again, as with all the other new administrative burdens, although the intent is beneficial, the amount of effort, expense, and real-world benefit provides little to the patients. The current structure of MOC involves requirements for licensure and professional standing, self-evaluation of medical knowledge, cognitive experience, and self-evaluation of practice. With some minor variations in the format, all 24 member boards of the American Board of Medical Specialties approved this initiative in 2006. Although everyone agrees with the principle of life-long learning, nearly a decade after 2006, there are rising concerns that the benefits of MOC are not commensurate with the cost, effort, and time away from practice. Many feel that knowledge gained by continuing medical education through specialty meetings is more effective and sustainable.

The frustration and stress relating to MOC has been highlighted in the literature. In an elegant editorial (2015) in *The New England Journal of Medicine*, Teirstein noted: "Boarded to Death—Why Maintenance of Certification is Bad for Doctors and Patients."[59] A Web-based petition gathered more than 19 000 signatures regarding current MOC requirements in internal medicine overseen by the American Board of Internal Medicine. A similar second petition gathered more than 6000 signatures. It seems that MOC has become a profitable revenue generator. For the financial year 2012, MOC generated nearly $55 million in revenue for the American Board of Internal Medicine. In a survey of the readers of the *The New England Journal of Medicine* in 2010, nearly 63% opposed MOC.[60] A similar survey of cardiologists noted that nearly 90% opposed the current burdensome structure of MOC.

There are several other administrative tasks and requirements that continue to add a major level of stress to physicians. Some of the other administrative burdens include compliance with extremely detailed requirements of Health Insurance Portability and Accountability Act, extremely variable licensing requirements for different states, and complexities involved in negotiations with employers, practice groups, employees, and others. It is almost certain that we will witness a continuing rise in administrative 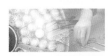 burden because of the evolving health care landscape. All of these administrative demands take the physician away from what he/she likes doing the most, the care of patients. This in turn contributes to the increasing national rate of burnout, which leads to increasing rates of depression, substance abuse, and suicide.

# Medical Student Debt That Transfers to Residency and Practice

The average medical student emerges from 4 years of medical school with a degree on light paper and debt, which is very heavy in its burden.[61,62] This debt is usually carried through residency (with or without forbearance) and into practice. The data provided by the American Association of Medical Colleges (AAMC) and the American Medical Student Association provide sobering figures that add to stress for any practicing physician or surgeon. The AAMC notes that for the 2014 graduates, the mean and median debt stand at $176 348 (increase by 4%) and $180 000 (increase by 3%), respectively. The percentage of students who owe more than $100 000, $200 000, and $300 000 stands at 79%, 43%, and 10%, respectively, with about 40% planning to enter the loan forgiveness or repayment program. With various permutations and combinations for repayment with or without forbearance, the AAMC notes the following: repayment (10-25 years, unless with a VA Educational Debt Reduction Program, which can drop it to 5 years), monthly payment ranging from $1600 to $3300, interest cost ranging from $108 000 to $303 000, and a total repayment value of $328 000 to $483 000 ($168 000 if participating in the VA Education Debt Reduction Program). Nearly 86% of the graduates carry some form of educational debt, which is 4.5 times higher than it was in 2003 and growing well beyond the consumer price index. Over the last 20 years, medical school tuition fees have increased by nearly 165% at private schools and 312% at public schools. This burden of debt is compounded by the fact that physician's salaries are declining at the same time. On an average a family physician could be paying an average of 8% to 15% of his/her income toward medical student educational debt. Although most physicians still earn more than most of those working in the United States, the rising burden of medical education debt, combined with declining salaries, is yet another contributing factor to BSAS.

# Workplace Productivity Pressures on Surgeons[63,64]

Surgeons are considered the economic engines of most hospitals and multispecialty practices because of superior revenue generation when compared with other specialties. The higher value of revenue generation by surgeons when compared with other specialties is well documented in the medical and mainstream literature. Merritt Hawkins, a national physician search firm, conducted a survey of hospital chief financial officers to quantify the amount of revenue generated 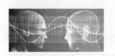 by 18 medical specialties.[63] The survey was conducted over a period of 12 months with the results published in 2016. It is noteworthy that surgical specialties constituted 3 out of the top 4 revenue-generating specialties. In an older study, Resnick et al[64] suggested that surgeon productivity directly related to hospital operating margin. They concluded that surgeons contribute significantly to the hospital margin and should be fully cognizant of that.

This reality of hospital margins and profits adds to the daily pressure on revenue generation. Although no specialty is immune to these financial pressures, surgeons tend to bear the brunt of it. Surgeons tend to be held to strict relative value unit productivity margins, which are assessed annually or even monthly. Detailed reports are frequently provided to physicians with line of sight toward their annualized targets. Inability 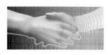 to meet the targets can lead to a strong sense of failure, a decrease in compensation or other penalties. Attempts to reach the predetermined targets can be very stressful and can influence surgeon's behavior and their practices.

## Loss of Professional Identity and Prestige

There is a general perception these days of a loss of professional identity, reputation, position in society, respect, and prestige among physicians. This is also worsened by the added perception of a loss of professional autonomy and the ability to chart the course of our own profession. It is clear that this feeling of despondency among surgeons is on the rise. Although very little may be published in the medical literature, there is an abundance of data in the general public's media attesting to this trend.[65–70]

Several reasons, real or perceived, may be contributing to this phenomenon. For centuries, being a physician was considered to be a noble profession, associated with a high standing and respect at work and in the general society. Physicians were empowered to always be able to control and influence the current status and the future path of their own profession, a basic tenet of the self-regulation foundation of the social contract. Most entered the profession with lofty ideals and a burning passion to serve the sick and infirm. The reasons outlined by applicants for entry into Medicine are impressive, lofty, idealistic, and poignant. Some enter the profession as a result of grave personal loss or tragedy. Some enter as a result of an epiphany that changes the entire course of their lives. Some have reasons that force them to abandon their current successful nonmedical profession to enter Medicine. The kaleidoscope of reasons outlined in personal statements are a panorama of burning desire and undying commitment to do nothing other than heal the sick and change the world.

The field of health care has changed significantly and will undoubtedly continue to change in the future. There is blurring of responsibilities and erosion of boundaries between physicians and the emerging cadre of nonphysician health care providers. The emergence and rise of nonphysician health care providers currently enhances medical practice and patient care and also contributes to the stress and burnout noted in physicians and surgeons. Mainstream publications[67] are noting how doctors may be "squeezed" out of

Medicine. Although this may be hyperbole, there is an element of truth in the rearrangement or reassignment of roles in health care delivery. Nonphysician health care providers make significant contributions to care delivery and will 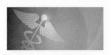 increasingly do so. What is needed is a seamless integration of these professionals. If done right and implemented with appropriate sensitivity, this, no doubt, will be of enormous benefit to the patients. Physicians may also feel that they are less involved or have less control in making decisions that affect their profession. This sense of loss is sometimes pervasive at the local, regional, and national level. Most feel that decisions regarding health care are made in political and regulatory halls far away from the environs of the sick by people who have never taken care of a patient or are not as experienced as physicians.

Another reason that may contribute to the rise of burnout, stress, and suicide is the emerging culture of an environment of blame directed toward physicians.[71-75] In a classic example highlighted in *The New England Journal of Medicine*, Catalyst section on Leadership, Shanafelt[75] noted that:

*"We tell physicians to get more sleep, eat more granola, do yoga, and take better care of yourself. These efforts are well intentioned," says Shanafelt. "The message to physicians, however, is that you are the problem, and you need to toughen up."*

*"We need to stop blaming individuals and treat physician burnout as a system issue," argues Shanafelt. "If it affects half our physicians, it is indirectly affecting half our patients."*

It may sometimes appear that many of the system-based ills affecting the profession are blamed on physicians themselves. Some of this may be true, but the vast majority of physicians wake up in the morning to exercise their rare privilege to take care of the sick and return home with the utmost satisfaction that is achieved on a daily basis. The proof for this lies in the fact that the vast majority of patients who walk into any hospital leave alive and that the overall health and longevity of the nation has improved significantly over the last century.

Physicians/surgeons also feel that while blame is squarely placed on them, any credit for good outcomes is evenly shared by everyone. Health care is a team effort and any credit or blame should be equally shared by all involved, a cause of consternation for physicians/surgeons. This recent trend of public shaming is emerging as another cause of burnout.[76-78] The culture of shaming physicians in public for unfavorable outcomes may have been transposed from the business culture in recent times. Most physicians are passionate about their work, practice ethically, and tend to be proud of their individual and professional reputation.

Most of these physicians are also highly successful during the entirety of their careers. To tarnish that in gross, public display for everyone including the nonphysicians to see does little for their morale. Although these efforts are laudable to weed out the rare "bad apples," they can contribute to decline in morale and add to the professional stress and burnout for the rest of the majority.

## Prevention and Management of Burnout, Substance Abuse, and Suicide

The current literature demonstrates the prevalence of BSAS. The first step toward limiting the toll the contributors may have on surgeons, and in turn on their surgical patients, is to acknowledge its prevalence. Acknowledging such factors does not weaken the reputation of surgeons but allows surgeons and the field of surgery as a whole to work toward advancement without the barriers brought about by their presence. There are steps that can be taken both independently and systematically to manage and prevent surgeons from experiencing BSAS. It is of utmost importance for all surgeons and managing bodies to take the steps necessary to prevent these contributors to promote a culture of optimal learning, physician wellness, and improved patient satisfaction and the best possible patient outcomes.

Burnout has been shown to affect quality of patient care, impair clinical judgment, and lead to medical errors. Dangerous consequences of burnout such as sleep disturbance, depression, chronic diseases, addiction, and suicide can be avoided by becoming more aware of burnout itself and being more proactive in preventing burnout before it damages the surgeon's professional life and personal well-being. Maintaining a balance between personal and professional life, regularly pursuing interests outside work, attending to important relationships, having spiritual connectedness, and staying healthy are a few ways to prevent burnout.[13]

Viewing the workplace, psychologist Frederick Herzberg's proposed the "two-factor" theory. His first factor "hygiene" includes salary, fringe benefits, status, and security. Absence of this factor causes dissatisfaction, but its presence does not guarantee professional satisfaction. He called his second factor "motivators," which includes challenges, personal growth, achievement, and recognition. The presence of the second factors leads to a greater overall sense of professional fulfillment.[79,80] In striving to maintain an environment that promotes these motivating factors, surgeons 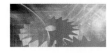 and managing bodies alike should work to reduce negative personal factors. This approach may improve the well-being of the surgeon and reduce stress.

Burnout increases the risk of depression resulting in an increased risk of suicide. Physicians and surgeons in particular are at higher risk of suicide.

Because of their medical knowledge and easy access to the means, they have higher rates of completed suicides as well. Screening tools should be implemented to identify surgeons at risk of burnout and depression.

Steps should also be taken to put programs into place to promote emotional health. One aspect of mental health most often noted in cases of burnout is stress. One of the most accessible and effective approaches to alleviate stress is physical exercise. Regular physical exercise has long-known positive effects on physical and mental health and is an important life skill and should be promoted for all physicians. A study done at Mayo Clinic found that exercise improves burnout scores and positively influences physicians' overall quality of life when performed on a regular basis.[81] Improvements in physicians' quality of life can directly correlate with improvements in patient care outcomes and satisfaction. Promotion of self-awareness and mindfulness training has also shown benefit in increasing the well-being of the physicians and improving the quality of patient interactions. Positive psychologic exercises, 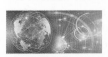 such as recognition and appreciation of gratitude and positive visualization, impart feelings of happiness and reduce depressive symptoms in participants.[82,83] Web-based cognitive behavioral therapy programs have shown to reduce suicidal thoughts in medical interns. These online programs are cost-effective and efficient for use in the medical field and may be accessed easily at the leisure of each individual physician.[84]

A health care provider who has endured psychologic and emotional trauma while experiencing an unexpected adverse patient outcome has been described as a "second victim." These second victims are vulnerable to the loss of confidence in their professional skills and knowledge; they may second guess themselves in their work, and develop anger or embarrassment, and make more medical errors. These emotional and psychologic effects are collectively termed "second victim syndrome." One of the strategies to support these victims is placing an emphasis on changing the professional environment from "culture of blame" to a "just culture" environment where the provider is not stigmatized from the blame and at the same time will get opportunities to learn from his/her mistakes.[85] Many medical institutions are currently moving toward just culture, as it supports improved physician and patient satisfaction, thus resulting in decreased physician burnout and medical malpractice claims. Providing institutional support from administrative leaders and establishing programs to assist health care providers in maintaining emotional and psychologic well-being is essential to help surgeons become more resilient to stress and provide better patient care.

Chemical addiction is another factor negatively affecting surgeons and, in turn, their patients, which must be dealt with on an individual and on a systems level. In a large national study conducted by Oreskovich et al, 15.4% of surgeons met diagnostic criteria for alcohol abuse or dependence.[21] A significant barrier to the management of these disorders or any other addiction comes from the reluctance to seek help due to the stigma regarding mental health and addiction. There are also barriers stemming from concerns that addiction will affect their credentials and jeopardize their medical license. A study done by Oreskovich et al[86] and supported by the ACS looked at the prevalence of alcohol use disorders among surgeons and concluded that the rate of alcohol use disorders among surgeons is the same or slightly higher than that among their counterparts in the general population. The study also found a strong association between burnout, depression, suicidal ideations, and career dissatisfaction. This study should serve as a model for other professional associations to destigmatize the disorders and encourage an active approach to identify and treat substance abuse and dependence and to promote the mental well-being of health care professionals.

Health programs available to physicians with substance use disorders have shown positive effects with favorable 5-year prognosis. In this study by Thomas McLellan et al[87] completion of a 60- to 90-day residential treatment program was followed by continued outpatient care. On completion of the outpatient care, return to work with continued participation in 12-step support groups was permitted. This was paired with random alcohol and drug testing and random visits by program staff at the workplace to improve successful outcomes. Such programs not only provide support to the physicians as needed to help attain abstinence, but they also provide assurance to hospitals, colleagues, and licensing boards that these physicians can return to their profession and care for their patients safely.

BSAS are all factors that negatively affect both personal and professional aspects of surgeons' lives and the patients they treat. These factors lead to lost time, money, and quality of care. Implementing, on an institutional level, a system of just culture as well as programs to help manage the stress and mental health aspects of surgical care that leads to these factors is essential to the well-being of the individual surgeons and the field of surgery as a whole. These implementations will also lead to improved patient satisfaction, outcomes, and a productive professional career.

---

## Summary

This chapter has attempted to outline the definitions of, quantify the burden of, and review some of the causes contributing to BSAS in surgeons. The solutions to address these trends are beyond the purview of this chapter. However, we have been able to briefly introduce some of the steps that may be taken toward the prevention and management of this set of professional challenges. It is evident that the incidence of BSAS is on the rise. The causes contributing 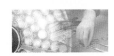 to this trend are multiple and permeate every level of the health care system from the individual in the operating room to the corridors of the federal government offices. Although we may not be certain of all the complex factors contributing to these trends, we as a professional need to assume ownership of these trends and address these issues expediently. Failure to do so will not only tarnish our noble profession but also injure the bright young men and women who will be the next generations of surgeons. This in turn will hurt our patients, who are the reason for our calling.

# References

1. Kaschka WP, Korczak D, Broich K. Burnout: a fashionable diagnosis. *Dtsch Arztebl Int.* 2011;108(46):781–787.
2. Depression: What is burnout syndrome? IQWiG (Institute for Quality and Efficiency in Health Care). https://www.ncbi.nlm.nih.gov/pubmedhealth/PMH0072470/. Accessed November 4, 2016.
3. Burisch M. *Das Burnout-Syndrom.* 4th ed. Heidelberg: Springer; 2010.
4. Michel A. Burnout and brain. *Observer–Association for Psychological Science.* https://www.psychologicalscience.org/publications/observer/2016/february-16/burnout-and-the-brain.html. Accessed November 4, 16.
5. ICD-10-CM Diagnosis Codes. http://www.icd10data.com/ICD10CM/Codes/Z00-Z99/Z69-Z76/Z73. Accessed November 4, 2016.
6. Golkar A, Johansson E, Kasahara M. The influence of work-related chronic stress on the regulation of emotion and on functional connectivity in the brain. *PLoS One.* 2014;9:e104550. doi:10.1371/journal.pone.0104550.
7. Freudenberger HJ: Counselling and dynamics: treating the end-stage person. In: Jones JW, ed. *The Burnout Syndrome.* Park Ridge, IL: London House Press; 1982.
8. Maslach C, Jackson SE. The measurement of experienced burnout. *J Occup Behav.* 1981;2:99–113.
9. Campbell Jr DA, Sonnad SS, Eckhauser FE. Burnout among American surgeons. *Surgery.* 2001;130(4):696–702.
10. Shanafelt TD, Balch CM, Bechamps GJ. Burnout and medical errors among American surgeons. *Ann Surg.* 2009;250(3):463–471.
11. Pulcrano M, Evans SRT, Sosin M. Quality of life and burnout rates across surgical specialties. A systematic review. *JAMA Surg.* 2016;151(10):970–978.
12. Kuerer HM, Eberlein TJ, Pollock RE. Career satisfaction, practice patterns and burnout among surgical oncologists: report on the quality of life of members of the Society of Surgical Oncology. *Ann Surg Oncol.* 2007;14(11):3043–3053.
13. Balch CM., Shanafelt TD, Sloan JA. Burnout and career satisfaction among surgical oncologists compared with other surgical specialties. *Ann Surg Oncol.* 2011;18(1):16–25.
14. Peckham C. Medscape Lifestyle Report 2016: Bias and Burnout. *Medscape.* January 13, 2016. Available at: https://www.medscape.com/slideshow/lifestyle-2016-overview-6007335. Accessed March 6, 2018.
15. The World Health Organization. *Substance Abuse.* http://www.who.int/topics/substance_abuse/en/. Accessed November 6, 2016.
16. National Institute of Drug Abuse. https://www.drugabuse.gov/about-nida. Accessed November 12, 2016.
17. The National Institute of Drug Abuse Media Guide. https://d14rmgtrwzf5a.cloudfront.net/sites/default/files/mediaguide_11_16.pdf. Accessed November 12, 2016.
18. McLellan TA, Skipper GS, Campbell M. Five year outcomes in a cohort study of physicians treated for substance use disorders in the United States. *BMJ.* 2008;337:2038.

19. Are C, Dhir M, Ravipati L. History of pancreaticoduodenectomy: early misconceptions, initial milestones and the pioneers. *HPB*. 2011;13(6):377–384.
20. Halsted W. Practical comments on the use and abuse of cocaine. *N Y Med J.* 1885;42:294–295.
21. Oreskovich MR, Kaups KL, Balch CM. Prevalence of alcohol use disorders among American surgeons. *Arch Surg.* 2012;147(2):168–174.
22. Oreskovich MR, Shanafelt T, Dyrbye LN, et al. The prevalence of substance use disorders in American physicians. *Am J Addict.* January 2015;24(1):30–38.
23. Centers for Disease Control and Prevention. *Definitions: Self-directed Violence.* http://www.cdc.gov/violenceprevention/suicide/definitions.html. Accessed November 12, 2016.
24. Centers for Disease Control and Prevention. *Suicide Facts.* http://www.cdc.gov/violenceprevention/pdf/suicide-datasheet-a.pdf. Accessed November 12, 2016.
25. The American Foundation for Suicide Prevention. Facts about physician suicide and depression. https://afsp.org/our-work/education/physician-medical-student-depression-suicide-prevention/. Accessed November 12, 2016.
26. Kessler D. Evaluating the medical malpractice system and options for reform. *J Econ Perspect.* 2011;25(2):93–110.
27. Bal BS. An introduction to medical malpractice in the United States. *Clin Orthop Relat Res.* 2009;467(2):339–347.
28. Mello MM, Chandra A, Gawande AA. National costs of the medical liability system. *Health Aff.* 2010;29(9):1569–1577.
29. Sekhar MS, Vyas N. Defensive Medicine: a bane to healthcare. *Ann Med Health Sci Res.* 2013;3(2):295–296.
30. Rothberg MB, Class J, Bishop TF. The cost of defensive medicine on 3 hospital medicine services. *JAMA Intern Med.* 2014;174(11):1867–1868.
31. New Gallup Poll Quantifies U.S. Physician Opinions on the Scope of Defensive Medicine Practices. http://www.jacksonhealthcare.com/media/194818/new_gallup_poll_quantifies_u.s._physician opinions on the scope of defensive medicine practices.pdf. Accessed November 12, 2016.
32. *A Costly Defense: Physician Sound off on the High Price of Defensive Medicine in the U.S.* http://www.jacksonhealthcare.com/media/8968/defensivemedicine_ebook_final.pdf. Accessed November 12, 2016.
33. What happens when doctors get sued. https://thedoctorweighsin.com/what-happens-when-doctors-get-sued/. Accessed November 20, 2016.
34. Workplace Safety and Health in the Health Care and Social Assistance Industry, 2003–2007. http://www.bls.gov/opub/mlr/cwc/workplace-safety-and-health-in-the-health-care-and-social-assistance-industry-2003-07.pdf. Accessed November 20, 2016.
35. Morrision JL, Lantos JD, Levinson W. Aggression and violence directed towards physicians. *J Gen Intern Med.* 1998;13(8):556–561.
36. Phillips JP. Workplace violence against health care workers in the United States. *N Engl J Med.* 2016;374(17):1661–1669.
37. Vellanki KH. The 2014 IHSSF crime survey. *J Healthc Prot Manage.* 2014;30(2):28–35.
38. Johns Hopkins Hospital: Gunman shoots doctor, then kills self and mother. http://abcnews.go.com/US/shooting-inside-baltimores-johns-hopkins-hospital/story?id=11654462. Accessed November 20, 2016.
39. Boston mourns surgeon killed by son of deceased patient. http://www.usatoday.com/story/news/nation/2015/01/21/boston-hospital-shooting/22096101/. Accessed November 20, 2016.

40. Barlow CD, Rizzo AG. Violence against surgical residents. *West J Med.* 1997;167(2):74–78.

41. Szeto GP, Ho P, Ting AC, Poon JT, Cheng SW, Tsang RC. Work-related musculoskeletal symptoms in surgeons. *J Occup Rehabil.* June 2009;19(2):175–184.

42. Davis WT, Fletcher SA, Guillamondegui OD. Musculoskeletal occupational injury among surgeons: effects for patients, providers, and institutions. *J Surg Res.* June 15, 2014;189(2):207–212.

43. Rambabu T, Suneetha K. Prevalence of work related musculoskeletal disorders among physicians, surgeons and dentists: a comparative study. *Ann Med Health Sci Res.* July 2014;4(4):578–582.

44. Soueid A, Oudit D, Thiagarajah S, Laitung G. The pain of surgery: pain experienced by surgeons while operating. *Int J Surg.* 2010;8(2):118–120.

45. Capone AC, Parikh PM, Gatti ME, Davidson BJ, Davidson SP. Occupational injury in plastic surgeons. *Plast Reconstr Surg.* May 2010;125(5):1555–1561.

46. Expert Advisory Group on Discrimination, Bullying and Sexual Harassment. Advising the Royal Australasian College of Surgeons. https://www.surgeons. org/media/22045685/EAG-Report-to-RACS-Draft-08-Sept-2015.pdf.   Accessed November 20, 2016.

47. Crebbin W, Campbell G, Hillis DA. Prevalence of bullying, discrimination and sexual harassment in Australasia. *ANZ J Surg.* 2015;85(12):905–909.

48. *Building Respect, Improving Patient Safety.* https://www.surgeons.org/ media/22260415/RACS-Action-Plan_Bullying-Harassment_F-Low-Res_FINAL.pdf. Accessed November 20, 2016.

49. Ling M, Young CJ, Shepherd HL. Workplace bullying in surgery. *World J Surg.* 2016;40(11):2560–2566.

50. National Training Survey 2013: Undermining. http://www.gmc-uk.org/NTS_2013_ autumn_report_undermining.pdf_54275779.pdf. Accessed November 20, 2016.

51. *Surgical Trainees 3X More Likely to Experience Bullying.* https://www.rcsed. ac.uk/news-public-affairs/press-and-media/press-releases/2014/may/surgical-trainees-3x-more-likely-to-experience-bullying. Accessed November 20, 2016.

52. Numann PJ. Workplace bullying in surgery. *World J Surg.* 2016;40(11):2569–2570.

53. *Factors Affecting Physician Professional Satisfaction and Their Implications for Patient Care, Health Systems and Health Policy.* http://www.rand.org/content/dam/rand/pubs/research_reports/RR400/RR439/RAND_RR439.pdf. Accessed November 12, 2016.

54. Sinsky C, Colligan L, Progmet M. Allocation of physician time in ambulatory practice: a time and motion study in four specialties. *Ann Intern Med.* 2016;6:epub ahead of print.

55. Shanfelt TD, Dyrbe LN, Sinsky C. Relationship between clerical burden and characteristics of the electronic environment with physician burnout and professional satisfaction. *Mayo Clin Proc.* 2016;91(7):836–848.

56. Doctors are burned out by busy work: study. *TIME Health Med.* http://time. com/4383979/doctor-burnout-electronic-health-records/. Accessed November 12, 2016.

57. Babbot S, Manwell LB, Brown R. Electronic medical records and physician stress in primary care: results from the MEMO study. *J Am Med Inform Assoc.* 2014;21:e100–e106.

58. World Health Organization Classification of Diseases (ICD). www.who.int/classifications/icd/en/. Accessed January 21, 2017.

59. Teirstein P. Boarded to death—why maintenance of certification is bad for doctors and patients. *N Engl J Med*. 2015;372(2).

60. Kritek PA, Drazen JM. Clinical decisions: American Board of Internal Medicine maintenance of certification program—polling results. *N Engl J Med*. 2010;362(15):e54.

61. Medical student education: debts, costs and loan repayment fact card. https://members.aamc.org/eweb/upload/2014%20DFC_%20vertical.pdf. Accessed November 20, 2016.

62. Medical student debt. http://www.amsa.org/advocacy/action-committees/twp/medical-student-debt/. Accessed November 20, 2016.

63. Murphy B. *Which Physicians Generate the Most Revenue for Hospitals?* http://www.beckershospitalreview.com/finance/which-physicians-generate-the-most-revenue-for-hospitals.html. Accessed November 20, 2016.

64. Resnick A, Corrigan D, Mullen J, Kaiser L. Surgeon contribution to hospital bottom line not all are created equal. *Ann Surg*. October 2005;242(4):530–539.

65. How American doctors lost their professional autonomy. http://www.forbes.com/sites/scottgottlieb/2014/05/16/how-american-doctors-lost-their-professional-autonomy/#1ef589cf4323. Accessed November 24, 2016.

66. The professional decline of physicians in the era of managed care. *New Engl J Public Policy*. http://scholarworks.umb.edu/cgi/viewcontent.cgi?article=1454&context=nejpp. Accessed November 24, 2016.

67. The future of medicine: squeezing out the doctor. http://www.economist.com/node/21556227. Accessed November 24, 2016.

68. The falling down professions. http://www.nytimes.com/2008/01/06/fashion/06professions.html. Accessed November 24, 2016.

69. Doctors and lawyers- no longer prestigious. http://business.time.com/2008/01/09/doctors_and_lawyers_no_longer/. Accessed November 24, 2016.

70. The professional status of physicians is at risk. http://www.kevinmd.com/blog/2011/07/professional-status-physicians-risk.html. Accessed November 24, 2016.

71. Is punitive culture contributing to physician burnout? http://www.kevinmd.com/blog/2016/02/punitive-culture-contributing-physician-burnout.html. Accessed November 24, 2016.

72. Fear of punitive response to hospital errors lingers. http://www.amednews.com/article/20120220/profession/302209938/2/. Accessed November 24, 2016.

73. Culture of safety lies in non-punitive leadership approach. http://www.hhnmag.com/articles/3389-culture-of-safety-lies-in-nonpunitive-leadership-approach. Accessed November 24, 2016.

74. Embracing a non-punitive culture for patient safety: http://www.marylandpatientsafety.org/html/education/solutions/2009/documents/Embracing_a_Non_Punitive_Culture_for_Patient_Safety.pdf. Accessed November 24, 2016.

75. Physician burnout: stop blaming the individual. *New Engl J Med, Catalyst*. http://catalyst.nejm.org/videos/physician-burnout-stop-blaming-the-individual/. Accessed November 24, 2016.

76. Best way to stop overprescribing antibiotics? Public shaming of course. http://arstechnica.com/science/2016/03/best-way-to-stop-overprescribing-antibiotics-public-shaming-of-course/. Accessed November 24, 2016.

77. The new and growing phenomenon of public shaming. http://www.physicianspractice.com/cultural-psychiatry/new-and-growing-phenomenon-public-shaming. Accessed November 24, 2016.

78. Bismark M, Paterson R. Naming, blaming and shaming? *Med Law.* 2006;25(1):115–125.
79. Herzberg F, Mausner B, Snyderman BB. *The Motivation to Work.* 2nd ed. New York: John Wiley; 1959.
80. Herzberg F. *Work and the Nature of Man.* Cleveland: World Publishing; 1966.
81. Weight CJ, Sellon JL, Lessard-Anderson CR, Shanafelt TD, Olsen KD, Laskowski ER. Physical activity, quality of life, and burnout among physician trainees: the effect of a team-based, incentivized exercise program. *Mayo Clin Proc.* December 2013;88(12):1435–1442.
82. Krasner MS, Epstein RM, Beckman H, et al. Association of an educational program in mindful communication with burnout, empathy, and attitudes among primary care physicians. *JAMA.* September 23, 2009;302(12):1284–1293.
83. Seligman ME, Steen TA, Park N, Peterson C. Positive psychology progress: empirical validation of interventions. *Am Psychol.* July–August 2005;60(5):410–421.
84. Finlay-Jones A, Kane R, Rees C. Self-compassion online. A pilot study of an internet-based self-compassion cultivation program for psychology trainees. *J Clin Psychol.* 2016.
85. Marmon LM, Heiss K. Improving surgeon wellness: the second victim syndrome and quality of care. *Semin Pediatr Surg.* December 2015;24(6):315–318.
86. Buhl A, Oreskovich MR, Meredith CW. Prognosis for the recovery of surgeons from chemical dependency: a 5-year outcome study. *Arch Surg.* 2011;146(11):1286–1291.
87. McLellan AT, Skipper GS, Campbell M, DuPont RL. Five year outcomes in a cohort study of physicians treated for substance use disorders in the United States. *BMJ.* November 4, 2008;337:a2038.

# Epilogue

Lloyd A. Jacobs, MD

PROLOGUE ▶ We have, in paragraphs interspersed in this writing, become aware of the substance problem with which Dr John Flynn has been wrestling. We have reached along with him a fork in the road. You, the reader, must recognize that you have both a stake in and an impact on his future.

An on-and-off Broadway play titled *Shear Madness* has the distinction of being called the longest running comedy by the *Guinness Book of World Records*. It is a whodunit; the mystery is the murder of the owner of the hair salon in which the play takes place. What is unique is that the play has 2 endings, ie, 2 outcomes. On any given night the audience does not know which will be presented. In many productions, the audience is asked to state their belief about the outcome of the mystery. So it is with the possible outcomes of Dr Flynn's substance abuse. There are 2 outcome scenarios: one that is more common in the past and one that is gaining traction but is still "the path less traveled."

In scenario A, Flynn finishes his training at an institution that is unaware of his problem. He begins practice but is made to move every 3 or 4 years when an episode occurs, which causes the leadership of the institution to threaten him. His career takes on a staccato quality until, in his mid-50s, he crashes and is forced into early retirement.

In scenario B, a colleague recognizes that something is wrong and confronts Flynn. Flynn accepts help. The chairman of his department is supportive, and the state board of licensure is punctilious but not harsh. After a period, Flynn is allowed to resume practice under supervision. Ultimately he experiences the exhilaration, which results from a career that is meaningful to him and his loved ones.

In his *Nicomachean Ethics*, Aristotle makes a distinction that helps in understanding the unique orientation of the surgeon even today. Aristotle distinguishes the observation and reasoning, which leads to knowledge from the type of reasoning that prompts to action. The latter is the subject of our ethics, and the choices of actions are termed "moral" choices. The surgeon, uniquely, occupies the realm of moral choice, choosing and performing acts in the world of reality. Such a stance presupposes a freedom of the will and the efficacy of actions to change the world. Although there are many occupations that act in this way, surgeons are quintessentially charged with moral choices and actions.

Surgeons are applied scientists, choosing between that which may improve a patient's well-being and that which is unlikely to do so. Aristotle distinguished the mental processes that causes one to know an intellectual product from the processes grouped under the heading of "phronesis," "prudence," or practical wisdom. Practical wisdom constitutes the sphere of ethics and informs the discipline of surgery.

Aristotle was scooped in the development of this distinction. The *Edwin Smith Papyrus* from Egypt entailed this distinction long before Aristotle and underscored the unique ethical base of the discipline of surgery. No other discipline demands the courage to act in reality, with one's hands, as the agent for another.

The *Edwin Smith Papyrus* is the world's oldest surgical textbook and arguably the world's oldest scientific document. It was purchased from an indigenous dealer in Egypt in about 1862 by the person whose name is now attached to it, one Edwin Smith, who was also a dealer in antiques. The manuscript itself is thought to date from about 1600 BC but is almost certainly a reproduction of documents that are much older, perhaps as old as the pyramids.

It should be noted that what Edwin Smith purchased was at least 3 documents, one of which he sold to Georg Ebers, that papyrus now bears his name. The document retained by Smith is, in fact, 2 very different documents.

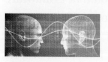
The surgical treatise is on the front of the papyrus; on its reverse is another very different content probably written later, which is similar to the document that had been sold to Georg Ebers. The Ebers Papyrus and the writing on the reverse of the Smith Papyrus have been described as "magico-religious." It consists of recipes and incantations for many diseases and has pejoratively been described as having little scientific basis or thought.

The main writing in the Smith document is different; it is well organized, clear, and experientially based. It would be specious for me to argue that surgery as a discipline is organized and clear, but that it is experientially based is incontrovertible and speaks of the unique nature of our discipline. The 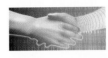 Edwin Smith textbook of surgery is a document of practical ethics in that it stresses the requirements of moral choice.

It is not my purpose to disparage the magico-religious writing in the Ebers' document or that on the reverse of the Smith document. Trauma surgery is in some ways easier to understand, at least in its etiology. Contrast a fracture with heart failure, for example. It is my intention to point out how different is the discipline of surgery from the whole of medicine and science. Even today the discipline stresses the craft of surgery; its knowledge base is heavily dependent on the accumulated experience of individuals.

The Smith textbook of trauma is remarkable for its careful descriptions of cases and the conclusions it reaches. What is even more remarkable is the ethical algorithm it presents and its emphasis on making a decision, which we, in retrospect, would recognize as a moral choice.

At the end of each clinical vignette, the surgeon is confronted with an algorithm with 3 pathways: to treat with expectation of success, to treat with reservations, or not to treat at all. The management of the expectations of patients and their surrogates is an obligation of the modern surgeon even currently. It is often said that knowing when not to operate is more difficult than the operative technique itself. The Smith document confronts both of these moral choices.

The Edwin Smith writing anticipates the Hippocratic physicians and their writings over several centuries in emphasizing the unique role of the surgeon. The Hippocratic Oath has served as a guide to the ethical physician and surgeon for centuries. It is clearly an anchor in the storm of change, which characterizes medicine currently. It contains, however, an enigmatic sentence that, I believe, testifies again to the uniqueness of the surgeons' work, as it states:

*"I will not use the knife, not even on sufferers from stone, but will withdraw in favor of such men as are engaged in this work."*

Surgeons are such men, and women too, I suspect, as are engaged in this work, notwithstanding the centuries-old discussion of the meaning of this sentence. In spite of suggested alternative meanings, I believe that the sentence means what it says: Surgeons are of a different class, intellectually, socially, and professionally. Surgeons possess and pursue phronesis and know-how, as well as knowledge.

Most surgeons and many laypersons are aware of the intermixing of the guilds of surgeons and barbers, which occurred throughout much of Europe in the late Middle Ages. Despite the obvious damage done by this mixing, the distinction is immortalized in the calling of surgeons in England "Mister" instead of "Doctor."

Harvey Cushing has justly been called the father of neurosurgery. Cushing's presidential address to the American College of Surgeons on 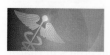 October 27, 1922 was titled "The Physician and the Surgeon."[1] In it, Cushing demonstrates the unique nature of the surgeon's intellectual, societal, and historical position. Although his purpose is to urge greater unity, his analysis of the distance between the disciplines is convincing. In a footnote to the essay, Cushing recounts a bit of history from about the end of the 19th century:

> *"…when a consultation on any important case was held, the surgeon was not as a rule permitted to be in the room where the physicians held their deliberations, but after the consultation was over, he was informed whether his services would be required or not."*

Clearly the surgeon has paid a high price for his artisanship, phronesis, and practical wisdom.

So surgeons are unique and different. No other discipline's acts and utterances, as an agent for someone else, are associated with the magnitude of import that the surgeon's moral choices entail. The discipline of surgery is the practice of an ethic, a deontological ethic deriving its authority from the venerable nature of the discipline itself.

The uniqueness of the discipline is reinforced by the ritual observance of an exercise called the mortality and morbidity (M&M) conference. It might better be called an ethics forum for surgeons. The ritualistic nature of this exercise is demonstrated by its weekly observance and its formulaic behaviors. It has often been observed that participants may sit in exactly the same seat for decades. There is an unmarked, unspoken area for medical students and one for residents. The faculty ghetto is similarly permanently circumscribed. The exercise is observed wherever modern scientifically based surgery is found and functions as an ethics forum.

This book has attempted to bridge the perceived gulf between the moral decision making in surgery and the psychic life and wellness of surgeons. The M&M conference serves exactly that; it is a forum for retrospective decision analysis and learning and also serves a number of invaluable psychologic functions. It elevates the discipline and supports its participants at once, if and only if it is successful in avoiding a pejorative and punishing tone.

It is important to distinguish the positive, reflective impact that this ethics forum may have on the well-being of the surgeon from the garden variety of egoism. In garden variety egoism, good causes may be served so that the doer may experience the self-adulation attendant to these actions. In the instance of the surgeon's moral choices and their impact on the surgeon's inner life, the force is derived from the deontological imperative to act as surgeons are required to act, and the sense of well-being is secondary. This distinction may be hairsplitting; however, the meaning of life derives from altruism, not from egoism.

The ethics forum we call M&M is often thought to be of ancient origin, when in fact it is an invention of the 20th century. Credit for its origin must be shared between 2 American surgeons, both of whom were groundbreaking innovators. Ernest Amory Codman, MD, FACS, was a maverick. Andrew Warshaw, MD, FACS, focused his 2014 presidential address to the American College of Surgeons on Codman. Codman's great contribution was an "end results" emphasis; it is fair to say that historically operative success had been variously measured and sloppily reported. Codman abhorred that and introduced careful categorization of end results and particularly of untoward results. We still use some of his nomenclature for operative complications.

It was Allen O. Whipple, MD, FACS, who initiated the weekly ethics forum now called M&M. He therefore, in my opinion, was the true originator of the ritual. He wrote:

*"Still another good idea was the holding of regular surgical conferences once a week to discuss the errors in diagnosis, the mistakes in technique and the infections of clean wounds and deaths, if any had occurred during the last week."*

All of the elements are here: the regular observance, the retrospective analysis, and the intersubjectivity. Whipple's contributions to our discipline were great; his name is immortalized for the operation pancreaticoduodenectomy, but his greatest contribution, in my opinion, was this ethics forum of regular observance and important psychologic impact, which we today call the M&M conference.

It may be well to list some of the psychologic and pedagogic functions of the ethics forum called M&M:

1. To building trust, cohesion
2. To provide a cautionary tale
3. To understand human error
4. To improve quality
5. To process regret
6. To consider end of life issues
7. To promote critical thinking

Chapter 46 in this book comprises a detailed analysis of the epidemiology of surgeon burnout. The problem is real and, in the opinion of many, has been neglected or purposefully marginalized. The statistics are convincing: depression, substance abuse, and suicide are occupational hazards of our discipline.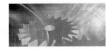

A plethora of solutions have been proposed. More tractable work schedules are frequently suggested. Strategies to increase personal resilience may be gathered under the heading of work-life balance and have included meditation and exercise or other health strategies. Recent work suggests that organizational change may be more efficacious than efforts aimed at individual resilience. In a recent article,[2] reductions in workload, changes in work evaluation methods, and increases in frontline participation in decisions were cited as having a salutatory effect.

More in keeping with the thrust of this book about ethics for surgeons are the impacts of ethical ambiguity and no-win situations in which no good outcome is possible. We have emphasized how common such situations are in the modern discipline of surgery. A loss of the sense of meaning in one's life is almost certain to produce some degree of burnout; indeed it may constitute a definition of burnout. It is not likely to be successful merely to advice that a surgeon maintain a sense of meaning. Institutional leaders can, however, promote frequent discussion of our discipline's venerable history and its legacy of connection to the altruism inherent in many traditions. The avoidance of a punishing culture is imperative. Ultimately, recognition that science provides only a glimpse of a reality wider than pure evidentialism reveals is essential.

The central notion of ethics, of moral decision-making, presupposes that humankind have some understanding of what is good or not good, and the freedom to choose between them. It is possible to argue for long from whence this understanding and freedom arise. Aristotle too, I believe, found these questions to be not only inscrutable but also trivial. He wrote that moral goodness results from habits that require cultivation. To become an ethical person requires the practice of ethical acts and utterances. Aristotle wrote:

*"Anything that we have to learn to do we learn by the actual doing of it."*

Surgeons are uniquely practitioners of moral actions, requiring continuous and conscious work of free will. Two precepts from the Hippocratic Oath apply. First, the Oath stresses beneficence toward those we teach. Our discipline has very often allowed our commitment to excellence to merge into harsh perfectionism, our self-confidence into hubris, and our perseverance into obsession. We must give greater value to the psychic well-being of those we teach.

Second, the Oath holds out a promise: If I do this, I may live and practice my craft with joy. This is also my wish for you.

# References

1. Reprinted in Cushing H. *Consecratio Medici*. Boston: Little, Brown and Company; 1928.
2. Panagioti M, Panagopoulou E, Bower P, et al. Controlled interventions to reduce burnout in physicians: a systematic review and meta-analysis. *JAMA Intern Med.* February 2017;177(2):195–205.

# ►Index

Note: Page numbers followed by "f" indicate figures and "t" indicate tables.